"The American people seem of at least two minds regarding the point at which common sense and diet intersect: those with no apparent interest in lengthening their lives and a counter-force that has wised up. But even those who perceive the wisdom of sensible living need practical instruction, which is precisely what *Long Life Now* offers."
—Steve Allen

"America needs *Long Life Now*. Americans need its information to start a personal revolution against the toxic poisoning of our planet."
—David Steinman, M.A., author
The Safe Shopper's Bible and
Diet For A Poisoned Planet

"The disastrous pressures fostered by industry, especially the petrochemical and pharmacological industries, seduces people into toxic life-style choices. Precise and cogent, *Long Life Now* strikes to the heart of the matter and makes the reader think."
—John Lee, M.D., author
What Your Doctor May Not Tell You About Menopause and *Optimal Health Guidelines*

"A must read."
—Dr. Earl Mindell, author
The Vitamin Bible and *The Herb Bible*

This book is printed on acid-free, elemental chlorine-free, 85% recycled paper with soy-based ink.

"Insightful, provocative and well-researched, *Long Life Now* is a valuable guide to maximizing your lifespan and filling your years with radiant health and the joy of living."

—Michael, Klaper, M.D., author
Vegan Nutrition: Pure And Simple and
Pregnancy, Children, And The Vegan Diet

"This is a blockbuster of a book which deserves a wide readership. In an easy-to-read style, he telegraphs the message that cancer and other degenerative diseases are truly preventable through a strategy of sensible diet and avoidance of chemical pollutants."

—Ralph Moss, Ph.D., author
Questioning Chemotherapy and *Cancer Therapy*

LONG LIFE NOW

Each chapter is built on previous chapters.
You will gain more from this book by reading
from the beginning.

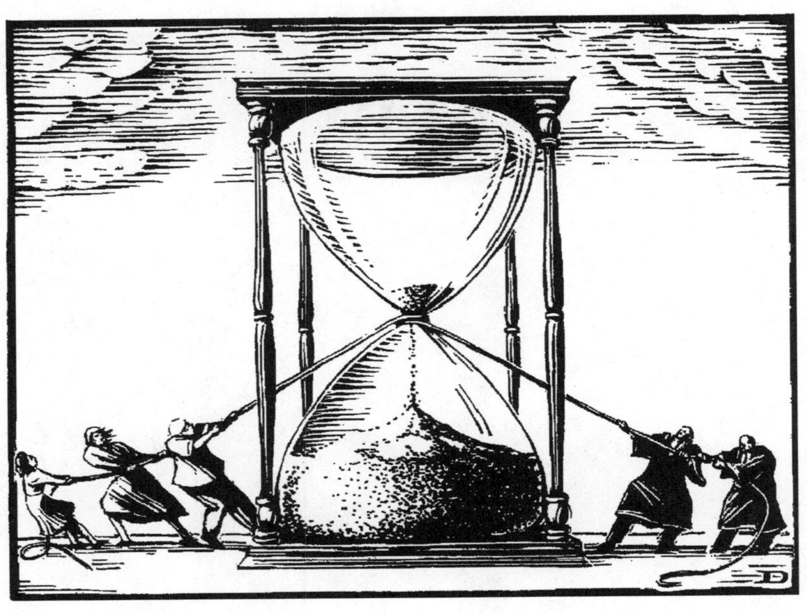

LONG LIFE NOW

STRATEGIES FOR STAYING ALIVE

First Edition

LEE HITCHCOX, D.C.

Celestial Arts
Berkeley, CA

Notice
The information in this book is intended as general reference only, not as a substitute for medical consultation or treatment. Those who are ill or taking medication should not make dietary changes without professional supervision.

Celestial Arts, P.O. Box 7123,
Berkeley, CA 94707

Cover illustration by Alan Okamoto

First Edition

Library of Congress Cataloging-in-Publication Data

Hitchcox, Lee, 1948–
Long life now : strategies for staying alive / Lee Hitchcox.
p. cm.
Includes bibliographical references and index.
ISBN 0–89087–763–7
1. Nutrition. 2. Nutritionally induced diseases. 3. Longevity.
I. Title.
RA784.H56 1995
613.2—dc20 95–19693
CIP

The paper used in this publication meets the requirements of American National Standard for Information Sciences—Permanence of Paper for Printed Library Materials, ANSI Z39.48–1984.

Permissions

Every effort has been made to trace the ownership of copyrighted material and to secure permission from the copyright holders. In the event of concerns over the use of copyrighted material, we regret the inadvertent error and will be happy to make the necessary corrections in future printings. Grateful acknowledgment is made for permission to reprint from the following:

Title hourglass illustration © Bob Dahm. Reprinted with permission.

U.S. capitol photo © Jim Johnson. Reprinted with permission.

Food label cartoon © Brian Duffy, *The Des Moines Register.* Reprinted with permission.

Macular degeneration illustration © Harriet R. Greenfield, M.A. Reprinted with permission.

Blood sugar chart adapted from *The Prevention Total Health System: Fighting Disease*, © 1984 Rodale Press, Inc., Emmaus, PA 18098. Reprinted with permission of the publisher.

Exercise chart adapted from *Geriatrics*, 48:62, 1993, © Advanstar Communications, Inc. Reprinted with permission of the publisher.

Prostate cancer chart adapted from Reddy, B., "Nutrition and its Relationship to Cancer," *Advances in Cancer Research,* 32:237, 1980, © Academic Press. Reprinted with permission of the publisher.

Breast/colon cancer charts adapted from Carroll, K., "Nutrition and Cancer: Fat," pg 445, *Nutrition, Toxicity, and Cancer,* Rowland, I.R., Ed., © CRC Press, Boca Raton, FL, 1991. Reprinted with permission of the publisher.

Hip fracture charts adapted from Hegsted, D., "Calcium and Osteoporosis," *Journal of Nutrition,* 116:2316, 1986, © American Institute of Nutrition. Reprinted with permission of the publisher.

Collagen illustration adapted from *Fountains of Youth,* © Ronin Publishing, Inc. Reprinted with permission of the publisher.

To
Carol, Grant, Jean,
and to those who seek and act before their time is up.

Acknowledgments
Hundreds of dedicated people contributed to this book. Special thanks to the guidance of Bethany Argisle, James Whitman, Leonard Rubin, Dana Buchanan, Steve Russell, Marge Thomas, as well as Joe Thornton (chlorine), John Lee (osteoporosis), Lilly Adams (Agent Orange), John Stauber (PR), Jeff Cohen (media), Ralph Moss (cancer), William Castelli (heart), Earl Mindell (additives), Bill Hirzy (EPA), Jeremy Rifkin (beef), Roy Walford (biological age), Alexander Leaf (Hunza diet), David Steinman and Samuel Epstein (pesticides), David and Elizabeth Armstrong (history), Jeff Taylor and Mike McGraw (USDA), Jack and Adrienne Samuels (MSG), Kenny Ausubel (seeds), John Yiamouyiannis and Robert Carton (fluoridation), Milan Param (chemical sensitivity), Chris Conran and Jack Herer (industrial hemp), Ralph Nader (GATT), T. Colin Campbell (China Study), Joan Price (exercise), Robert Charm (humor), John and Mary McDougall, Robert Siegel, Julian Whitaker, Howard Lyman, Covert Bailey, Burton Goldberg, Francis Moore Lappe, Dean Ornish, John Robbins, Patricia Bragg, Mollie Katzen, Harvey and Marilyn Diamond, Michael Klaper, Jennifer Raymond, Neal Barnard, Nathan Pritikin and Jack LaLanne (inspiration).

Special thanks to the agents and publishers who turned down *Long Life Now* since there is no such thing as good writing, only good rewriting. And lastly, I wish to acknowledge the voices within to which the credit for this book truly belongs. May it serve humanity.

LONG LIFE NOW Contents

Each chapter is built on previous chapters.
You will gain more from this book by reading
from the beginning.

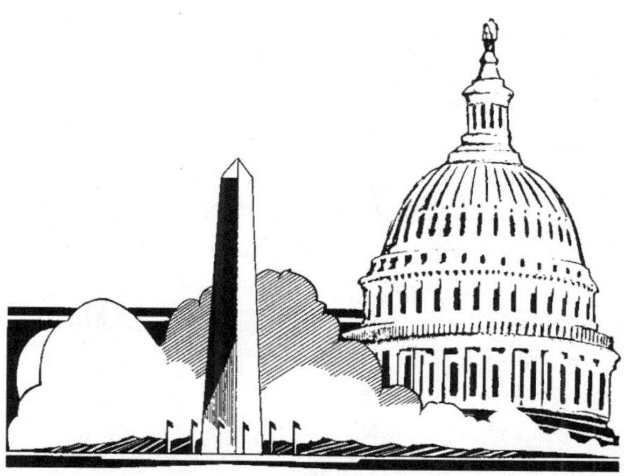

Introduction

On the evening of April 4, 1968, Martin Luther King, Jr. was shot while standing on a balcony of the Lorraine Motel in Memphis. Washington, D.C. quickly erupted in flames. The events that followed would touch my life.

I was only 19 at the time when my Army company was suddenly transformed into a riot control unit. We were crammed into trucks filled with tear gas grenades and shipped off. Rumbling down the beltway in a green serpentine convoy stretched out for miles, my unit soon arrived in Washington.

After days of guarding burnt-out buildings, we were given leave to visit the Washington Monument. Two friends and I gazed at its lofty splendor for our first time. Bragging and bravado challenges were tossed about. After not enough discussion, we raced up the stairway to the top, hearts pounding and drunk with our youthful prowess. We could do anything.

I vowed to return someday and climb those 898 steps again. Years passed and, at age 36, I did return to Washington with that promise in mind. Feeling fit and lean after months of hard training, I was ready. Finally the big moment arrived. While wearing running clothes and pumping adrenaline, I approached the Monument with great ceremony.

Surprise! The stairway was closed and had been closed for years. It seems there were too many 30- and 40-year-old men having heart attacks attempting to climb the stairs. Red warning signs were posted and promptly ignored. The government eventually closed the stairway forcing people to use the elevator. The Washington Monument has long served as a powerful symbol of our nation. To me, it's a symbol of our nation's ill health. As long as the stairs remain closed to prevent heart attacks, there's much work to be done.

In 1988, James Garner (spokesperson for the Beef Industry) suffered a heart attack and underwent quintuple-bypass surgery.[1] While in the hospital, someone sent him a vegetarian cookbook with a note wishing him a "speedy and lasting recovery." Mr. Garner held a press conference claiming that cigarette smoking, rather than diet, caused his medical condition.

During the 1960s, the American Medical Association accepted $18 million from tobacco companies to conduct research on the industry's behalf.[2] Ian MacDonald, M.D. and Henry Garland, M.D. disputed the *Surgeon General's Report* that smoking causes cancer. Ironically Dr. Garland reportedly died of lung cancer and Dr. MacDonald incinerated himself while smoking in bed.[3]

During the Vietnam War, autopsies of teenage American soldiers showed evidence of atherosclerosis while the arteries of Vietnamese soldiers remained clear.[4] Doctors reported similar findings during the Korean War.[5] At the time, I saw no connection between diet and health.

After the war, the herbicide Agent Orange became a concern. My CBR (Chemical, Biological, Radiological) warfare training failed to address long-term consequences. The government claimed that those exposed to Agent Orange had no higher cancer rates than the general population. This was not reassuring. More Americans die of cancer each year than were killed in World War II, Korea and Vietnam combined.[6]

The following luminaries have inspired millions, each in their own way, and on their own terms…

Author	Book	Cause of Death
Stuart Berger	The Immune Power Diet	Heart attack age 41 (1994)
Jim Fixx	The Complete Book of Running	Heart attack age 52 (1984)
Rachel Carson	Silent Spring	Breast cancer age 56 (1964)
Wolfman Jack	Have Mercy	Heart attack age 57 (1995)
Anthony Sattilaro	Recalled by Life	Prostate cancer age 58 (1989)
Robert Mendelsohn	Confessions of a Medical Heretic	Heart attack age 61 (1988)
Euell Gibbons	Stalking the Wild Asparagus	Heart attack age 64 (1975)
Paavo Airola	How To Get Well	Stroke age 68 (1983)
Nathan Pritikin	Live Longer Now	Leukemia age 69 (1985)
Adelle Davis	Let's Eat Right To Keep Fit	Bone cancer age 70 (1974)
J.I. Rodale	Health Finder	Heart attack age 72 (1971)
Georges Ohsawa	Zen Macrobiotics	Heart attack age 72 (1966)
Norman Cousins	Anatomy of An Illness	Heart attack age 75 (1990)
Linus Pauling	Cancer and Vitamin C	Prostate cancer age 93 (1994)

Jeff Smith (The Frugal Gourmet) has undergone open-heart surgery.[7] Julia Child (The French Chef) battled breast cancer.[8] To die a needless and pointless death during the prime of life is the ultimate indictment of our time. Over the years, I've lost loved ones to preventable illness and now share the vision of many: to vanquish cancer, heart disease and the other bitter legacies of civilization.

Science and technology have made unprecedented strides in expanding our knowledge of degenerative diseases. But now, as the dawn of the 21st century draws near, virtual immunity is within reach. The program within this book has been researched and presented without compromise. *Long Life Now* is dedicated to turning this vision into reality.

—Lee Hitchcox, D.C.

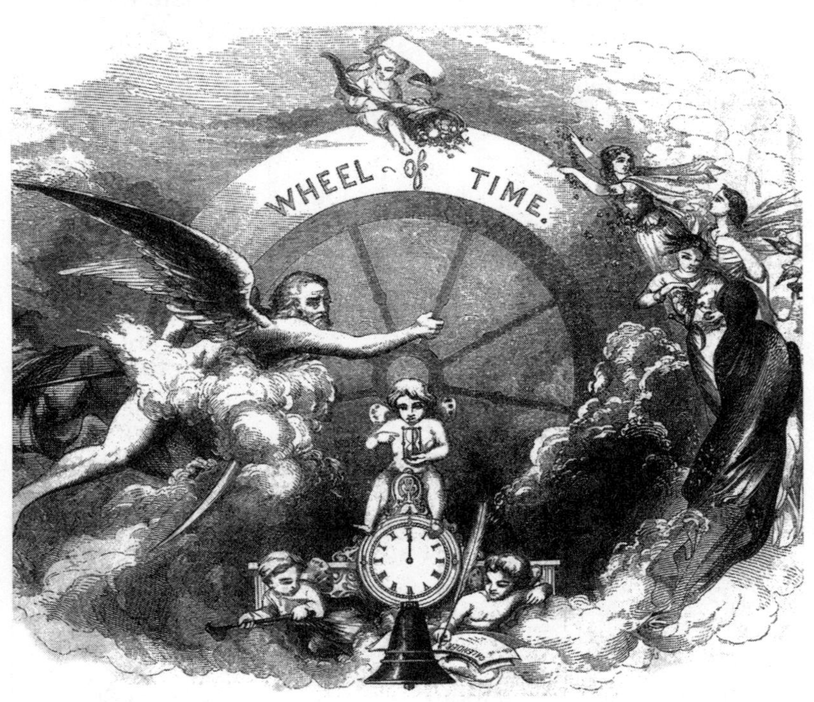

CHAPTER 1
New Thinking

". . . re-examine all you have been told at school or church or in any book, dismiss what insults your soul, and your very flesh shall be a great poem."

—Walt Whitman
Leaves of Grass preface, 1855

"A physician can sometimes parry the scythe of death, but has no power over the sand in the hourglass."

—Hester Lynch Piozzi
letter, Nov. 12, 1781

Most of us are resigned to lead ordinary lives. Secure in the daily routine of job, commute and the week's laundry, there's no reason to question the balance. There are those who dream of something more: wild secret fantasies of intrigue and adventure in some faraway exotic paradise, indulging in the pleasures of life while riding off into the crimson-red sunset. And then there are the select few who live their dreams.

Most of us are resigned to the predictable future of growing old with everyone else, with its attendant consequences of Alzheimer's, incontinence and nursing homes. There are those who dream of something more: wild secret fantasies of prolonging youth and dancing 'til dawn immune from illness, unencumbered by the ravages of time. And then there are the select few who live their dreams.

There will be 1 million American centenarians by the year 2040. If your goal is to soar with the eagles—to reach for and grasp a full active life well beyond 100—then you must seek information and act on it before your time is up. And you must realize there is more to this game than diet alone, especially when vested financial interests do not share your goals.

Americans dread growing old and many seek tools for slowing the aging process. They accept the preposterous notion that aging can be slowed. This movement will change forever the demographics of our nation. The resulting transformation of government, science, industry and medicine will herald a new day for this rich but troubled society. Only rarely do forces coincide to transform the world as we know it. That time is now.

Our nation now faces enormous medical and environmental challenges: cancer, pesticides, air/water pollution, deforestation, topsoil depletion, global warming, acid rain, birth defects and a 50% drop in human sperm count. Seemingly insurmountable problems remain insurmountable until they're addressed. Eradicating these conditions, I believe, requires three conversions:

- Change our diet from animal-centered to plant-centered.
- Change our economy from petrochemical-based to plant-based.
- Change our government from lobby-centered to people-centered.

Each is an integral strategy for staying alive. The combined influence of these actions has the power to reshape national institutions and policies on a scale unprecedented in U.S. history.

NUTRITION

Most people eat what they were brought up to eat, and old habits die hard…until a dreaded disease threatens their life or that of a loved one. Few are able to change their diet **before** the diagnosis is made. Books help.

Nutrition books based on theory line the bookstore shelves like ever-changing sentinels. Readers struggle through the labyrinth by skimming chapters and translating code words while searching for which diet to trust. The stakes are high: how long you'll live.

> *"Be careful about reading health books. You might die of a misprint."*
>
> —Mark Twain (1835–1910)

There are places on this planet, cultures noted for their extreme longevity, where people live past 100 free of disease. Their diet may be the foundation for slowing the biological aging process—the holy grail of scientific endeavor.

The U.S. has over 30,000 diets on public record, more than any other nation. All diets fall into three general categories:

- Weight Loss Diet: that period of time before you gain all the weight back.
- Treatment Diet: short-term program to correct a medical condition.
- Maintenance Diet: long-term program to preserve health.

In *Long Life Now,* the word "diet" refers to maintenance diet. Important note: this program is not designed for infants. Breast milk is high in cholesterol and 56% fat which is needed for the infant's central nervous system development. Most infant formulas contain only one-fifth the essential fat of breast milk.[1] This diet is not designed for children, who need less fat than infants but more fat than adults. Children on very low-fat diets show failure to thrive. The province of this book encompasses optimal nutrition applied to normal healthy adults.

We live in a time of great transition marked by a disquieting sense of pain. Much suffering stems from an industrial system that promotes alienation, isolation and superficial distraction. Many feel alienated from nature, isolated from each other and distracted by the media. From a corporate standpoint, heaven forbid if people ever question their core beliefs and take back their personal power. Even worse if they ever organize at the grassroots level and take back their national power. And God help us if they ever do both.

One of the harshest economic realities of our time is the conflict-of-interest that contributes to mortality in America:

- Dow Chemical sells pesticides and anti-cancer drugs.
- DuPont and Union Carbide sell pesticides and medical diagnostic equipment.
- General Electric operates hazardous waste sites and sells mammography machines.
- ICI-Zeneca, the founding sponsor of Breast Cancer Awareness Month, sells pesticides and anti-cancer drugs.[2]

It's often tempting to ignore pesticides since they seem beyond our control. No one wants to hear that foods are polluted with cancer-causing chemicals and there's nothing we can do about it. But in fact, there's a great deal we can do about it.

MANIFESTO FOR CHANGE

Americans are told they can "lower cancer risk" by cutting their fat intake to 30%. They are not told the full story. Fats and pesticides are independent causes of cancer.

- Israeli breast cancer rates dropped sharply in recent years despite an increase in dietary fat; Israeli pesticide exposure continues to decline.
- American breast cancer rates climbed sharply in recent years despite a drop in dietary fat; American pesticide exposure continues to worsen.

Cutting cancer risk involves more than taking consumer action at the personal level to lower fats. It also involves citizen action at the national level to reduce pesticides. National pesticide reform requires fundamental policy change in the following six areas:

- Pesticide laws
- Risk assessment
- Cancer programs
- Farm subsidy programs
- National media
- Campaign finance laws

These are the six pillars of the pesticide industry infrastructure. By understanding each pillar and their interconnected links, the public can collapse this powerbase like a house of cards. National pesticide reform also involves closing the U.S. government's five revolving doors:

- National Cancer Institute (drug industry)
- Food and Drug Administration (drug industry)
- Department of Agriculture (meat/dairy industries)
- Environmental Protection Agency (polluters)
- Congress (Washington lobbies)

Each revolving door stands as a testament to the betrayal of public trust—formidable adversaries to democracy. We as a people deserve better. By taking national level action, citizens can make a difference in the lives of all generations to come. Each revolving door and pillar is addressed in the chapters that follow.

THE INFRASTRUCTURE

"This is 1990, and you have a choice. Society says: 'Hey, we've got cash, and we'll pay for a million dead cows and chickens tonight. We want them raised en mass, living wing to wing, nose to nose, eating their own crap and pumped with chemicals. We want them knifed to death, squawking and mooing in the night. We want their blood flowing down drains, their hides in one pile, their guts in another. Here's the cash; have them here by Wednesday.'"[3]

—Ted Nugent, musician

The U.S. food production and distribution system is a $625 billion dollar industry employing 21 million people, the largest business in North America.[4] Next largest is the chemical industry. Both businesses intertwine with the medical industry through pesticides and pharmaceuticals. The oil companies supply raw materials from which pesticides and drugs are made. Each industry intimately contacts government through campaign contributions. Together they account for nearly half the nation's GNP.

In this age of unprecedented complexity, it's difficult at times to fully grasp the issues at hand, especially when there's a war on. Grim institutions of the American diet—hospitals, slaughterhouses, nursing homes—exist as monuments to the old way of thinking, a way of life under siege. Lives and livelihoods are both on the line.

Millions of Americans struggling for survival with broken bodies and shattered dreams stand as living tributes to industry's bitter price. The price is too high. The sheer weight of evidence seen in the stark light of science can no longer be ignored. Profound changes are taking hold and industry's greatest fear is for ordinary citizens to begin asking questions.

No system cloaked in deception, no matter how powerfully entrenched or how vast its resources, can survive the wrath of truth. Medical knowledge doubles every 8 years and the empire's fate is sealed: study by study, brick by brick. When truth and knowledge join, no desperate clutch on the past can shield deception from the brilliance of its light.

As the drama and battles unfold before us, their passing will bring the dream of a better life and hope for a better tomorrow. Medical destiny is now a matter of choice.

CORPORATE FRONT GROUPS

"You can only win the ecology wars if you set out to destroy the environmental movement once and for all...We're going to destroy them, like they're trying to destroy you."[5]

—Ron Arnold, speaking to ranchers
Center for the Defense of Free Enterprise

Be wary of grass root organizations with hidden agendas and green sounding names. Groups representing special interests often wave false flags. Examples:

- Abundant Wildlife Society of North America; American Animal Welfare Foundation (cattle and fur industries)[6]
- American Council on Science and Health; Responsible Industry for a Safe Environment (pesticide industry)[7]
- Food Facts Coalition (meat industry)[8]
- Food Watch (agribusiness farming)[9]
- U.S. Council for Energy Awareness (nuclear industry)[10]
- National Wetlands Coalition; Environmental Conservation Organization; Wilderness Impact Research Foundation (pro-development)[11]
- Workplace Health & Safety Council (anti-worker safety)[12]
- Citizens for Sensible Control of Acid Rain; Information Council for the Environment (coal industry)[13]
- Clean Air Alliance; Coalition for Vehicle Choice (auto and oil industries)[14]
- People for the West (mining industry)[15]
- Citizens Coalition for Sustainable Development; We Care; Evergreen Foundation; Mothers' Watch; Yellow Ribbon Coalition (timber industry)[16]
- Animal Health Institute (animal drug industry)[17]
- Committee Against More Taxes and Bureaucracy (tobacco industry)[18]

- Society for Environmental Truth; Accuracy in Media (pro-corporate media)[19]
- Citizens for the Environment; Friends of the Rivers; Wise Use; Putting People First; Committee for a Constructive Tomorrow; Global Climate Coalition; Consumer Alert; National Legal Center for the Public Interest; Alliance for America; Institute for Justice; Reason Foundation (anti-environmental)[20]

The children represent our greatest hope for sustainable stewardship of this planet and for healing the mistakes of generations past. It is the goal of *Long Life Now* to help keep the parents alive so their children can be launched.

U.S. HEALTH-CARE

"The destiny of countries depends on the way they feed themselves."

—Anthelme Brillat-Savarin, 1825

Since the Industrial Revolution beginning in 1848, Western society has fundamentally altered the biological basis of human existence—diet and environment—from which health arises. Chronic disease is now considered normal. Well people are disappearing.

Despite its armamentarium of powerful drugs and aggressive treatment strategies, conventional medicine demonstrates scant progress against the growing specter of resistant infections, autoimmune disorders and environmental afflictions of unknown origin.

Heart attack patients, after undergoing heroically complex surgical procedures, are served the same abysmal foods that brought them to the hospital in the first place. President Bush was served steak on the night of his heart scare. U.S. soldiers returning from the Persian Gulf War were welcomed back with first-class medical treatment, ice cream and hot dogs. America has the world's most expensive health-care system, yet we rank 16th in life expectancy. No intervention with drugs or surgery can erase a lifetime of self abuse.

Each year, nearly 400,000 Americans undergo heart bypass surgery for blocked coronary arteries. Most patients believe surgery will correct their problem. However, it is an immutable law of biology that a disease caused by a detrimental diet cannot be corrected by surgery. We ignore this principle at our peril.

- Following heart bypass surgery, 50% of bypassed arteries clog up within 5 years.[21]
- Following balloon angioplasty, 33% of dilated arteries clog up within 4–6 months.[22]

Each heart bypass operation replaces only 6 inches of an arterial system but leaves the other 60,000 miles of total length. In most cases, these procedures do not improve survival.[23]

By treating symptoms with drugs or surgery while ignoring the underlying cause (diet), treatment often becomes an expensive exercise in futility. During recent doctor strikes in Canada, England, Israel and America, the death rates actually fell.[24] Dubious and mercenary procedures lie at the core of America's health-care crisis.

In 1985, the National Research Council recommended that U.S. medical schools include more courses in nutrition. Since that time, the number of medical schools offering nutrition courses has dropped.[25] U.S. medical schools receive large endowments and grants from pharmaceutical companies.

THE PRACTICE OF MEDICINE

Most physicians practice early detection or treatment to the exclusion of prevention. Doctors know that a 10% fat diet can prevent or reverse degenerative disease, yet few make this recommendation. There are several possible reasons:

- Insurance coverage – there is no realistic reimbursement for nutritional counseling.[26]
- Tradition – doctors are not comfortable requiring behavioral change.[27]
- Compliance fear – doctors are afraid people won't do anything if the changes are too drastic.
- Peer review fear – doctors don't wish to practice differently from their colleagues.
- Expectations – patients expect doctors to perform procedures, but successful prevention means no procedures performed.
- Lack of nutrition education – most physicians receive less than 3 hours of nutrition during medical school.[28]

- High-tech training – MDs trained in high-tech procedures think nutrition is beneath them. Real doctors don't talk about food.
- Personal eating habits – fewer than 20% of doctors have improved their own diets.[29]
- Economics – moderate fat recommendations (20–30% fat) insure the continuing supply of cancer and heart disease patients. Patients generate profit.

During the 1950s, dentists became so successful in promoting prevention (dental hygiene) that their efforts resulted in fewer cavities, fewer patients and a tougher environment to make a living. Several dental schools have since closed. This economic lesson is not lost on the medical profession.

> "*. . . most physicians don't think about prevention—they want to treat disease.*"[30]
>
> —Jeffrey Blumberg, USDA
> Human Nutrition Research Center on Aging

PARABLE IN THE GRASS

Place a 10-pound red brick on a lawn and the grass under the brick will turn yellow and eventually die. This brick represents our diet. The government places a second brick on top of the first, representing pesticides and additives. The government brick is painted green, the color of GRAS (Generally Recognized As Safe), and we now have 20 pounds bearing down.

Several blades of grass are mad as hell and aren't going to take it anymore. They replace the red brick label (Beef & Saturated Fat) with a new label (Chicken & Vegetable Oil) and the situation is unchanged. Twenty pounds by any other name is still 20 pounds and the grass is still dying.

Several grass doctors try vitamins, herbs and fancy fertilizers. Others examine the family history and genetic background. Failing this, the grass may be told it's a psychological problem and referred out for group grass therapy. Meanwhile the government stands ready to commission another study and use more green paint. The problem can only be corrected by removing both bricks.

"You the individual can do more for your health and well being than any doctor, any hospital, any drug, any exotic medical device."

—Surgeon General's Report

George Washington is said to have died after his physician took 3 quarts of his blood to treat a sore throat. Three U.S. presidents—Washington, Garfield, McKinley—died from medical treatments that did more harm than good, treatments administered by the best doctors of the day. The ultimate responsibility for health lies with you alone. The path to long life cannot be taken by surrendering to another the power to call the tune.

The healthiest, longest-lived people on earth have no access to modern medicine. They practice prevention. Profound social changes will occur when it's no longer considered normal to die young. The medical profession, pesticide industry, cattle ranchers and general public all share the same philosophical aspirations for a better world. There is, however, disagreement over the best way to get there.

ALL HAT AND NO CATTLE

Despite their education and training, physicians, chiropractors, dietitians and government scientists have a track record of dying from the same degenerative diseases as everyone else because they have the same diet as everyone else. You can do better.

- Chiropractors receive an average of 71 hours of nutritional training.[31]
- Registered dietitians receive more training although one-third eat at fast-food places once a week.[32]

"Most dietitians have been trained to teach people not to restrict their diet unnecessarily. Giving up meat and/or dairy products goes against the grain. . ."[33]

—George Eisman, R.D.

The American Dietetic Association (ADA) publishes studies by the National Dairy Council,[34] receives funding by the National Live Stock and Meat Board, and joined McDonald's in promoting their "Happy Meals."[35]

"We provide them [ADA] with funding, and they help us by promoting sound, balanced information."[36]

—Donna Schmidt
Meat Board public relations director

Powerful special interests often influence national organizations. Protect yourself by recognizing corporate tentacles, tactics and marketing practices. Do not gracefully surrender your youth by falling prey to deception. To beat the system, don't play by the company rules.

DIETARY ADVICE

Experts have advised people what to eat for over 2,000 years.

"Your food shall be your medicine and your medicine shall be your food."

—Hippocrates, 424 B.C.
founder of medicine

"Prepare simple meals, chew well, sup lightly."

—Leonardo da Vinci

"To lengthen thy life, lessen thy meals."

—Benjamin Franklin

"Chew your liquids and drink your food."

—Mahatma Gandhi

Expert nutritional advice carries an air of reasonableness that often masks deeper more vexing issues. Everyone, it seems, has a different opinion. At a time when contradictory studies and dueling authorities on both sides are the norm, it's little wonder why controversy prevails.

The airwaves are now awash in oat bran commercials, claims, counterclaims and hype—as are we. Wading through the muddled piles gets pretty slippery when droppings of nutritional nuggets lie thick on the ground. The best defense is to realize that dietary advice originating from government agencies and prestigious national institutions is, in fact, economically-driven. As always, the devil is in the details, not the headlines.

SOCIAL PROGRAMMING

"The key words are balance, variety and moderation."
—National Live Stock and Meat Board
Exploring Meat and Health

Since the late 1800s, public relation professionals within the food industry have profoundly influenced America's meat-based culture, shaping it to their own image. Social programming runs deep, as a cursory glance at our language reveals:

- Bring home the bacon, not worth beans, full of beans
- Meat of the matter, meat and potatoes, meat market
- Meaty, no bull, beefcake, cheesecake, beefy, cheesy
- Beef it up, hamming it up, high on the hog, bone up
- Bone to pick, cut to the bone, no bones about it
- Pork barrel politics, hog wild, whole hog, hot dog
- Fat of the land, fat chance, trim the fat, chew the fat
- Breadwinner, big cheese, buttering up the boss
- My bread and butter, buttercup, creamed
- Gravy train, the rest is gravy, cream of the crop
- Peaches and cream, rich creamy taste, milkrun
- Milking the crowd, land of milk and honey
- Milk of human kindness, cry over spilled milk
- Chicken out, no spring chicken, talking turkey
- Cold turkey, cold fish, other fish to fry, fishy
- A real honey, honey bun, jelly belly
- Sweetheart, sweet talk, sweet success, sweet life
- Pie in the sky, piece of cake, take the cake, caked on
- Egged on, shell out, good egg
- Salt of the earth, worth its salt

Corporations spend hundreds of millions each year on advertising, their most powerful social programming force. The ideals of a nation are reflected in its advertising slogans:

Beef

- Real food for real people, beef gives strength
- Good news for people who like to eat
- Nutrition you can sink your teeth into
- Nothing satisfies like beef
- Eat light with beef, be a star with beef

Dairy Products
- Everybody needs milk, milk is good fast food
- Milk is nature's most perfect food
- Milk has something for everybody
- Milk does your body good
- You never outgrow your need for milk
- Calcium the way nature intended
- The backbone of every woman's diet

Pork
- The other white meat, America is leaning on pork

Eggs
- The incredible edible egg, four a week is OK

Sugar
- Nature's energy food, pour on the energy
- There's no real substitute for real sugar

Vegetable Oils
- Does your heart good, eat to your heart's content
- A taste you can take to heart, make it his oil for life

Chemical Companies
- Better living through chemistry
- A hand in things to come

Infant Milk Formulas
- First choice, the best start in life

Nursing Homes
- Be as free as you want to be
- Your passport to new experiences

> *"A drum makes a loud noise because it is empty."*
> —Peruvian proverb

SACRED BELIEFS

When social programming and dietary advice converge, the unholy alliance creates hardening of the attitudes: sacred beliefs accepted as gospel, carved in stone and brought down from the mountain as divine nutritional commandments.

Hospitals and nursing homes are filled with people impaled on the sword of blind conviction. True believers live and die by their impenetrable beliefs—major players in a most dangerous game. Examples:

Belief: If you're healthy, you can eat anything in moderate amounts. Low-fat diets are unnecessary for most people.

Reality: Low-fat diets are unnecessary if you're happy living no longer than most people.

Belief: The Japanese are genetically immune to cancer and heart disease.

Reality: The Japanese lose their "immunity" to these diseases when they immigrate and begin eating Western food.[37]

Belief: Americans are genetically predisposed to cancer and heart disease. Elevated blood cholesterol runs in families.

Reality: The English language also runs in families but it's not genetic. Chronic disease owes no allegiance to nationality.

Belief: Nutrition is bunk. My grandmother ate Twinkies and Ding Dongs, yet lived to be 90 while working everyday.

Reality: Your grandmother was lucky to die without chronic disease or institutionalization. Many older Americans are not so fortunate.

Belief: Living beyond age 90 is just not worth it.

Reality: When the elderly say this, it's probably true—for them. Biological age is everything.

> *"I would really question how anybody could say that vegetarianism is a growing belief. Man is by nature a carnivore."*[38]
>
> —John McBride, spokesperson
> Livestock Marketing Association

The national norm is changing. By the year 2000, the majority of Americans may be largely vegetarian for health reasons.[39]

DISINFORMATION

Major industries know quite well that contentious issues are often adjudicated in the court of public opinion. Corporate public relations firms manipulate public opinion using various deceptive practices. In 1990, the National Dairy Board hired a PR firm to promote growth hormones in milk. The firm infiltrated an anti-hormone conference by planting the audience with "housewives" who appeared to favor injecting cows with hormones.[40]

In 1993, the American Cancer Society rebutted Bill Moyer's "Frontline" documentary on pesticide risk. The cancer society downplayed the risk by following guidelines drafted by the pesticide industry's PR firm.[41] Pesticide supporters cited the American Cancer Society's position.

The California Department of Agriculture claims that counties with the highest exposure to pesticides have the lowest breast cancer rates.[42] This position conflicts with current evidence. The increased cancer risk among farmers is well documented,[43] and children of California farmworkers are twice as likely to be born with deformed limbs.[44]

The Ad Council's Partnership for a Drug-Free America receives funding from the alcohol, tobacco and pharmaceutical industries.[45] Consequently their public-service ads ignore America's real drug problems. Legal drugs kill hundreds of thousands each year, compared to a few thousand dying from illegal drugs.

Monsanto Corporation, which ranks among the 10 worst polluters, recently joined Earth Day USA[46] and Business for Social Responsibility.[47] The greenwashing of corporations placates the public while pollution continues unabated. The co-optation of advocacy groups mutes their voice.

Corporations often hire "third party" scientists to argue their case before the media. The American Council on Science and Health (ACSH) represents itself as an independent and objective science institute, yet their positions closely follow those of its sponsor:[48]

- The ACSH (funded by pesticide makers) promotes pesticides.
- The ACSH (funded by Burger King) promotes fast foods.
- The ACSH (funded by Monsanto, Coca-Cola and PepsiCo) promotes saccharin and NutraSweet.

- The ACSH (funded by the Malaysian palm oil industry) promotes tropical oils.
- The ACSH (funded by Monsanto) promotes growth hormones.

The ACSH downplayed the risk of toxic chemicals during TV and *Fortune* magazine interviews with no disclosure of funding sources.[49] Stephen Sternberg, director of ACSH, headed the Shell Chemical Ad Hoc Committee of Pathologists which claimed that the pesticides aldrin and dieldrin were *not* carcinogenic.[50]

Hard science and sober risk assessment play decisive roles in molding public perception. But when vast fortunes and careers rest on the latest scientific research, questionable practices abound. Science today has more than its share of junk science.

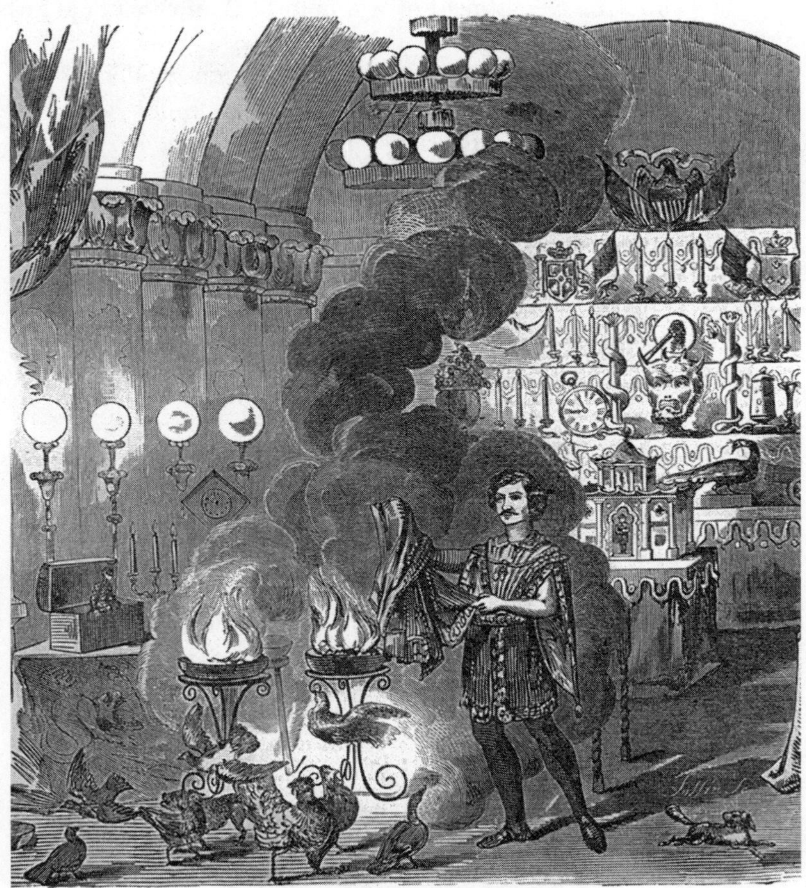

MACALLISTER, THE CELEBRATED WIZARD AND MAGICIAN.

Junk Science

"There's no reason to believe that anyone trained in the scientific method is going to be influenced by the source of payment for his or her endeavors. There are undoubtedly a few exceptions . . ."[51]

—Dr. Elizabeth Whelan, president
American Council on Science and Health

The field of nutrition is neither precise nor elegant. Long considered the troubled stepchild of science, nutrition inhabits a complex realm of tenuous assumptions, conflicting theories, shifting political winds and opposing economic positions.

An enduring law of nature states that anything can be proven given enough creativity on the part of the interpreter. Exactitude in science can be, at times, less than forthcoming when biased research overlooks ugly little facts. The elegant precision of logic and the measured guidance of reason are irretrievably lost when culture, prejudice and the funding process all converge.

We all want to know the truth—not truth mutated beyond recognition. Pre-planned agendas and politics have no place in this quest. Every profession has its price, and the price of expertise is an intimate relationship with the profession's darker side. Science is no exception.

"It is difficult to get a man to understand something when his salary depends on his not understanding it."

—Upton Sinclair

Not all science is as pure as its polished carapace would have us believe. Both the Bible and nutritional research have been cited for just about everything. You can find scientific evidence to make any point or sell any product, depending on who paid for the study.

During the Alar scare, for example, the apple industry claimed a person must eat 28,000 Alar-treated apples each day for 70 years to increase cancer risk. By seasonally adjusting the temperature, you can prove Canada has no winter. By cloaking value judgments with a veneer of objectivity, researchers from opposing camps often reach conflicting conclusions based on the same data. Consider the following two studies published in the *British Medical Journal:*[52]

- Calcium supplementation in the diet: not justified by present evidence, 1989
- Calcium supplementation in the diet: justified by present evidence, 1990

From this it appears the experts change their minds every week…or so it seems. Small wonder why people are throwing up their hands, not knowing what to believe. Don't give up and consult the tabloids quite yet. There is a better way.

> *"Get your facts first, and…then you can distort 'em as much as you please."*
>
> —Mark Twain

FACTS

- 99% of cancer patients have eaten potatoes.
- 99% of heart attack patients have eaten potatoes.
- 100% of potato eaters born in 1842 are dead.

Do these findings suggest potatoes to be a health hazard? That depends on the **interpretation**, an arduous and often murky undertaking at best. The following examples shed light on the creative interpretations employed by medical researchers:

EXAMPLE #1

The Nurses' Health Study of 89,494 nurses showed no relation between fat intake and breast cancer risk.[53]

Medical Interpretation:

- Low-fat diets do not reduce breast cancer risk.

***Long Life Now* Interpretation:**

- 25% fat diets do not reduce breast cancer risk. Total fat intake ranged from 25% to 45% of calories.
- This study (funded by the NIH) ignored most of the human race which eats far less fat and has a much lower cancer rate.

The dairy industry was reportedly involved in at least part of this study.[54] Other private funding sources were not disclosed.

EXAMPLE #2

A study of 111 patients with elevated cholesterol levels showed only a slight reduction in those eating low-fat diets.[55]

Medical Interpretation:[56]

- Low-fat diets have only a minor effect on blood cholesterol.

***Long Life Now* Interpretation:**

- 30% fat diets have only a minor effect on blood cholesterol.
- This study (funded by Merck Laboratories) ignored the Lifestyle Heart Trial in which patients on 10% fat diets showed much larger cholesterol reductions.[57]

Project LEAN is a national campaign to reduce fat intake from present levels to 30% of calories. The notion of calling 30% fat diets "lean" shows how prejudiced our society has become. Better nutritional studies are blocked by the personal eating habits of many scientists.

> *"I really like hamburgers. I have to make an effort not to go to Burger King or McDonald's too often."*[58]
>
> —William Evans, Ph.D.
> USDA Human Nutrition Research Center

EXAMPLE #3

A study of 79 heart disease patients found no difference in coronary artery narrowing in those receiving cholesterol lowering therapy.[59]

Medical Interpretation:[60]

- Lowering blood cholesterol does not reduce heart disease risk.

***Long Life Now* Interpretation:**

- Lowering blood cholesterol with drugs from 213 to 159 mg/dl does not reduce heart disease risk, especially when saturated fat intake remains at 8%.
- This study (funded by Bristol-Myers Squibb) ignored 80% of the human race which has cholesterol levels under 150 without drugs and will never have a heart attack.

EXAMPLE #4

Calorie restriction is the only technique that consistently extends the lifespans of mice and rats.[61]

Media Interpretation:[62]

- Calorie restriction is the key to longevity.

***Long Life Now* Interpretation:**

- The restricted-calorie rodents live longer than their free-eating neighbors who gorge themselves on grotesquely abnormal amounts of food.

Dr. Ronald Hart of the National Center for Toxicological Research, advocates human calorie restriction and dropped his own weight from 270 to 185 pounds.[63] However, ideal body weight does not rise with age; it remains level starting at age 20. Did Dr. Hart weigh 270 pounds at age 20? If not, then his program of calorie restriction is actually closer to calorie normalization.

EXAMPLE #5

Chinese women who consumed dairy products had 20% denser bones than Chinese women who did not.[64]

Media Interpretation:[65]

- For strong bones, eat more dairy products.

***Long Life Now* Interpretation:**

- This study compared Mongolian Chinese women to non-Mongolian Chinese women; genetic differences may have influenced the result.[66]

- This study (funded by Bristol-Myers) did not control for exercise level which may have influenced the result.[67]

Mona Calvo, Ph.D., nutritionist with the FDA, cited this study as a reason for consuming dairy products.[68] Dr. Calvo's research is funded by the National Dairy Council.[69]

EXAMPLE #6

Healthy subjects who consumed MSG (monosodium glutamate) had no more reactions than those who consumed a placebo.[70]

FDA Interpretation:[71]

- MSG is perfectly safe.

***Long Life Now* Interpretation:**

- The placebo group was given NutraSweet (aspartane) which causes the same reactions in sensitive people as MSG.[72]
- This study (funded by the MSG industry) fails to show the safety of MSG and should not be used to convince regulators that MSG is safe.

"Facts do not cease to exist because they are ignored."
—Aldous Huxley
Proper Studies

EXAMPLE #7

Prostate cancer is more common in North America than in Asia. Men who migrate from Asia to North America retain their low risk, but their sons acquire prostate cancer at a higher rate.[73]

Medical Interpretation:[74]

- Prostate cancer may have both genetic and environmental components.
- No practical recommendations for prevention are indicated.

***Long Life Now* Interpretation:**

- Prostate cancer may have environmental components only.
- Asian diets may help prevent prostate cancer.

EXAMPLE #8

A study of 110 osteoporosis patients showed a decrease in vertebral fractures in those receiving fluoride therapy.[75]

Medical Interpretation:[76]

- Fluoride therapy reduces vertebral fractures and is safe to use.

Long Life Now **Interpretation:**

- This study focused only on vertebral fractures and ignored hip fractures which increase with fluoride therapy.[77] The drug's safety has not been demonstrated.
- This study was funded by the Public Health Service (which is mandated to promote fluoride)[78] and the University of Texas Southwestern Medical Center (which holds patent rights to this drug).[79]

CORPORATE JUNK SCIENCE

The Boeing Company of Seattle was recently sued by several workers after they developed symptoms of multiple chemical sensitivity (MCS) from a common exposure. Boeing responded by funding a clinical study which examined this issue.[80] The study was deeply flawed.[81]

The control group was chosen from a musculoskeletal pain clinic and most of the MCS group didn't have MCS.[82] The researchers concluded that immunological tests are useless in evaluating MCS patients and psychological symptoms are a central component.[83] Before this study was published, Boeing used it for cross-examination during a deposition.[84] When a company funds research which they use in their own legal defense and when they alone have access to the unpublished results, serious concerns ought to be raised within the legal, medical and scientific communities.

Impartial studies rarely spring from researchers influenced by their desire for financial gain. Pharmaceutical companies pay clinical investigators up to $1 million a year for drug studies, and the researchers realize their jobs depend on desired results.[85] Each year at least 125,000 Americans die from adverse reactions to prescription drugs, and another 10 million suffer lesser adverse effects.[86] Tainted science spawns therapeutic misadventures.

Monsanto conducted reportedly fraudulent studies on two of its most profitable products: Agent Orange (2, 4, 5–T) and PCBs (polychlorinated biphenyls).[87] By delaying the banning of these chemicals, Monsanto made millions in extra profits. The EPA conducted a criminal investigation of Monsanto's research.[88]

The polystyrene industry conducted studies in response to concerns over polystyrene packaging leaching chemicals into food. This research concluded that some styrene in food may be natural, and not from the packaging.[89]

The widespread and inherently seductive nature of conflict-of-interest is not adequately addressed by most academic institutions and biomedical journals.[90] This sad commentary on professional integrity calls into question the authority of dubious scientific endeavors. Nothing short of full financial disclosure can halt the pernicious specter of industry-sponsored research.

RESEARCH GUIDELINES

Not all studies are worth the paper they're printed on, and only the critical appraisal of data can tell the tale. Most people are no more inclined to interpret research than to decipher the Dead Sea Scrolls—yet the flood of conflicting studies continues unabated. The following guidelines can help you cut through it:

- Champion healthy skepticism. Rarely is a study immune from criticisms leveled against it. Conclusions are often revised in light of new information.

- Don't let the headlines change your whole life. Wait and see if the new study can pass the test of time. To be accepted, new studies must be duplicated several times.

- Large studies over several years are more reliable than small short-term studies. Animal research may not be transferable to humans.

- Be especially wary of studies that try to sell you something. Examples:

  – Alcohol reduces heart disease
  (funded by the alcohol industry).[91]

  – Seafood lowers blood pressure and blood fats
  (funded by the seafood industry).[92]

– Red meat improves iron absorption (funded by the beef industry).[93]

– Milk improves iron absorption (funded by the dairy industry).[94]

– Soybeans lower blood cholesterol (funded by the soybean industry).[95]

– Walnuts lower blood cholesterol (funded by the walnut industry).[96]

– Drugs lower blood cholesterol better than diet (funded by the pharmaceutical industry).[97]

– Olive oil lowers breast cancer risk (funded by Greece).[98]

– Caffeine doesn't cause osteoporosis (funded by the coffee industry).[99]

– Pesticides don't cause cancer (funded by the chemical industry).[100]

> *"Worship the spirit of criticism...it always has the last word."*
> —Louis Pasteur (1822–1895)
> French chemist

BOVRIL

IS THE GUARANTEED PRODUCT OF

PRIME OX BEEF.

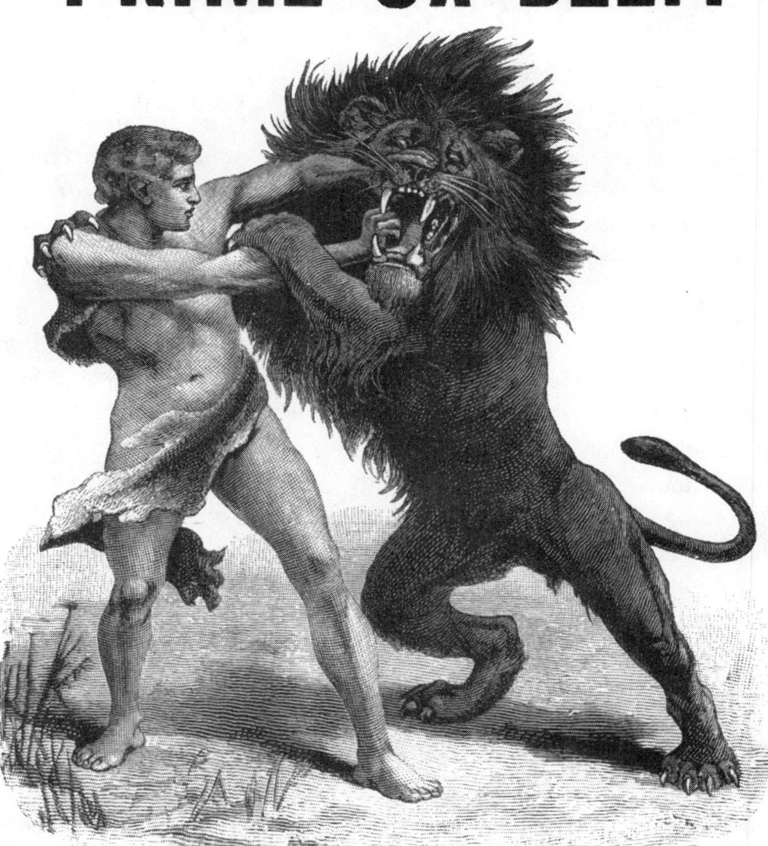

BOVRIL GIVES STRENGTH.

Advertisement, circa 1894

CHAPTER 2
Dietary Components

"The prevention of disease today is one of the most important factors in the line of human endeavor."
—Charles H. Mayo, M.D.,
Collected Papers of the Mayo Clinic and Mayo Foundation, 1913

"The power of nutriments reaches to the bone and to all parts of bone, to sinew, to vein, to artery, to muscle, to membrane, to flesh, fat, blood, phlegm, marrow, brain, spinal marrow, the intestines and all their parts."
—Hippocrates, 400 B.C.

The U.S. holds the dubious distinction of consuming more meat than any other nation with 70% of its protein from animal sources. Less fortunate nations forego that luxury and their low chronic disease rates contrast sharply with ours.

There's a parallel between our nation and the Roman Empire: the Romans ate themselves to death. Emperor Claudius I regularly served banquets of pork-stuffed sea urchins, roast deer, jellyfish, flamingo and parrot. Emperor Heliogalalus preferred camels' feet, ostrich brains and conger eels fattened on Christian slaves.

The Roman upper class suffered from lead poisoning because their aqueducts, water pipes, wine vessels and glazed cooking pots all contained lead. Meanwhile the poorer folks enjoyed good health by doing without banquets and lead pipes.

Lest one believe that such indiscretions are a quaint oddity of the less enlightened and distant past, consider the billions spent by industrialized nations in waging war on degenerative disease—cancer, heart disease, osteoporosis—afflictions rare in developing countries. Consider also Scotland's national dish of haggis: minced sheep heart, lungs, liver and mutton, all cooked inside a sheep's stomach. Glasgow, Scotland, has the world's worst heart attack rate.

In 1795, the British Navy began stocking ships with limes containing vitamin C to ward off scurvy. The U.S. eradicated diseases of deficiency (scurvy, rickets, pellagra, beriberi, goiter) during the early 1900s. Modern diseases of affluence arise primarily from dietary excess, not deficiency. The notion of excess doesn't sit well in corporate circles since it doesn't sell products.

- Heart disease is not caused by aspirin, oat bran, niacin, or fish oil deficiency.
- Cancer is not caused by beta carotene, vitamin C, olive oil, or shark cartilage deficiency.
- Osteoporosis is not caused by calcium, magnesium, boron, or estrogen replacement deficiency.
- Premature aging is not caused by chromium picolinate, bee pollen, royal jelly, coenzyme Q-10, Pycnogenol, melatonin, or kombucha mushroom deficiency.

Health does not spring from magic bullets or soundbites. To focus on products while ignoring the underlying cause is a formula ripe with failure. Isolated nutrients are no substitute for the thousands of undiscovered essential components which whole foods likely contain. Isolated nutrients are no substitute for changing the diet.

Studies report that increasing fruit and vegetable intake can cut cancer and heart disease risk by 35–50%. Therein lies the seeds of dangerous advice: that the way to counteract dietary intemperance is to eat **more** of something else. The underlying cause (excess fat and protein) is seldom addressed due to aggressive marketing by the meat and dairy industries.

In America, health is a business and most businesses operate by giving the public what they want. National institutions advocate 30% fat diets while assuming anything less is "unrealistic and culturally unacceptable." Such cosmetic advice is arrogant. Consumers have a right to the information they need to make informed decisions.

No one wants their life cut short. No one wants to waste away in a nursing home as a stagnant pond of body fluids, bedsores and clogged conduits tethered to an IV pole. Immunity from chronic illness requires building a fortress of knowledge, hardened against the vagaries of artful deception, ornamental government recommendations and deeply-instilled aberrations that corporations would have you believe. The foundation rests firmly on dietary components.

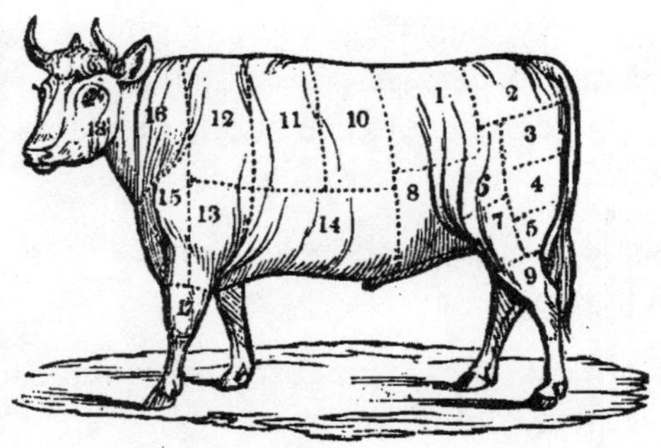

Proteins

"For its merit I will knight it, and then it will be called Sir-loin."
—King Charles II
to a fine cut of beef

"If a person accepts the theory that a low-fat diet will help prevent cancer, beef should probably be in that person's diet."
—National Cattlemen's Association
12 Myths About Beef

"Beef is the backbone of the American diet and always has been. To think that meat of all things causes cancer is ridiculous."[1]
—John Morgan, president
Riverside Meat Packers, 1976

In 1982, John Morgan died of colon cancer.[2] This caused a bit of a marketing problem.

The FDA claims that "Americans have the safest food supply in the world." Not all Americans share this confidence. While in office, President Reagan hired cattlemen to raise special "natural" beef without drugs or hormones.[3] His efforts to protect the health of his family were not successful. Ronald Reagan lost part of his colon and Nancy Reagan lost one of her breasts to cancer.

The problem wasn't the chemicals in beef, it was the beef itself. The cancer risk from chemicals pales compared to the lifetime risk from excess fat and protein. Few Americans have the financial means to raise "natural" beef, but most do consume meat everyday.

The USDA spends $4.7 million each year on the school lunch program. Current guidelines mandate that protein requirements be provided by meat, poultry, fish, or beans. These requirements seem more concerned with industry profits than with human dietary needs. The 1992 guidelines of the National Academy of Sciences do not include animal products as a necessary part of a healthy diet.[4]

GETTING ENOUGH PROTEIN

> *"To obtain too little protein is a mark of carelessness or ignorance."*[5]
>
> —Adelle Davis
> *Let's Eat Right To Keep Fit*

Many believe that large amounts of protein are needed for optimum health. But in our society, the real danger is too much protein, not too little.

> *"And people who eat more meat have higher blood cholesterol levels and higher blood albumin levels, which is a function of protein intake. As blood levels of albumin and cholesterol go up, the diseases we tend to get in the West—cancer, heart disease, and diabetes—also start going up. It's quite remarkable."*[6]
>
> —Dr. T. Colin Campbell
> China Health Project

The World Health Organization recommends 10–15% of calories from protein but most Americans consume 18%.[7] The actual human requirement for protein is far less:

- American Journal of Clinical Nutrition: 4%[8]
- World Health Organization: 6%[9]
- National Research Council: 8%[10]

Excess protein is broken down into nitrogen waste products (urea, uric acid, creatinine, ammonia) which are excreted in the urine. Over a lifetime, the kidney tissue deteriorates from the increase in flow and pressure. By age 80, most Americans have lost 33–50% of their kidney function and excess protein appears to be the prime cause.[11] People with kidney disease are placed on low-protein diets.

Excess protein contributes to osteoporosis,[12] cancer,[13] gout,[14] kidney stones,[15] rheumatoid arthritis,[16] and heart disease.[17] A lower protein diet is an **advantage**, not a disadvantage.

Most American men consume 100 grams of protein each day but need only 20–42 grams.[18] No diet is healthy if it supplies more protein than the body needs.

PROTEIN COMBINING

> *"The protein in most grains and legumes is incomplete because it does not contain all of the essential amino acids...They must be consumed with other foods that complete their amino acid mix and balance."*
>
> —National Live Stock and Meat Board
> *Exploring Meat and Health*

This notion originated from rat research during the 1940s and has since proven false.[19]

> *"Protein combining is unnecessary."*[20]
>
> —Francis Moore Lappe
> *Diet for a Small Planet*

The World Health Organization's protein requirements are based in part on the following chart:

Protein From Foods (grams per 3,000 calories)[21]

Amino Acids	Daily Requirement	Wheat	Beans	Broccoli
Tryptophan	0.5	1.4	1.8	3.8
Phenylalanine	0.6	5.9	10.9	12.2
Leucine	2.2	8.0	17.0	16.5
Isoleucine	1.4	5.2	11.3	12.8
Lysine	1.6	3.2	14.7	14.8
Valine	1.6	5.5	12.1	17.3
Methionine	0.2	1.8	2.0	5.1
Threonine	1.0	3.5	8.5	12.5
Total	37.0	120.0	198.0	338.0

This chart shows why it's virtually impossible to eat enough calories to maintain weight without getting enough protein—including all 8 essential amino acids—even if only one food is eaten. It's easy to get too much protein.

The protein requirement of older adults ranges from 0.57–1.25 grams per kg per day.[22] The study which reported older adults needing the higher protein level was funded by Kraft General Foods and the USDA.[23]

Contrary to claims by the meat and dairy industries, excess protein leads to disease. Most of our early protein charts were based on the protein requirements of rats, which are higher than those of humans.[24] (Human breast milk is 5% protein; rat's milk is 49% protein.)

All starch-based diets are packed with protein. As a percentage of calories, potatoes are 11% protein, wheat 16%, beans 26%, and broccoli 45%. For comparison, beef is 30% protein. Those who ignore the Four Food Groups by eating less meat live longer. This realization, although bad for the hamburger lobby, is essential for optimal health.

In 1977, the U.S. Senate Select Committee on Nutrition and Human Needs issued its initial report. The committee's original recommendation to eat less meat was later modified in the final report to eat less saturated fat—due to lobbying pressure by the meat industry.

> *"The American Dietetic Assn., the American Heart Assn., the National Heart, Lung and Blood Institute, and other organizations generally recommend 5–7 oz. of lean, trimmed meat daily."*
>
> —National Cattlemen's Association
> *12 Myths & Facts About Beef Production*

America's blind belief in meat is exemplified by Smoky's Tavern & Steakhouse in West Fargo, North Dakota. Smoky's offers a 3¼ pound sirloin steak. Those who eat it receive an "I Ate a 52 oz. Steak" T-shirt colored in "manly red." Those who can't finish it receive an "I Almost Ate a 52 oz. Steak" T-shirt in "baby blue."[25]

> *"Moderation—not elimination—is the key."*[26]
> —National Live Stock and Meat Board

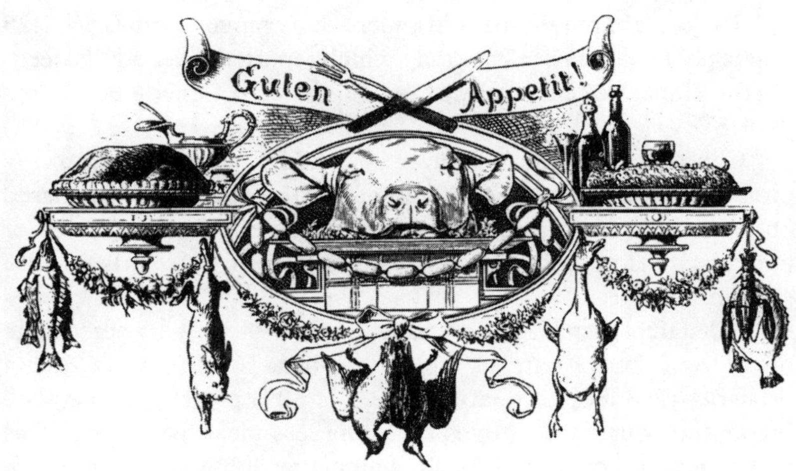

Fats

"Our greatest concern is our excessive intake of dietary fat and chronic diseases such as coronary heart disease, some types of cancers, diabetes, high blood pressure, strokes and obesity."

—C. Everett Koop, M.D.
Surgeon General's Report

"We're afraid that people won't make any change if it's too drastic."[27]

—Scott Grundy, M.D., director
National Cholesterol Education Program

In 1869, on the eve of the Franco-Prussian War, Emperor Napoleon III held a contest. Since butter was in short supply, a prize would be offered for the best butter substitute. French chemist Mege-Mouries won the contest by combining skim milk and suet (melted beef fat). He called his new product oleomargarine. The artificial fat industry was born.

Of all lascivious unmentionables in American cuisine, nothing tops fat. No other coveted enticement crosses social boundaries with such abandon. Superbowl connoisseurs favor chips, dip, Haagen Dazs and steak on a forklift. Others prefer somewhat richer fare: flaming soufflé pesto with clarified consommé, wild mushroom caviar on chocolate mousse, bourbon cheesecake and chateaubriand. For hardened cases, heart bypass surgery and chemotherapy are the preferred alternatives to diet and lifestyle changes.

Food	% Fat Calories
Potatoes	1%
Spaghetti	3%
Beans	4%
Jack-in-the-Box Cheeseburger	66%
Girl Scout Cookies, Tagalongs	67%
Sugar-Free Eskimo Pie	77%
T-Bone Steak	82%

Chronic diseases account for 85% of U.S. health-care costs with excess fat the prime culprit—contributing to more deaths than cigarettes, alcohol and HIV infections combined.[28] But blazing a trail through the thicket of misinformation surrounding fat is not easy. Political chicanery and mischief laden much dietary advice. The use of "heart-healthy" vegetable oil is a prime example:

> *"Puritan is made from canola oil, the vegetable oil lowest in saturated fat. It is an excellent choice to help meet present dietary recommendations for reducing saturated fat and cholesterol intake."*
>
> —American College of Nutrition

Such advice does a disservice. Total fats cause the most damage. Switching from butter to vegetable oil does nothing to lower fat intake since all vegetable oils are 100% fat.

The immune system naturally produces anti-cancer agents (interferon, interleukin). Vegetable oils suppress immune function and increase cancer risk more than animal fats.[29] Vegetable oils can be therapeutic in treating rheumatoid arthritis and other autoimmune diseases marked by overactive immune systems, but are not recommended for those with normal or suppressed immune function.

Most Americans consume 37% of their calories from fat. Americans are urged to eat a "low-fat" diet ranging from 5–30% of calories. The American Heart Association recommends 30%; the

World Health Organization recommends 15–30%.[30] The actual human requirement for fat is far less:

- American Journal of Clinical Nutrition 0.7%[31]
- World Health Organization 3%[32]
- Nathan Pritikin 5-10%[33]
- John McDougall 5-10%[34]
- Roy Walford 8%[35]
- Dean Ornish 10%[36]

If a person consumes 37% fat while needing only 3%, their body will be forced to deal with the excess. Of all dietary transgressions, excess fat burdens the body with the greatest load. All forms of fat are linked to cancer.[37] In China, the fat intake ranges from 6–24% of calories. Chinese cancer rates are lowest in the 6% fat regions.

> *"Cancer is most frequent among those branches of the human race where carnivorous habits prevail."*
>
> —*Scientific American*, 1892

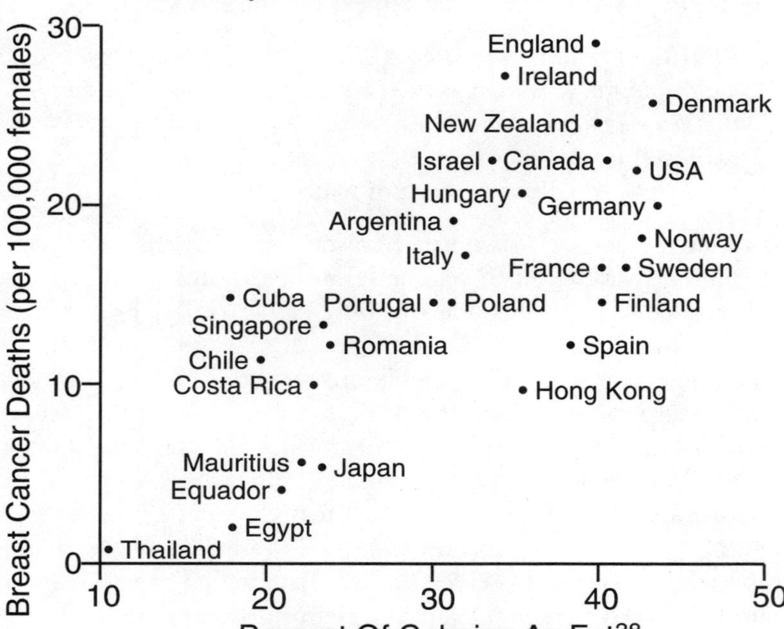

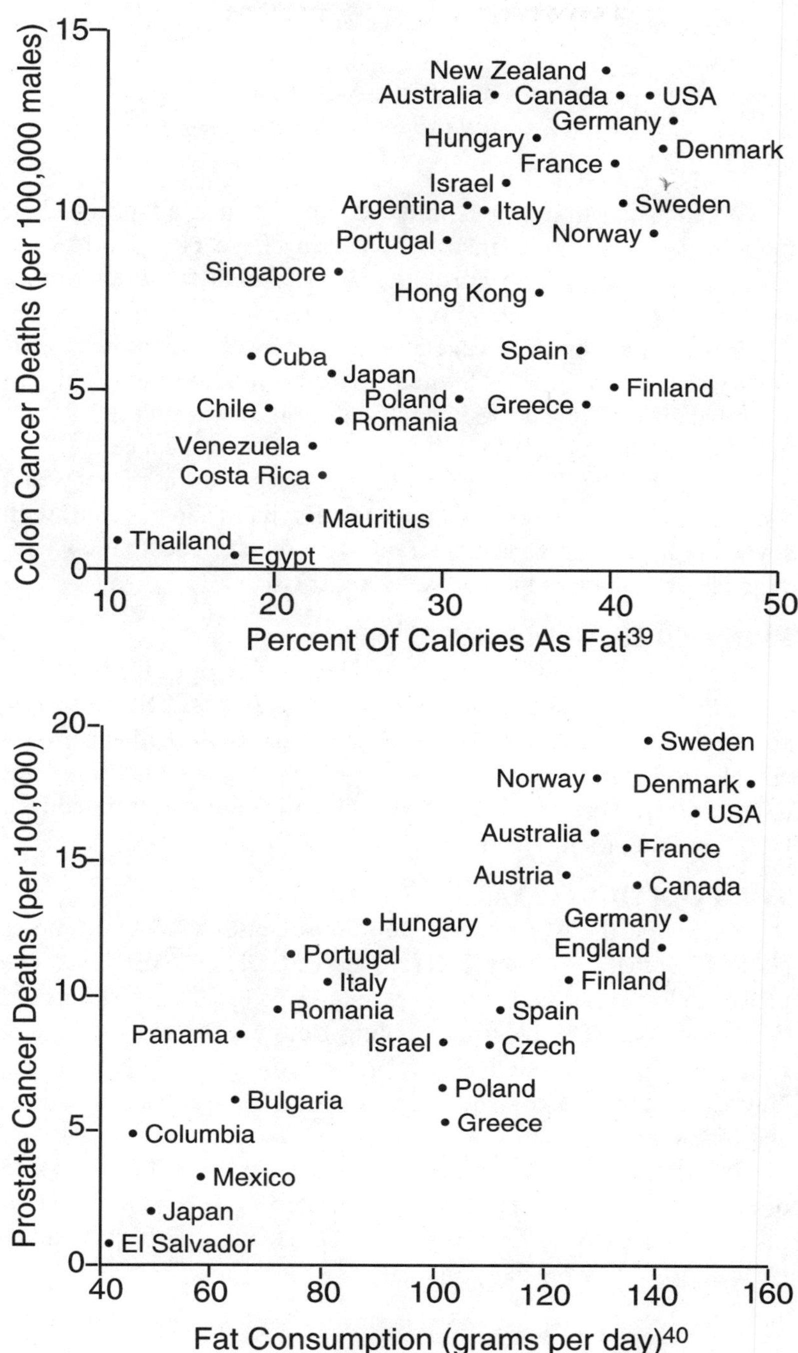
Colon Cancer Deaths (per 100,000 males)
15
10
5
0
10
20
30
40
50
Percent Of Calories As Fat39
New Zealand
Australia
Canada
USA
Germany
Hungary
Denmark
France
Israel
Argentina
Italy
Sweden
Portugal
Norway
Singapore
Hong Kong
Spain
Cuba
Japan
Finland
Poland
Greece
Chile
Romania
Venezuela
Costa Rica
Mauritius
Thailand
Egypt
Prostate Cancer Deaths (per 100,000)
20
15
10
5
0
40
60
80
100
120
140
160
Fat Consumption (grams per day)40
Sweden
Norway
Denmark
USA
Australia
France
Austria
Canada
Hungary
Germany
Portugal
England
Italy
Finland
Romania
Spain
Panama
Israel
Czech
Poland
Bulgaria
Greece
Columbia
Mexico
Japan
El Salvador

"To date, reported links between diet and cancer have been mostly hypothetical."

—National Cattlemen's Association
12 Myths About Beef

FATS AND CANCER

When Asian immigrants move to the U.S. and adopt our diet, their breast cancer incidence rises within 10 years.[41] Worldwide, the risk of breast cancer correlates directly with fat intake (total, saturated, polyunsaturated, monounsaturated).[42]

In laboratory studies, vegetable oils promote tumors more efficiently than animal fats.[43] Switching from saturated fat to polyunsaturated oil raises cancer risk.[44] Vegetable oils drive cholesterol from the blood to the colon, where it contributes to colon cancer.[45]

"Heart-healthy" fats equal cancer-unhealthy fats. In recent years, food companies have replaced tropical oils (palm and coconut) with soybean oil, and fast-food restaurants have replaced beef tallow with vegetable oil. Both factors elevate cancer risk.

FATS AND HEART DISEASE

When immigrants move to the U.S. and adopt our diet, they develop heart disease at the same rate as Americans.[46] Studies show vegetable oils to be strongly associated with artery damage.[47] Atherosclerosis is not stopped by switching from butter (saturated fat) to corn oil (polyunsaturated fat) or olive oil (monounsaturated fat). Only lowering total fat stops the progression.

THE POLITICS OF FAT

Each year the American Dietetic Association (ADA) promotes National Nutrition Month (March) EAT RIGHT AMERICA. The idea is to lower fat intake from present levels to 30%. In support of this effort, the ADA received funding from McDonald's, the Beef Industry Council, the National Live Stock and Meat Board, NutraSweet, Coca-Cola, the Sugar Association, Nabisco, Sara Lee, and Sandoz Pharmaceuticals.

In 1993, a scientific conference concluded that low-fat diets (30% or less) are not necessary to lower cholesterol levels, and that very-low-fat diets (25% or less) offer no advantages. This conference was sponsored by the dairy industry.[48]

Belief: 10% fat diets cause deficiencies in fat-soluble vitamins.

Reality: Fat-soluble vitamin deficiency (A,D,E,K) does not exist in humans on a varied low-fat diet.[49] Our society is plagued by diseases of excess, not deficiency.

Belief: 10% fat diets cause deficiencies in essential fatty acids.

Reality: Essential fatty acid deficiency (arachidonic, linoleic, linolenic) does not exist in humans on a varied low-fat diet.[50]

Belief: Low-fat diets are dangerous.

Reality: Non-fat diets are dangerous; 10% fat diets are not.

Belief: Low-fats diets are culturally unacceptable; 10% fat diets are too drastic.

Reality: Culturally unacceptable is losing a breast, prostate or colon. Drastic is cutting a foot-wide hole in someone's chest.

> *"They say now if you cut down on fat, you can live 4 months longer—no doubt in a bed, under an oxygen tent, with a needle in the arm. Who cares about that?"*[51]
>
> —Jeff Smith, author
> *The Frugal Gourmet*

Cutting fats to 30% may add only 4 months to life.[52] Dr. Ornish's study demonstrates that 10% fat diets can extend life for years and add much to its quality.[53]

> *"Prolongation of an extremely low-fat diet for more than 3 months can lead to immunosuppressive problems like viruses and multiple food allergies and chemical sensitivities."*[54]
>
> —Ann Louise Gittleman, author
> *Beyond Pritikin*

Thousands of people on the Pritikin, Ornish and McDougall programs experienced no such difficulties.[55] In civilizations down through the ages, from the Mexican Aztecs to Chinese Dynasties, low-fat diets have stood the test of time.

VEGETABLE OIL

It takes 13 ears of corn to produce one tablespoon of corn oil. Processed oil concentrates the fat-soluble pesticides. Most vegetable oils are bleached and extracted with hexane. Chemical solvents can remain in the final product and "cold pressed" oils offer no assurance of quality.

Vegetable oils are pure fat and vulnerable to rancidity from heat, light, air and time. This includes all oil-based capsules. Manufacturers often remove the vitamin E for sale separately, which further increases rancidity. Vegetable oils are no health food.

HYDROGENATED FATS

Hydrogenation is the process of adding hydrogen atoms to vegetable oil. Hydrogenation prolongs shelf life, solidifies oil, and converts the structure of fat from the natural cis form to the unnatural trans form.

Trans fats do not exist in nature. They combine with cell membranes, disrupt cellular functions, interfere with essential fatty acid metabolism, and contribute to heart disease and cancer.[56] Trans fats must be labeled on all vegetable oils sold in Canada, but not in the U.S. Most Americans consume 5–15% of their total calories from trans fats.[57]

FISH OIL

Blood cholesterol was lowered in some fish oil studies;[58] in other studies, cholesterol was raised.[59] Fish oil lowers vitamin E in the body and suppresses immune response.[60] The body uses its own vitamin E reserves in metabolizing rancid fish oil.

HIDDEN FATS

Mono- and diglycerides (found in Entenmann's "fat-free" foods) are partial fats which convert into full fats (triglycerides) during digestion.[61] Lecithin is a two-thirds fat molecule (phospholipid) which also converts into full fats. Lecithin adds to the body's fat burden and does not emulsify cholesterol.

> *"We must always think about things, and we must think about things as they are, not as they are said to be."*
>
> —George Bernard Shaw

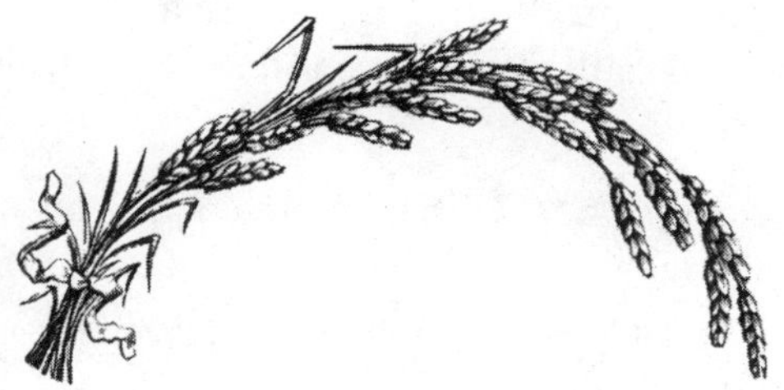

Carbohydrates

"White flour is a wholesome food and has a proper place in the well balanced, adequate diet."[62]

—American Medical Association

"The millers who impose white bread upon the nation have worked an evil . . . Woe to this nation unless it re-establish the fundamentals of nutrition which white flour and other denatured foods have broken down."[63]

—Harvey Wiley, M.D.
original FDA Commissioner

"You can travel 50,000 miles in America without once tasting a piece of good bread."[64]

—Henry Miller

Between 800 B.C. to 200 A.D., Rome ruled Europe by commanding the greatest army the world had ever seen: the Roman legion. The most elite infantry units were the centurions equipped with body armor, helmet, shield and thrusting sword. Despite their 85-pound burden, centurions endured forced marches and dealt the decisive blow on enemy ranks. Whenever possible, they discarded meat in favor of corn and grains. The human body works best on starch.

The primary purpose of food is to provide fuel for the body's metabolism. Carbohydrates are the most efficient fuel. The World Health Organization recommends 55–75% of calories from carbohydrates. Most Americans consume 45% (mostly white flour and sugar).[65]

Not all carbohydrates are created equal and wise food choices depend on knowing which is which. Dairy products contain simple sugars (lactose, galactose, glucose), the only carbohydrates found in the animal kingdom. Beef, chicken, fish and eggs contain no carbohydrates. All carbohydrates can be divided into four major groups:

1) Simple Sugars: All fiber removed and no nutrients other than empty calories (except honey and molasses). Simple sugars are absorbed more quickly than other carbohydrates. Examples:

Simple Sugars	**Natural Sugars**	**Sugar Alcohols**
• Sucrose	• Honey	• Sorbitol
• Fructose	• Molasses	• Mannitol
• Glucose	• Maple Syrup	• Maltitol
• Lactose	• Corn Syrup	• Xylitol
• Galactose	• Rice Syrup	• Dulcitol
• Maltose	• Barley Malt	

2) Synthetic Long-Chain Sugars: All fiber removed and no nutrients other than empty calories. Synthetic sugars are absorbed more slowly than simple sugars but more quickly than starches. Examples:

- Maltodextrin
- Polydextrose
- Polycose
- Glucose Polymers

These are often found in sports drinks, food bars, protein powders and fat-free ice cream. Contrary to label claims, synthetic sugars are not complex carbohydrates.

3) Refined Complex Carbohydrates (Starches): Most fiber and nutrients removed during processing. Examples:

- White Four
- White Rice
- Cornstarch

4) Unrefined Complex Carbohydrates (Starches): Contain proteins, fats, vitamins, minerals and fiber. Lower in calories, more filling and more slowly absorbed than other carbohydrates. Examples:

- Whole Grains
- Vegetables
- Beans

Numerous terms describing carbohydrates range from deceptive to straightforward. Understanding these terms is critical for optimal health.

SUGAR TERMS

Informed consumers will be wary of the following ingredients:

- Sucrose (white sugar) – composed of one fructose and one glucose molecule. The refining process includes bleaching agents, anti-caking treatments and filtering through charred cattle bones. Sucrose has an unlimited shelf life.
- Brown sugar (kleen raw or turbinado) – 96% sucrose with molasses added.
- Powdered sugar (confectioners sugar) – sucrose with cornstarch added.
- Fructose (levulose or fruit sugar) – usually made from cornstarch. Fructose enters the cells more slowly than other sugars and without using insulin.
- Glucose (dextrose) – often made from cornstarch. Glucose is the main blood sugar and basic fuel for the body.
- Maltose (malt sugar) – composed of two glucose molecules.
- Lactose (milk sugar) – composed of one galactose and one glucose molecule. Most adults lack the enzyme needed to breakdown lactose.
- Polydextrose – 89% dextrose, 10% sorbitol and 1% citric acid.
- Sucanat – evaporated sugarcane juice.
- Honey – minuscule nutrients and more calories per teaspoon than sucrose.
- Molasses – 65% sucrose and a by-product of sugarcane refining. Molasses contains more nutrients (iron, calcium), more contaminants (pesticides, lead) and more sulfur dioxide than other sugars.

In 1919, a storage tank in Boston Harbor suddenly ruptured spilling over 2 million gallons of molasses. The resulting molasses wave, cresting at 50 feet, swallowed 8 buildings and killed 21 people.[66]

FLOUR TERMS

Flour contains less fiber, fewer nutrients and more absorbable calories than whole grains. The weevil beetle, which normally thrives on wheat, cannot survive on white flour.

- Flour, Wheat Flour, Unbleached Flour – white flour.
- Bleached Flour – white flour treated with benzoyl peroxide or chlorine.
- Enriched Flour – white flour with added thiamin, niacin, riboflavin and iron.
- Whole Wheat Flour – most nutrients and fiber retained during processing.

REFINED GRAIN TERMS

- Macaroni – white flour and egg whites.
- Noodles – white flour and egg yolks.
- Ramen Noodles – white flour, often deep-fried.[67]
- Spinach Pasta – 97% white flour, 3% spinach.
- Buckwheat Soba – mostly white flour.
- Durum Flour – white flour.
- Semolina Flour – white flour.
- Couscous – durum or semolina flour, rolled into granules.
- Farina – wheat endosperm.
- Seitan – wheat gluten.
- Polenta – course cornmeal (corn grits), without bran or germ.
- Maize – refined cornmeal, without bran or germ.
- Polished Rice – white rice.
- Basmati Rice – quick-cooking, long-grain white rice.
- Parboiled Rice (converted) – partially precooked white rice.
- Instant Rice – completely precooked white rice.

BREADS

In ancient Egypt, where bread baking began as a profession, anyone caught altering the traditional bread would be hung from their thumbs by the bakery gate. Things are a bit different today: chlorine, formaldehyde and pesticides are among the 80 additives allowed in bread without disclosure. Some breads stay indented after being squeezed due to chemicals added to make the loaf hold more water. This enhances both the shelf life and profit margin.

WHOLE GRAIN TERMS

- Whole Wheat Berries – original form before refining. Hard Red Winter variety will last for 10 years without refrigeration.
- Cracked Wheat – toasted and crushed.
- Bulgar – steamed, dried and cracked wheat.
- Hulled Barley – bran and nutrients retained.
- Buckwheat Kasha – hulled and toasted kernels.
- Buckwheat Groats – hulled and untoasted kernels.

Country	Rice Consumption[68] (per person per year)
USA	18 pounds
Japan	158 pounds
China	365 pounds
Burma	421 pounds

In China, the word "restaurant" means "house of rice." Three whole grains (rice, wheat, corn) feed 90% of the world's population. In the U.S., livestock consume 70% of all grain.

> *"Everything you see I owe to spaghetti."*[69]
> —Sophia Loren

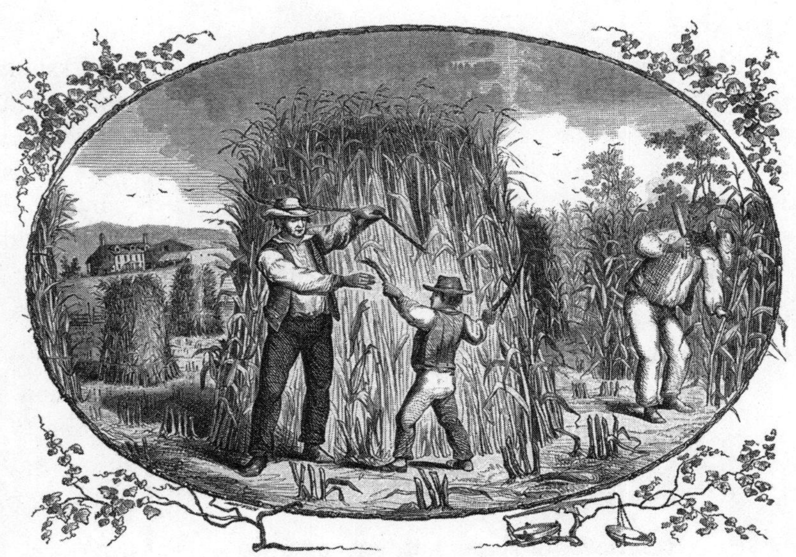

Additives

"Never eat anything whose listed ingredients cover more than one-third of the package."
—Joseph Leonard

"All, as they say, that glitters is not gold."
—John Dryden
The Hind and the Panther

Dating back to Egyptian pharaohs, additives were used to enhance the color, flavor and preservation of food. Soldiers in ancient times were paid off in salt. Things are somewhat more complicated today. Modern processed food bears little resemblance to the unrefined state from which it emerged.

A visit to the supermarket provides convincing evidence that people will eat just about anything. Most Americans consume about 10 pounds of additives each year, not counting sucrose, dextrose, salt and corn syrup.[70] More than 3,000 additives are used in foods. Some are listed as ingredients, others are not. Strange things happen when hundreds of chemicals combine in the body. It's impossible to predict precisely the interactions or long-term consequences.

All additives fall into two general categories:

1) **Direct Additives** (deliberately added to food).
- Nutrients – vitamins, minerals
- Preservatives – nitrates, benzoic acid, antioxidants
- Processing aids – thickeners, fillers, emulsifiers
- Flavorings – MSG, salt, sweeteners
- Colorings – bleaches, coal tar

2) **Indirect Additives** (not deliberately added to food).
- Residues – pesticides, hormones, drugs
- Packaging – lead from soldered cans, dioxins from bleached paper containers, chemicals from microwaveable styrofoam

BEEF

About 80% of U.S. agricultural pesticides are used on only four crops—corn, soybeans, cotton, wheat—major components of livestock feed. Corn grown for cattle feed is allowed to contain more pesticides than corn grown for human consumption. Beef has the highest herbicide level of any U.S. food.[71]

Half the U.S. antibiotics are given to livestock, either by food or injection.[72] This practice contributes to antibiotic-resistant bacteria. Most hamburger meat comes from spent dairy cows, the most heavily medicated farm animals. Modern beef production methods often include the following novel ingredients:

Cattle Feed
- Hydrolyzed poultry feathers, straw, cardboard and sawdust
- Ground newspaper mixed with molasses
- Plastic pellets, sewer sludge and ammonia
- Cottonseed oil mash (pesticide saturated)
- Chicken feces, sheep and cattle remains (high protein)
- Cement dust (makes cattle thirsty)

Hormones
- Estrogen, estradiol, testosterone, progesterone

Antibiotics
- Penicillin, tetracycline, sulfamethazine, streptomycin

Direct Additives
- Sodium-nitrate, nitrite, sulfite, BHA, BHT

U.S. cattle may be infected with a new strain of "mad cow disease," also called bovine spongiform encephalopathy (BSE).[73] In humans, it's known as Creutzfeldt-Jakob disease, an incurable and fatal form of dementia. BSE can be contracted by eating infected animals. The USDA allows the practice of feeding dead cattle to living cattle.

> *"Responding to the challenges of our competitive free-market system, cattlemen use efficient production methods to provide consumers with a safe and wholesome product."*
>
> —Beef Promotion and Research Board
> *Cattle and Beef: The American Industry*

ICE CREAM

As one of civilization's most complicated foods, ice cream contains over 1,600 chemical additives without disclosure.

Ice Cream Chemical	Flavor	Other Uses[74]
Aldehyde	Cherry	Dyes, plastic, rubber
Piperonal	Vanilla	Kills lice
Amyl butyrate	Banana	Oil paint solvent
Benzyl acetate	Strawberry	Nitrate solvent
Ethyl acetate	Pineapple	Leather and textile cleaner
Butyraldehyde	Nut	Rubber cement
Isoamyl acetate	Pear	Paint remover, shoe polish

> *"Ice cream is a healthful food made from milk and cream along with other good things."*[75]
>
> —National Dairy Council

> *"Ice cream was made by God—are you going to tell me there's something wrong with it?"*[76]
>
> —Bill Cosby

Ruben Mattus, the founder of Häagen-Dazs, sold his ice cream company in 1983 before undergoing open heart surgery.

FOOD IRRADIATION

Food irradiation (equivalent to 30 million chest X-rays) is being promoted as the ideal solution to bacteria contamination and foodborne illness. The nuclear, poultry and meat industries stand to reap sizable profits. However, this technology does have a price.

Food irradiation produces radiolytic products including benzene, formaldehyde, peroxides and benzopyrene quinones. According to the FDA, these products exist in nature and are harmless to people in the amounts consumed.[77] But irradiation also produces a different class of compounds called unique radiolytic products which do not exist in nature. These have not been tested for safety. No study cited by the FDA can justify the safety of food irradiation.[78]

Irradiation kills bacteria which emit smells warning that food has spoiled. Food is not sterilized by irradiation and the surviving organisms are radiation-resistant.[79] In one study, 80% of children fed irradiated wheat developed abnormal blood cells (polyploidy lymphocytes) associated with leukemia.[80] When irradiated wheat was discontinued, the blood cells returned to normal. In another study, Chinese fed irradiated foods developed abnormal chromosomes.[81] Irradiated sugar damages human chromosomes, and several animal species have died eating irradiated foods.[82]

ABC-TV's 20/20 aired a show on food irradiation, which concluded that scientific concerns were scare tactics. The wife of the show's executive producer is president of a PR firm representing the nuclear industry.[83] To help prove that food irradiation is safe, proponents may wish to volunteer for a human study in which half eat irradiated foods and half eat non-irradiated foods.

Food irradiation may be called "electronic pasteurization" or "picowaved." Irradiated whole foods will be identified with a flower-shaped symbol, but irradiated ingredients and processed foods may be sold without disclosure.[84] Breads made from irradiated wheat need not be labeled. Food irradiation can be stopped (as in 29 other countries) with a government ban or with a national consumer boycott following mandatory labeling.

GENETICALLY-ENGINEERED FOOD

The biotech industry has the power to change forever the world's food supply. Dozens of biotech companies (DuPont, Monsanto, Eli Lilly) are field-testing 678 gene-altered crops.[85] Combinations include potatoes spliced with chicken genes, tomatoes spliced with fish genes, corn spliced with virus genes, and pigs spliced with human genes. Thousands of bacteria, insect and animal combinations are being planned. Bioengineering transgresses the species barrier, a boundary heretofore inviolate.

The first gene-altered food for sale in the U.S. (Calgene's Flavr Savr Tomato) contains a marker gene that confers resistance to the antibiotic kanamycin.[86] The FDA admits that antibiotic-resistant genes can reduce the benefit of prescribed antibiotics.[87] Mixing genes could increase pesticide use if resistance is transferred to nearby weeds.[88] Virus genes can recombine with other viruses to create more virulent strains.[89] It is difficult to recall new life forms.

All new technologies carry unknown risks. EMS (eosinophilia-myalgia syndrome), the disease responsible for 38 deaths and 1,500 injuries from the use of tryptophan, was caused by genetically-altered bacteria.[90] A second biotech accident has also occurred: researchers inadvertently transferred brazil nut genes containing an allergen into soybeans.[91]

In 1992, the FDA announced it will not regulate gene-altered foods. Manufacturers may sell bioengineered foods without safety testing or disclosure. With such potential for harm, the FDA's cavalier attitude is not in the interest of public health. A recent survey found that 85% of Americans want genetically-engineered foods to be labeled. Labeling confers information and accountability; lack of labeling encourages abuse.

> *"For most people around the country, if the FDA approves a product, they believe it to be safe. They accept the judgments of groups like the FDA and the AMA. That's what we're counting on."*[92]
>
> —Robert Shapiro, president
> Monsanto Chemical Co.

ALUMINUM

Only nine elements compose 99.25% of the earth's crust. Aluminum is number three (after oxygen and silicon). Hidden aluminum sources pervade the American diet: salt (silicoaluminate), cake mixes (aluminum phosphate), and pickles (alum). Ubiquitous aluminum lurks in shampoo, antiperspirants, antacids, cookware and drinking water.

Alzheimer's disease occurs only in Western countries. Aluminum, a cumulative neurotoxin, concentrates in the senile plaques and neurofibrillary tangles in the brains of Alzheimer's patients.[93]

Communities with elevated aluminum in their drinking water have a higher prevalence of Alzheimer's.[94] The progression of Alzheimer's was slowed in one group of patients receiving an aluminum binding agent.[95] With the rising prevalence of Alzheimer's among older Americans, a personal strategy for avoiding aluminum accumulation seems prudent.

ASPARTAME

As the most popular artificial sweetener in history, aspartame (NutraSweet, Equal, Spoonful) is consumed by more people than any other synthetic chemical in the world.[96] Industry portrays aspartame as an innocuous food additive with no adverse effects. Such a position seems difficult to justify.

Aspartame is composed of methanol (methyl alcohol), aspartic acid and phenylalanine. Methanol is a known neurotoxin and cumulative poison.[97] At high temperature, methanol breaks down into formaldehyde and formic acid, both known to cause reactions in sensitive individuals.[98] In high doses, aspartame damages brain cells and induces brain tumors.[99] The FDA has received more adverse reaction reports due to aspartame than any other food additive.[100]

In 1981, the FDA approved aspartame using flawed studies from the manufacturer.[101] FDA Commissioner Authur Hayes approved aspartame despite its known risks.[102] In 1983, Hayes left the FDA to join a public relations firm for G.D. Searle Company, the maker of aspartame.[103] Searle is now owned by Monsanto. The American Dietetic Association openly endorses aspartame, and provided a free public information hotline, funded by Monsanto.[104]

FAT SUBSTITUTES

- **Simplesse** by Monsanto
- **Caprenin** by Proctor & Gamble
- **Trailblazer** by Kraft General Foods
- **Olestra** by Proctor & Gamble

Simplesse and Trailblazer are derived from egg whites and dairy protein (casein). Caprenin is derived from fatty acids. Olestra (sucrose polyester) is an undigestable molecule never seen before in the food supply. The long-term effects of fat substitutes are unknown.

ARTIFICIAL COLORS

The FDA contends that artificial colors are no less desirable than natural ones. Yet nothing edible in nature has the color of a maraschino cherry. Artificial colors (U.S. certified colors) carry the prefix FD&C, signifying their use in foods, drugs and cosmetics. Example:

- Official Name: FD&C Yellow No. 5
- Common name: Tartrazine
- Technical name: 5-oxo-1-(p-sulfophenyl)-4-[(p-sulfophenyl) azo]-2-pyrazoline-3-carboxylic acid, trisodium salt

Tartrazine (used in candy, pickles and junk food) has been shown to induce hyperactivity in children.[105] Cheese, butter and ice cream may contain artificial colors without disclosure.[106] (The dairy industry has a strong Washington lobby.)

Never eat anything you can't pronounce, anything which must be explained, or anything with a longer life expectancy than you. According to funeral directors, American corpses are decomposing more slowly due to the greater use of food preservatives.[107]

> *"I want nothing to do with natural foods. At my age, I need all the preservatives I can get."*[108]
> —George Burns

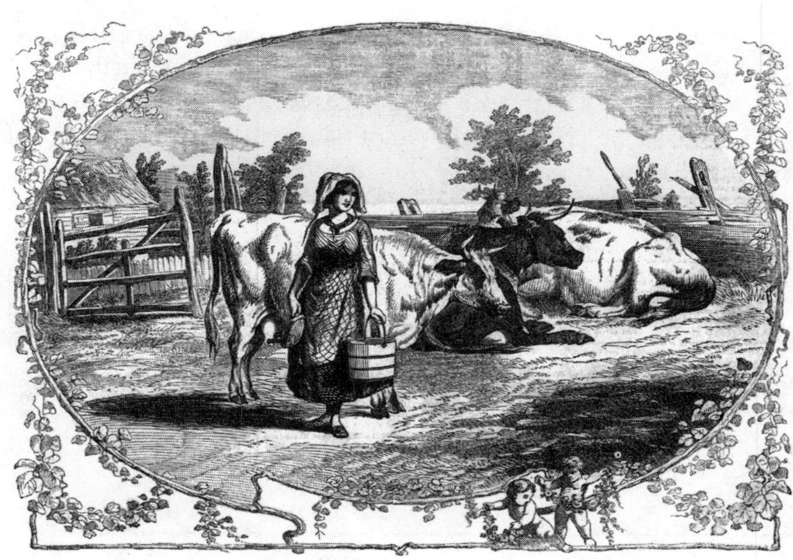

Dairy Products

"The American Heart Association recommends adults have two or more cups of low-fat milk products a day."[109]
—National Dairy Board

"Dairy products are among the most nourishing foods, and a fitting complement to almost any meal."[110]
—Editors of *Prevention*

History is unclear when humans first started milking domesticated animals. Iran was the first to domesticate goats around 7000 B.C.; Greece began cattle production around 6000 B.C.; an Elamite seal from 2500 B.C. shows a goat being milked.

The U.S. and Scandinavian countries are the world's top milk consumers. Dairy products (excluding butter) supply major nutrients in the American diet: calcium (75%), proteins (20%), fats (11%), and total calories (10%).[111]

Lactose is the principal carbohydrate of dairy milk. Most adults undergo a gradual decline in the intestinal enzyme (lactase) needed to break down milk sugar (lactose). This decline begins in early childhood, increases with age, and produces a litany of ills in sensitive individuals. Among North American adults, lactose intolerance occurs in 79% of Native Americans, 75% of blacks, 51% of Hispanics, and 21% of Caucasians.[112] Yogurt contains 40% less lactose than cow's milk but more glucose and galactose.

Casein is the principal protein of dairy milk, comprising about 80% of protein calories. Whey and lactalbumin are minor proteins. Cheese and buttermilk contain casein but no lactose; goat's milk contains lactose but no casein.[113]

Removing the fat from dairy products concentrates the protein and lactose content. Dairy fat contributes to heart disease by being 66% saturated.[114] Clarified butter (ghee) is more saturated than regular butter. Cow's milk generates more stomach acid than any other food.

Comparing Milks (values for 8 ounces)[115]

	Calories	% Fat Calories
Cow (whole, 4%)	150	51%
Cow (low-fat, 2%)	120	35%
Cow (low-fat, 1%)	100	22%
Cow (skim)	85	4%
Buttermilk (1%)	100	18%
Goat (whole)	168	54%
Soy (regular)	100–213	22–60%
Soy (low-fat)	100–140	13–18%
Rice (regular)	130–203	2–21%
Rice (almond flavored)	272	23%

Dairy protein is the leading cause of food allergies.[116] Dairy products are implicated in the cause of insulin-dependent diabetes,[117] cataracts,[118] multiple sclerosis,[119] prostate and ovarian cancers,[120] intestinal blood loss,[121] lymphoma,[122] rheumatoid arthritis,[123] iron deficiency anemia,[124] lymph node enlargement,[125] osteoporosis,[126] and female infertility.[127]

The pasteurization of milk (high temperature) generates trans fats which integrate into cell membranes. The homogenization of milk (fat globules evenly distributed) increases oxidation and atherosclerosis. Raw milk keeps for 3 days; processed milk keeps for 11 days. Raw milk sours; processed milk rots. Dairy milk may be an unfortunate substitute for human milk in infancy or a risky food source thereafter, or both.

Small quantities of undigested proteins are absorbed through the human intestinal tract on a regular basis.[128] Undigested proteins can migrate from the blood into breast milk. Mothers of colicky infants were found to have cow protein antibodies in their breast milk.[129]

If undigested proteins from dairy products can be absorbed, then so can other substances. It's therefore wise to consider the other substances that dairy products may contain.

Dairy Products May Contain Pesticides:

The FDA Total Diet Study found pesticides in 70% of U.S. cheese. No milk available on the U.S. market is free of pesticide residues.[130] The U.S. allows twice the heptachlor level in milk as the World Health Organization. [131]

Dairy Products May Contain Drugs:

According to the General Accounting Office, up to 82 drugs are used in dairy cows but the FDA only tests for four. Milk may contain traces of 80 different antibiotics.[132]

Dairy Products May Contain Infectious Agents:

Including E. coli, listeria, tuberculosis, pus, salmonella,[133] bovine leukemia virus,[134] and bovine immunodeficiency virus (BIV).[135] Both viruses can infect other species and BIV has infected at least one human.[136]

Dairy Products May Contain Contaminants:

Including dioxins and PCBs.[137] Roughly 12% of rendered cattle are fed to dairy cows.

Dairy Products May Contain Hormones:

The FDA has allowed bovine growth hormone (BGH) to be sold in milk without disclosure since 1985.[138]

BGH increases udder infections and the need for antibiotics.[139] BGH elevates insulin growth factor in milk which may cause allergic and gut tissue reactions in humans.[140] Insulin growth factor in the presence of casein is not destroyed by the digestive system.

The American Medical Association and Monsanto jointly produced a 20 minute TV show promoting BGH. The program features the American Dietetic Association, which was paid $100,000 by Monsanto to field phone calls from concerned consumers.[141]

The four BGH manufacturers (Monsanto, Eli Lilly, American Cyanamid, Upjohn) contributed at least $1.3 million to congressional candidates.[142] Genentech, the biotech company that developed BGH for Monsanto, was a major funder of Clinton.[143] The FDA official who approved the use of BGH (without labeling) was a former Monsanto attorney.[144] BGH will likely cost taxpayers $510 million by 1999 in dairy price support programs.[145]

> *"There is no crisis regarding milk safety, and we have no evidence to warrant consumer concern."*[146]
>
> —Gerald B. Guest, director
> FDA Center for Veterinary Medicine

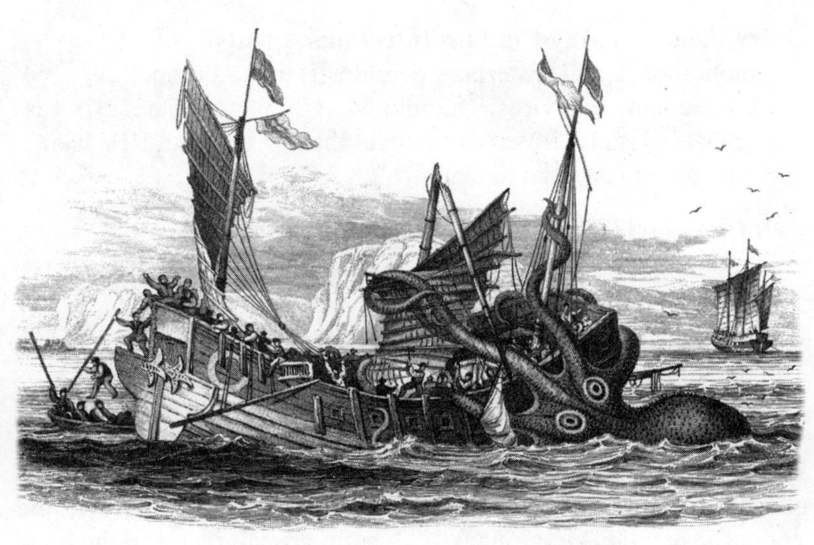

Seafood

"You can drink the polluted Great Lakes waters over a lifetime and not get as much chemical contamination as you'd get from eating one fish meal."[147]

—Jeffery Foran, environmental expert
George Washington University

"If it swims, it's edible."[148]

—Bill Demmond, vice president
Inland Seafood Corp.

In times past, coal miners brought canaries into the mines to check for pockets of poisonous gas. Sudden death signaled a warning. Today there's a new kind of canary. The following sign was posted on a Santa Monica fishing pier in response to fish measuring the highest DDT level in the nation:[149]

WARNING

Eating fish caught in Santa Monica Bay may be harmful to your health because of chemical contamination. You should not eat the fish called White Croaker, King Fish, or Tom Cod.

Fish concentrate chemicals by breathing the polluted water in which they swim. One pound of fish from Lake Ontario can contain all the toxins from 1.5 million quarts of polluted water.

The EPA estimates fish can concentrate PCBs (polychlorinated biphenyls) up to 9 million times the amount in the water.[150] Current PCB levels in humans will remain detectable for the next six generations.[151] Most PCBs in the American diet originate from fish.[152] Seafood is not always a prize catch.

PRACTICE SAFE SEAFOOD

Seafood shipped long distances may be treated with antibiotics, chlorine, sulfites and sodium phosphate without disclosure.[153] With no mandatory federal inspection program, seafood may be highly contaminated with industrial chemicals (PCBs, dioxins), pesticides (DDT), and heavy metals (mercury, lead). No other food presents such a broad range of contamination.

Contaminated seafood affects beef, chicken and eggs since PCB-tainted fish meal is routinely fed to livestock and chickens.[154] Livestock consume half the world's fish catch.[155]

Great Lakes coho salmon exceed the government's PCB safety limit by 70-fold.[156] New Jersey and New York health departments have advised women of childbearing age to avoid certain species of fish since chemicals could harm a developing fetus or breastfeeding infant.[157] A Wayne State University study found that mothers who ate 2–3 Great Lakes fish per month had babies with smaller heads, slower movements and short-term memory problems.[158]

> *"[Great Lakes fish should not be eaten by] children or by men or women who ever plan to have children."*[159]
>
> —Genesee County Medical Society, Michigan

Pollution emasculates fish. We spend about $50 million each year stocking the Great Lakes because the males of certain species never reach full sexual maturity. Rainbow trout have hatched with bisexual organs. Chemicals accumulate in fatty tissue throughout the life of fish or shellfish. Older, larger fish usually pose a greater hazard.

There are two basic approaches for dealing with contaminated seafood:

- Government Approach. Eat a wide variety of seafood.
- *Long Life Now* Approach. Select your seafood wisely.

Safe seafood selection is made easier with the following guidelines:

- **Avoid seafood caught from the major pollution hot spots:**
  – Niagara River, Hudson River, Long Island Sound, NY
  – Chelsea River, Boston Harbor, Salem Harbor, MA
  – San Francisco Bay, San Diego Bay, Santa Monica Bay, CA
  – Chester River, Baltimore Harbor, MD
  – James River, Chesapeake Bay, VA
  – Puget Sound, WA; New Orleans, LA
  – Black River, OH; Black Rock Harbor, CT
  – The Great Lakes; Hamilton Harbor, Ontario

- **Avoid Predatory Fish:** High on the food chain; accumulate methyl mercury (swordfish, marlin, shark, tuna, bass, pike).

- **Avoid Bottom Feeders:** Vulnerable to toxic sediment; develop fish cancers (catfish, carp, flounder).
- **Avoid Migratory Fish:** Vulnerable to coastal pollution (striped bass, bluefish, mackerel, salmon, Atlantic sturgeon).
- **Avoid Farm Raised Fish:** Fish farms may use hormones, antibiotics, vaccines and pesticides without disclosure[160] (catfish, carp, trout, salmon).
- **Avoid Shellfish:** Especially vulnerable to coastal pollution (oysters, clams, mussels, scallops, crab, lobster).
- **Avoid Freshwater Fish:** The same group that pregnant and nursing women are advised to avoid.

At this point, only the safest fish are left: small, low-fat, offshore, ocean varieties (sole, snapper, cod, haddock, pollock, ocean perch, halibut, grouper, monkfish, orange roughy).

> *"Treat a fish just like you love it, and release it. Let it live and if you want something to eat, you can get a hamburger at McDonald's later, or at the Cattle Crossing Cafe."*[161]
>
> —Jimmy Carter
> speaking to schoolchildren

Vitamin Wars

"[It is] not in our policy to jeopardize the financial interests of the pharmaceutical companies."[162]
—Dr. Charles Edwards
former FDA Commissioner

"Excess and deficiency are equally at fault."
—Confucius, XI .15

Throughout recorded history people have treated themselves for various ailments using common and not-so-common substances: herbs, potions, mystical elixirs and strange concoctions steeped in botanical lore. The tradition continues today.

Wheel a shopping cart down the aisle of any supermarket and consider the vitamins and minerals shouting their presence in everything from orange juice to cereal. Venture into any natural food store and peruse the curious offerings of coenzymes, carotenoids, flavonoids and exotic root extractions. Ponder the herbal-based, enteric-coated, micro-encapsulated thermogenic energy precursors. A virtual cornucopia of chemical delights awaits the initiated.

Roughly half the U.S. population takes some form of dietary supplement either as a pill, capsule, liquid, or powder. Consumers utilize this $4 billion dollar industry to care for their own needs without any help from government. The FDA would like to change all that. FDA swat-teams frequently raid health food stores and clinics as officers break down doors with guns drawn. These high-profile media events, however, often overlook the underlying issues.

As our population ages, there's a growing economic imperative for the need to prevent chronic illness. Opposing this trend are those lucrative enterprises that profit from orthodox medical procedures.

Dietary supplements are non-patentable and the pharmaceutical industry's primary competitor. From the consumer standpoint, supplements are an inexpensive way to achieve and maintain health. From the drug company standpoint, supplements cut into their profits. Both sides are positioned for an economic showdown.

In 1989, the National Research Council released a 768-page study which found no health benefits from supplements.[163] This conclusion was widely reported:

"US Says No To Vitamin Pills: They Won't Help, May Hurt."[164]

However, the media did not report that this study was funded by Occidental Petroleum, the Kaiser Foundation and other private organizations, not the U.S. government. These organizations profit from conventional medical procedures, as do the researchers who conducted the study.

TRYPTOPHAN

As the most effective producer of serotonin currently known, L-tryptophan (an amino acid) has given millions of people relief from pain, insomnia and depression. It was cheap, safe, without side-effects and sold over-the-counter. But it also cut into the sales of Valium, Halcion, Prozac, Xanax, Codeine, Dalmane and other prescription drugs.

During the late 1980s, contaminated tryptophan was linked to an outbreak of EMS (eosinophilia-myalgia syndrome) and traced to a single Japanese company (Showa Denko).[165] The FDA banned tryptophan from the market following 38 deaths due to EMS. Although the contamination problem was corrected and tryptophan continues to be used in hospitals and infant formulas, the ban remains in effect. Drug companies have profited handsomely since the ban.

PROFITEERING

Dr. Richard Wurtman is an MIT professor and FDA expert witness. In testifing before Congress, he urged that all amino acids be banned from the market. Dr. Wurtman reportedly owns over 20 medical use patents for amino acids—patents which would yield windfall profits only if amino acids were made available by prescription-only.[166]

A revolving door exists between the FDA and the drug industry. FDA officials often emerge from drug companies and return to them after leaving government service. In 1992, over 150 FDA officials owned stock in the drug companies they regulated.[167] This arrangement seems less than exemplary in serving the public interest.

The FDA regulates supplements under authority of the Dietary Supplement Health and Education Act. Before its passage, the FDA Task Force made the following recommendations:[168]

- Establish a Dietary Supplement Limit (DSL) for each vitamin and mineral which would be the maximum daily intake that the FDA deems safe.
- Classify those supplements that exceed the DSL as unsafe food additives and remove them from the market.
- Regulate all amino acids and products containing amino acids as drugs.

Regulating all products containing amino acids as drugs would be difficult since half of NutraSweet is phenylalanine, an amino acid. These proposals would have replaced most supplements with "nutriceuticals"—patentable, profitable and available by prescription-only. The FDA Task Force reached this position after considering various issues:

> *"The Task Force considered...what steps are necessary to ensure that the existence of dietary supplements on the market does not act as a disincentive for drug development."*[169]
>
> —FDA Task Force executive summary

The FDA claims they harbor no bias against supplements and that they're acting in the best interest of public health. You must decide this for yourself.

> *"The American public does not have the knowledge to make wise decisions...FDA is the arbiter of truth. Trust us. We will tell you what is good for you."*[170]
>
> —David Kessler, M.D.
> FDA Commissioner

ARGUMENTS FOR TAKING SUPPLEMENTS

- Most American food is processed and deficient in nutrients.
- The soil is depleted from modern farming practices.
- Drugs, birth control pills, stress, pollution and junk food each increase the need for nutrients.

- Immune function is enhanced by vitamins C and E in amounts above the RDA.
- Most cancer patients have low levels of anti-oxidants.
- Multivitamins decrease the risk of birth defects.
- Beta-carotene can slow atherosclerosis.[171]

ARGUMENTS AGAINST TAKING SUPPLEMENTS

- Foods provide all the nutrients anyone need. Supplements give a false sense of security.
- It's a waste of money to make your urine and palms turn different colors. Americans have the most expensive urine in the world.
- Long-lived societies (Hunzas, Okinawans) don't take pills.
- Megadoses of vitamins A, D, B6 and niacin can cause liver and nerve damage.
- Bonemeal, dolomite and oyster shells may contain lead and mercury.
- Yeast contains purines which may cause food allergies and gout.
- Excess iron may increase heart disease and cancer risk.[172] Iron is toxic and should not be taken by men or nonmenstrating women.
- Calcium tablets may promote gallstones and urinary track infections.[173]
- Zinc tablets may contribute to heart disease, colon cancer, immunodeficiency and Alzheimer's.[174]
- Vitamin C in the presence of high body iron stores may increase heart disease risk by oxidizing LDL cholesterol.[175]
- Excess beta-carotene may cause birth defects, orange skin, low white cell counts and reduced levels of vitamin E.[176]
- Excess magnesium may increase heart disease risk.[177]

VITAMIN B12 AND VEGETARIANS

Like some insidious creature chained in the basement, the B12 issue has haunted vegetarian circles for years because it's the only scientifically valid criticism of a plant-based diet. And the issue isn't going away.

Vitamin B12 is an essential nutrient needed to prevent pernicious anemia and irreversible neurological damage. Vitamin B12 is produced only by bacteria, not by plants or animals, and is the only vitamin containing a mineral (cobalt). Colon bacteria supply small amounts, however, B12 is not absorbed from the colon.

The human body tenaciously holds B12 reserves for 3–6 years, and the minimum requirement is only 0.1 micrograms per day.[178] Higher B12 absorption occurs when reserves are low so that intake can be sporadic without causing a shortage. B12 deficiency can be confirmed by a low B12 blood level (under 300 pg/ml) combined with elevated methylmalonic acid and homocysteine.[179]

Vitamin B12 comes in two basic forms:

- Cobalamin – naturally occurring in food.
- Cyanocobalamin – commercially available form with cyanide added as a stabilizer. (This type is not found in nature.)

The biologically active forms of B12 are found predominantly in animal products. Plant foods are essentially devoid of B12, especially in countries with adequate sanitation practices. Many believe in vegetarian sources of B12: yeast, spirulina, sourdough bread, sea vegetables, sauerkraut, and fermented soyfoods (tempeh, miso). However, there are no reliable vegetarian B12 sources because the vitamin is either:[180]

- Non-existent or negligible.
- Not absorbed by the human body.
- A non-active B12 analogue (corrinoid).

Consuming a B12 analogue may cause vitamin B12 deficiency. Between 5–30% of the reported B12 in foods may be analogues. Labels showing the B12 content of foods and supplements cannot be trusted since the manufacturers are required to use inaccurate testing methods (USP assay).[181]

Should vegetarians take vitamin pills to supply their B12? Even the experts change their mind on this issue:

> *"Do not use vitamin pills to supply your requirements. These pills contain breakdown products of B12, which have an anti-B12 effect and can cause B12 deficiency . . . ."*[182]
>
> —John McDougall, M.D.
> *The McDougall Plan*, 1983

> *"Therefore, I suggest that after you've been off animal foods for a few years, you take a B12 vitamin pill periodically."*[183]
>
> —John McDougall, M.D.
> *The McDougall Program*, 1990

There are no known long-lived societies using supplements for their essential nutrients. There are no known long-lived societies on a strict vegan vegetarian diet.[184] The China Health Study found no vegan vegetarians.

It is therefore recommended that the optimum diet include small quantities of low-fat animal products for the sole purpose of supplying vitamin B12. Even Mahatma Gandhi drank goat's milk (doctors orders) and was considered a lacto-vegetarian.[185]

The New Four Food Groups (grains, beans, fruits, vegetables) presented by the Physicians Committee for Responsible Medicine has bearing on the B12 issue:

> *"The Four Food Groups, as we presented it, wasn't trying to say what the totality of the diet should be. It only said what the basis, the foundation of the diet should be... So if a person has a bowl of ice cream once a month, that isn't violating the New Four Food Groups."*[186]
>
> —Neal Barnard, M.D., president
> Physicians Committee for Responsible Medicine

The notion of "animal sources of B12" is blasphemy to most vegan vegetarians, just as "vegetarian sources of B12" is heresy to most dietitians. As the B12 controversy rages on, it's worth considering that the world's longest-lived people consume 1% of their calories from animal products. *Long Life Now* is based on that diet.

TYPES OF VITAMINS

1) Synthetic Vitamins (Isolated)

Vitamin A – palmitate (from palmitic acid)
Vitamin C – ascorbic acid (from corn starch or sorbitol)
Vitamin C with rosehips – 98% ascorbic acid, 2% rosehips
Vitamin D – ergosterol or calciferol
Vitamin E – dl alpha tocopherol

Derived from chemicals or highly processed foods. Synthetic vitamins in fortified cereals may not be well absorbed.[187]

2) Natural Vitamins (Isolated)

Vitamin A – fish oil or vegetable oil source
Vitamin C – acerola, rosehips or bioflavonoids
Vitamin D – fish oil source
Vitamin E – d alpha tocopherol or mixed tocopherols

Derived from less processed foods. Natural vitamins may be coated with shellac since the FDA considers it a natural ingredient.[188] Most capsules contain gelatin, a natural ingredient from cattle hooves. Some pills dissolve slowly; others never dissolve. One man took calcium tablets for years. When his septic tank was cleaned, the bottom was caked with little white pills.[189]

Most natural and synthetic vitamins are manufactured by one of nine sources: Roucell, Eastman Kodak, Hoffman LaRoche, Pfizer, Takeda, Henkel, BASF Wyandotte, Rhone-Poulenc, and Tanabe. Individual vitamin companies use their own labels.

3) Food Bound Vitamins (Non-Isolated)

These vitamins contain proteins, lipids, carbohydrates and fiber. There is limited evidence that food bound vitamins may have greater bioavailability, absorption and retention than other types.[190] Most food bound vitamins are produced by one of two sources: Bio Foods and Grow Company.

GREEN SUPERFOODS

Spirulina algae, blue-green algae and chlorella algae are often touted as "the perfect food." Let's conduct an experiment. Place two people inside a large glass cube. Feed one person only rice and the other only algae. After 6 months, the rice-eater will be thriving but the algae-eater will be dead from kidney failure. (Algae is 58–65%

protein.) Algae is an excellent source of trace minerals, chlorophyll, enzymes and other nutrients, but is **not** the perfect food.

Each nutrient has a safe window between necessity and toxicity:

- Widest safety range: water soluble vitamins (B and C).
- Narrowest safety range: ultratrace minerals (boron, nickel, copper, silica, chromium, selenium, molybdenum, vanadium and germanium).

The minerals especially must be kept in balance since increasing the intake of one mineral can reduce the absorption of another:

Intake	Absorption
Sodium ↑	Potassium ↓ Calcium ↓
Phosphorus ↑	Zinc ↓ Calcium ↓ Magnesium ↓
Zinc ↑	Copper ↓ Iron ↓ Calcium ↓
Calcium ↑	Zinc ↓ Copper ↓ Iron ↓ Magnesium ↓
Iron ↑	Zinc ↓ Chromium ↓ Calcium ↓

True health does not arise from ancient formulations channeled by Tibetan masters, mystical botanicals from Incan temples, miracle herbs from the Peruvian Amazon, or extractions of Canadian pine tree bark. True health comes from within. Nutritional supplements work best as a supplement, rather than substitute, for food.

> *"I take 100 liver and yeast tablets, 75 kelp, plus zinc, potassium, dolomite, selenium, bonemeal, vitamins E, C, A and D… I put them in a blender with about 8 ounces of warm water, and then I gulp the whole thing down . . . ."*[191]
>
> —Jack LaLanne, 1979

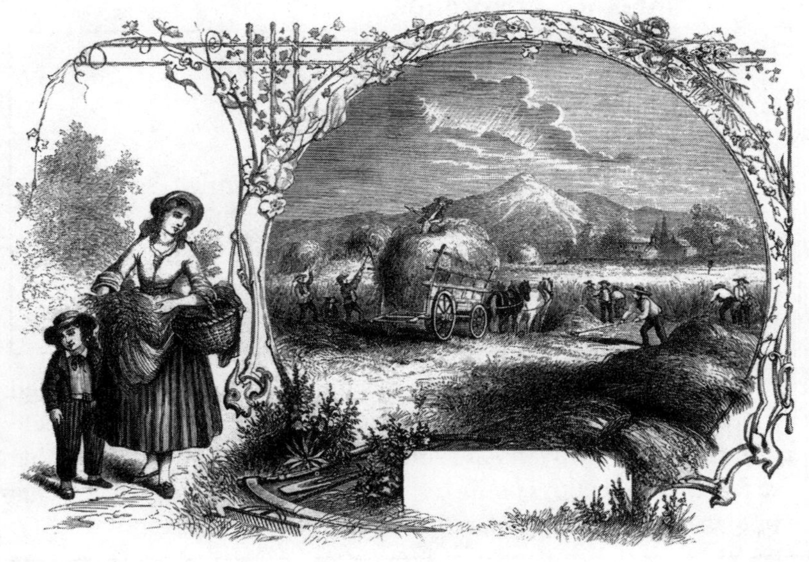

CHAPTER 3
Diets Past and Present

"The simple fact is that our diets have changed radically within the last 50 years... These dietary changes represent as great a threat to public health as smoking."
—Sen. George McGovern, 1977
Senate Select Committee on Nutrition

"We learn from history that we learn nothing from history."
—George Bernard Shaw

During World War I, Denmark was blockaded and threatened by a food shortage so severe that the Danish government imposed drastic measures to avoid starvation. Alcohol, meat and white flour production was halted. Grain was diverted directly to Danish citizens. People consumed more whole grains, fruits and vegetables because nothing else was available. Consequently the death rate fell by 34% and Denmark became one of the healthiest nations in Europe. When the war ended and eating habits returned to normal, cancer and heart disease returned to prewar levels.[1]

Similar changes occurred in Norway, Holland, England and Wales during World War II. As meat consumption dropped, so did the death rate. When the war ended and meat consumption rose, the death rate followed.[2] After WW II, Russians increased their consumption of saturated fats and Japanese began eating meat. In both countries, heart disease climbed.

Few events are as stressful as war. History suggests that diet overrides stress as the major factor leading to degenerative disease. Food is our most intimate contact with the environment and ultimately determines our capacity to thrive.

JAPAN VS. CHINA

For thousands of years, traditional eating patterns in Japan and China were mostly vegetarian. That similarity is fast disappearing under pressure of modern times. Since 1950, Japanese meat, egg and milk consumption has risen over 8-fold. Cancer is the leading cause of death in Japan, and breast cancer will likely become the most common disease among Japanese women by the year 2000.[3]

Year	Japanese Fat Intake
1949	7%
1991	25%

The average Japanese fat intake is currently 25%, but this figure is skewed since older Japanese eat 15% fat while younger Japanese consume closer to 40%. (McDonald's and Kentucky Fried Chicken play a part.) Japanese fat farms are now commonplace. Japanese and American children are comparable in obesity and cholesterol levels.

In certain isolated rural areas of Japan, it's become common for elderly parents to outlive their children (who die of cancer or stroke). They even have a name for it—Sakasabotokei— parents burying their children.[4] In Japan, diet and disease risk depend upon **generation**.

In 1983, Chinese-Oxford-Cornell researchers began the largest study ever conducted on diet and disease: the China Health Project.[5] Chinese cancer rates were found to vary by several hundred fold between different regions. The average fat intake in Beijing and other Chinese cities was 15% in 1983; today it's 30%. In the booming Guangdong province, Pizza Hut restaurants sell 5,000–6,000 pizzas daily. A weight-loss club recently opened in the northeast city of Shenyang. Animal products supply 6% of total Chinese calories (range 0.1–59%).

As areas of China become more affluent and as meat consumption rises, degenerative diseases closely follow. In traditional rural areas, cancer and heart disease are virtually unknown. In China, diet and disease risk depend upon **region**. Not surprisingly, the American Meat Institute claims that findings in the China Health Project are groundless.[6]

U.S. HISTORY

- **1850:** Diets were mostly whole grains, fruits, vegetables and very-free-range chickens. Heart disease – rare; Cancer – rare
- **1870:** Cattle barons conquered the Great Plains by financing the buffalo hunters. Railroads shipped cattle to distant markets.
- **1880:** Minnesota flour mills produced white flour using steel rollers. For the first time in 4,000 years, people could eat grain totally stripped of nutrients.
- **1900:** Eating patterns shifted with meat replacing grains. Cause of death: Heart disease – No. 4; Cancer – No. 8
- **1919:** World War I ended. Chlorine gas converted to drinking water treatment.
- **1945:** World War II ended. Chemical warfare weapons converted to chemotherapy. Pesticides, artificial fertilizers and hydrogenated oils introduced.
- **1990:** Over 100,000 new chemicals injected into the food supply since 1945. Cause of death: Heart disease – No. 1; Cancer – No. 2

Cancer is projected to overtake heart disease by the year 2000—due in part to major dietary changes.

- Sugar consumption since 1910: increased 33%[7]
- Grain consumption since 1910: decreased 50%[8]
- Animal product consumption since 1910: increased 40%[9]

Year	Sugar Consumption (per person per year)
1700	4 pounds
1800	20 pounds
1978	120 pounds
1994	137 pounds

AVERAGE AMERICAN DIET

"If someone wants to cut...fat, they can order their Whopper without mayonnaise."[10]

—Michael Evans, spokesperson
Burger King Corp.

"You can find your way across the country using the burger joints the way a navigator uses stars."[11]

—Charles Kuralt
former news anchor

Cutting across lines of age and class, food choices exact a heavy toll: the obese mother with one breast; the blind diabetic with one leg; the bedridden senior with a collapsed spine; the orphaned child with a father dead of heart disease. Each indictment issues from a single source: the average American diet.

There was a time when American cuisine was thought to be the healthiest in the world. This myth, like others propagated by conglomerates with heavy advertising budgets and light consciences, was based on mythology. The American diet has made surgeons, cattle ranchers and nursing home owners independently wealthy.

During the past 20 years, Americans have cut their fat intake by switching from beef to chicken and fish. Americans ate more poultry per capita than any other country in 1992, and stood only behind Argentina and Uruguay in beef consumption.[12]

Year	Chicken Consumption (per person per year)
1975	26 pounds
1992	46 pounds
2005	94 pounds

Dominating all other lifestyle factors, nutrition determines both the quality of life and life itself. Understanding exactly what Americans eat is the first step towards optimal health.

Animal products comprise 44% of the calories, 70% of the protein, and 66% of the fat in American diets.[13] Our eating habits contrast sharply with those of rural Chinese:[14]

	Carbohydrates	Fats	Proteins	Fiber
USA	45%	37%	18%	11 grams
China	77%	15%	8%	34 grams

American Diet	Male	Female
Carbohydrates	287 grams	177 grams
Proteins	100 grams	68 grams
Fats	91 grams	61 grams
Cholesterol	450 mg	300 mg

Most Popular American Foods[15]

- Coke, Pepsi
- Kraft processed cheese
- Campbell's soup
- Budweiser beer

Top Fat Sources[16]

- Oil, lard, butter, margarine, shortening (44%)
- Red meat, poultry, fish (34%)
- Dairy products, eggs (15%)

Top Calorie Sources[17]

- Milk, cheese
- Margarine
- Beef
- Soft drinks
- White flour
- Sugar

According to the USDA, Americans consume 61–91 grams of fat daily. According to the United Nations, Americans consume 163 grams of fat daily.[18] Different data gathering methods account for the apparent discrepancy. The USDA uses diet surveys; the UN uses food supply data (annual food production, plus imports, minus exports, expressed per person). The UN overestimates fat intake by not considering wasted food. Either way, it's excess fat.

WHAT AMERICANS EAT (per person per year)[19]

Food	1,300 lb.
Red Meat	112 lb.
Poultry	63 lb.
Seafood	15 lb.
Eggs (number)	236
Milk and Cream	234 lb.
Cheese	26 lb.
Ice Cream	23 lb.
Fats and Oils	68 lb.
Sugar	147 lb.
Candy	22 lb.
Artificial Sweeteners	25 lb.
Salt	15 lb.
Food Additives	10 lb.
Soft Drinks	47 gallons
Coffee	68 gallons
Pop Corn	56 quarts
Doughnuts	756
Cakes, Cookies, Chocolate	60 lb.
Potato Chips	7 lb.

The U.S. diet has shifted in recent years toward a reduction in saturated fat. As a result, surplus beef fat is now available at a lower price. Kansas State University is conducting research to convert this surplus beef fat into diesel fuel.[20]

One has to admire their creativity in adapting to changing dietary preferences. However, considering the inordinate amount of grain, topsoil, water, pesticides, raw materials and fossil fuel needed to produce 1 pound of beef, this project seems a less-than-optimum use of our natural resources.

About 65% of America's agricultural land is used for livestock feed. From the vantage point of an alien spacecraft, cattle might appear to be the dominant species on earth since they occupy most of the planet's land area and consume most of the world's resources.

"I've run more risk eating my way across the country than in all my driving."

—Duncan Hines
Adventures in Good Eating

Environmental groups claim that each pound of beef requires 2,500 gallons of water to produce, but the Cattlemen's Association claims only 200 gallons per pound. The Cattlemen's Association excludes rainfall from the calculation; environmental groups include it.

FOOD GRAB BAG

- Cholesterol Heaven – estimated surplus grease generated by New Orleans restaurants: 2 million gallons per year.
- Lard Heaven – estimated lard eaten by the average American family of four: 300 pounds per year.
- Smog Heaven – estimated pollutants from charbroiling meats in Los Angeles: 4 tons per day (vaporized cholesterol).[21]
- Pizza Heaven – estimated pizza eaten by Americans: 90 acres per day.[22]
- McDonald's now has fast-food shops in 18 U.S. hospitals.[23]
- The School Lunch Program once included catsup as a certified vegetable.
- Official snack food of the Olympics: Hostess.
- Official bread of the Olympics: Wonder.
- Favorite lunch of Richard Nixon: Cottage cheese and catsup.
- Favorite snack of Ronald Reagan: Jelly Belly jelly beans.
- Favorite snack of George Bush: Pork rinds (fried hog skin).
- Favorite snack of Bill Clinton: Baby Ruth candy bars.
- Desert option on board Air Force One: red Jell-O, marshmallows and mayonnaise.[24]
- Beef eaten by each American: 7 steers per lifetime.[25]

> *"The nutrition neurotic is characterized by...the loss of faith in modern processing; and the fear that conventional foods cause degenerative diseases."*[26]
>
> —American Medical Association

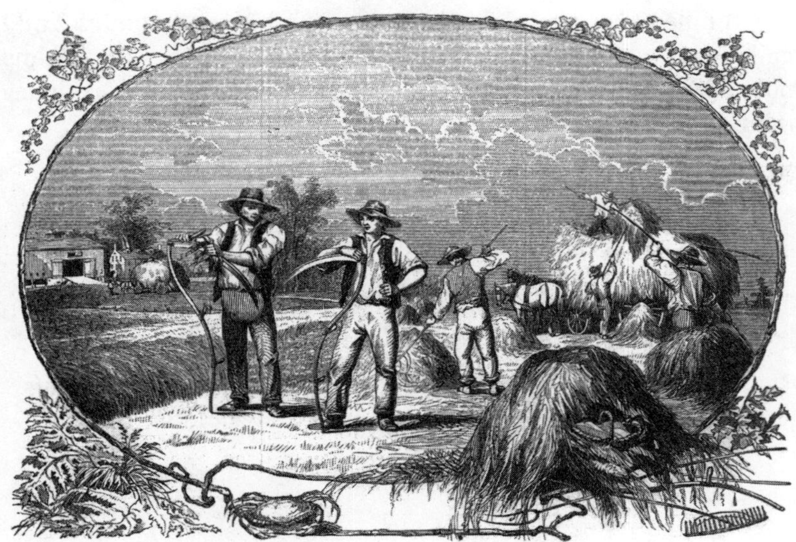

Choices

"It should be recognized that both vegetarian and nonvegetarian diets have the potential to be either beneficial or detrimental to health."[27]

—American Dietetic Association

"Every food philosophy has its dogma and its devils, its sin and its salvation."[28]

—Annemarie Colbin

"If you're not interested in things going on around you, well, you're probably not eating enough red meat."[29]

—Julia Child

The American diet is under attack from all quarters and for good reason: nutrition and health cannot be separated. We are deeply rooted in the culture that raised us and that culture is changing. America is undergoing a shake-out period. The evolution of national norms is no easy task and major social reform rarely occurs without a fight. Changing of the national diet is no exception.

Well-entrenched battlelines separate consumers from special interests, with both sides driven by the instinct for self-preservation. Propaganda abounds, as do dubious ideologies seldom sullied by facts or logic. Cutting through the clutter requires understanding what the choices are.

Choice #1: USDA Basic Four Food Groups (1956)

Milk Group 2 or more servings	Meat Group 2 or more servings
Vegetable–Fruit Group 4 or more servings	Bread–Cereal Group 4 or more servings

Balance, variety, moderation! This diet was promoted courtesy of the American agriculture lobby. Cheese is included in both the Milk and Meat Groups. Animal product consumption has no upper limit.

Choice #2: New Four Food Groups[30]

Fruit Group 3 or more servings	Bean Group 2–3 servings
Vegetable Group 3 or more servings	Whole Grain Group 5 or more servings

Diet proposed by the Physicians Committee for Responsible Medicine, an organization dedicated to prevention.[31]

Choice #3: USDA Food Guide Pyramid (1992)

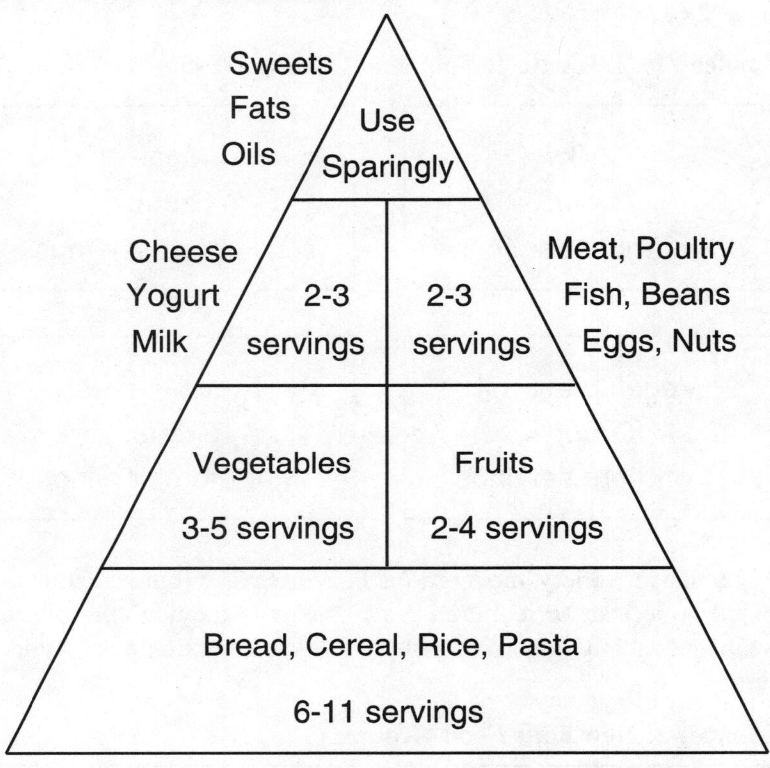

The USDA is mandated to promote the consumption of animal products. The release of this pyramid was held up for more than a year because of pressure from the meat and dairy industries.[32]

> *"We wanted to avoid a good-food, bad-food ranking and the de-emphasis of meat."*[33]
>
> —Gary Wilson, spokesperson
> National Cattlemen's Association

Choice #4: National Dietary Guidelines

- American Heart Association
- American Medical Association
- American Dietetic Association
- American Cancer Society

National organizations often recommend 30% fat, 300 mg of daily cholesterol, and four eggs per week. These guidelines reflect efforts by industry to maintain the status quo but fail to greatly lower heart disease or cancer risk. The guidelines simply don't go far enough.

> *"By working closely with other organizations, such as the AMA and the ADA, we were able to get a responsible, credible message to consumers."*[34]
>
> —National Live Stock and Meat Board

The Cattlemen's Association and the Beef Industry Council pay for dietary brochures distributed by the American Heart Association.[35]

Choice #5: Bodybuilder Diet

Bodybuilders consume proteins from wide ranging sources: soy powders, egg albumen, dairy casein, liquid amino acids, poultry, fish and red meat. Competitive bodybuilders often achieve that "cut-up and ripped" look using a two-step dietary program:

- **Bulk Up:** Gain weight by increasing protein and carbohydrate calories.
- **Pre-Competition:** Maintain protein intake while decreasing carbohydrates and fluids.

Warning: Americans lose kidney function and bone density with age. Protein accelerates that loss. A long-term price can be paid even without taking steroids. Andreas Cahling (Mr. International), Bill Pearl (four-time Mr. Universe), Edwin Moses (World Champion 400 meter hurtles), and Dave Scott (Ironman Triathlon winner) are all vegetarians.

Choice #6: Mediterranean Diet

During the 1960s, the people of Crete had the lowest heart disease rate in the industrialized world despite their 40% fat diet. Their secret was a mostly vegetarian diet and the liberal use of olive oil (monounsaturated). Advocates of this diet recommend switching fats without reducing total fat intake.

The idea that one can load up on fat and stay healthy is false, seductive and dangerous. During the 1960s, breast cancer rates in Greece were twice as high as in Japan.[36] Breast cancer rates in Italy and Greece are now 2–3 times higher than in Japan. Obesity is a national problem in several Mediterranean countries. This diet is heavily promoted by the olive oil, wine and nut industries.[37]

Choice #7: French Diet

The French Paradox has long confounded researchers. France has the lowest heart disease rate of any industrialized nation (other than Japan) despite their gourmet sauces, rich cheeses and buttered goose liver. No culinary mediocrity here. However, the French have eaten 39% fat diets since 1988; Americans have eaten 39% fat diets since 1950.[38] The French live 1.6 years longer than Americans; heart disease is still the leading cause of death in France and the rate is rising. France may be under reporting their heart attack deaths by listing them as death by "natural internal event."[39]

The French consume more garlic and vegetables, fewer trans fats, more cheese and less milk than Americans. Cheese fat may be less damaging than homogenized milk fat because cheese is complexed with minerals and poorly absorbed.

Red wine elevates HDL (good cholesterol), thins the blood and acts as an antioxidant. The more red wine consumed the cleaner the arteries will be, but the greater the risk of cancer, hypertension, stroke, alcoholism and liver disease. France has the world's highest incidence of liver cirrhosis. In 1979, Paris had the highest overall cancer rate of any city in the world.[40] A high price to pay for 1.6 extra years.

"Lunch kills half of Paris, supper the other half."
—Montesquieu
Varietes

Choice #8: Eskimo Diet

The Inuit Eskimos (meaning "raw meat eaters") subsist on fish, seal, walrus, polar bear, and beluga whale blubber. They bruise easily, are slow to form blood clots, develop fatal nose bleeds, and have virtually no heart disease. Their traditional diet consists of:[41]

Meats	Fats	Proteins	Calcium
90%	50%	30–35%	2,200 mg

The Eskimos have one of the world's highest rates of hemorrhagic stroke, osteoporosis, obesity, and one of the shortest life spans. They apparently die from other causes before cancer or heart disease have time to develop. The fat tissues of Inuit mothers contain the world's highest known levels of organochlorine pesticides.[42]

Choice #9: Stone Age (Paleolithic) Diet

The Stone Age diet rests firmly on the assumption that human nutritional needs—after 10,000 years of agriculture and 200 years of industrialization—are still adapted to the prehistoric past. Preagricultural hunter-gatherer societies consumed:[43]

Meats	Fats	Proteins	Calcium
35%	21%	33%	1,750 mg

Although Paleolithic life expectancy was less than 23 years (due to high infant mortality and occupational hazards), older forebears were likely free of degenerative diseases. Our remote ancestors ate whatever was available, plant or animal.[44] Paleolithic evidence provides little support for a vegan vegetarian diet.

Choice #10: Japanese Diet

The traditional Japanese meal includes rice, noodles, soy sauce, tofu, miso soup, vegetables and condiments of fish. The Japanese have the longest life span in the industrialized world, an advantage which diminishes with age.

Life Expectancies

	At Birth[45]	At Age 65[46]	At Age 75[47]
Japan	79	18.4	10.1
U.S.A.	75	16.8	10.4

Traditional Japanese consume up to 15,500 mg of sodium daily—contributing to their high rates of hemorrhagic stroke and stomach cancer.[48]

> *"[In Japan] cancer is the cause of roughly 1 death in 4; heart attack and strokes each 1 in 5, and respiratory illness 1 in 12. One male in every 52 kills himself (for women, suicide is 1 in 70)."*[49]
>
> *—Asia Week*

Choice #11: Macrobiotic Diet

Macrobiotic philosophy (meaning "large life") integrates the Taoist doctrine of Yin and Yang balance into daily food selection.[50] Based on the Japanese diet, Macrobiotics stress unrefined foods locally-grown according to climate and season.[51] Although healthy, this diet is quite restricted. Most fruits, avocados and nightshade plants (potatoes, tomatoes, eggplants, peppers) are avoided.

Most current evidence supports low-fat, high-fiber diets in the prevention and treatment of cancer. Prostate and pancreatic cancer patients on Macrobiotic diets outlived those on regular diets.[52]

Choice #12: Raw Food Diet

Raw food diets (living foods) center on uncooked vegetables, sprouts and fruit. Fats are added to provide enough calories since all cooked starches are excluded (grains, beans, potatoes). *The Hippocrates Diet* raw food program is 24% fat.[53] Epidemiological studies suggest this may be less than ideal for long-term health.

On the other hand, raw foods preserve the nutrients destroyed by cooking (enzymes, chlorophyll, water-soluble vitamins) and may be therapeutic for short-term cleansing.[54] The world's longest-lived people eat 80% of their vegetables raw—not 100% of their calories raw.

Choice #13: Vegetarian Diet

Vegetarian diets may be high in fat by over using rich vegetable foods (avocados, olives, tofu, nuts, seeds, peanut butter, oils). Vegetarian diets can be divided into several subgroups:

- Vegan Vegetarian: no meat, poultry, fish, eggs, or dairy. (There are no known long-lived societies on a strict vegan diet.)[55]
- Lacto Vegetarian: includes dairy or goat's milk products.
- Ovo Vegetarian: includes eggs.
- Pesco Vegetarian: includes seafood.
- Poulo Vegetarian: includes poultry.
- Semi Vegetarian: includes occasional meals using animal products as a condiment.
- Low-Fat Vegetarian: fats are limited to 10% of calories.
- Low-Fat Semi Vegetarian: the diet of people noted for their extreme longevity.

Choice #14: No Pain Vegetarian Diet

- Lacto-Ovo-Pesco-Poulo-Häagen Dazso-Chocolate Chipo-Twinkieo-Vegetarian.

> *"Part of the secret to success in life is to eat what you like and let the food fight it out inside."*
> —Mark Twain

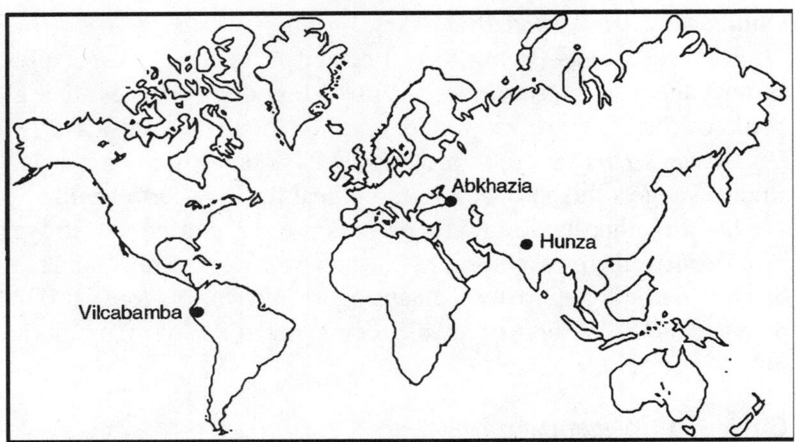

Longevity Centers

"There is no biological reason why human beings should not reach the age of 150."[56]

—Dr. Alexis Carrel
Rockefeller Institute

"Life has lengthened considerably since I was born; and there is no reason why it should not lengthen 10 times as much after my death."

—George Bernard Shaw
Back to Methuselah

In traditional cultures throughout the world, heart disease, cancer and osteoporosis are virtually unknown. Fully 80% of the human race avoids the degenerative conditions so common among older Americans. What we consider normal is not normal at all. The prevention of both diseases of affluence and diseases of poverty will allow the extension of human lifespan to near its biological limit.[57]

In remote mountainous regions, there exist cultures noted for extreme longevity, their ancient ways shrouded in secrecy or largely forgotten. The elders in these communities stand as living testaments to our biological potential. By studying these cultures, common factors can be applied to our own society. The three most famous longevity centers are:[58]

- The Hunza Valley in the Himalayan Mountains, northwest Pakistan (Kashmir)
- The Vilcabamba Valley in the Andes Mountains, southern Ecuador
- The Georgian Republic in the Caucasus Mountains, former Soviet Union (between the Black and Caspian Seas)

Centenarian Profiles		
	American	**Hunza**
Environment	Nursing home	Mountain region
Activity	Sedentary	Strenuous activity
Physical Condition	Cancer, stroke, heart disease	Comparatively symptom free
Mental Condition	Alzheimer's, wasting senility	High mental acuity
Social Position	Burden to society, disdain from youths	High social status, envy from youths
Outlook	"It's just not worth it living past age 90."	"Everyday is a gift beyond age 100."

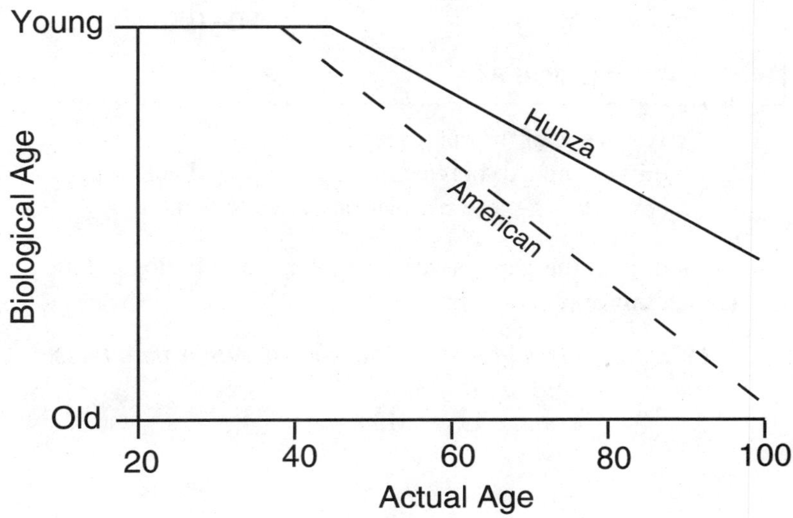

"Let death find us on horseback or planting cabbages."
—Andre Maurois

LONGEVITY CENTER FACTORS

- Low-fat starch-centered diet. Food, water, air and soil free of toxic chemicals.
- Active lifestyle, daily exercise, never retire.
- No dependence on medical technology.
- The young expect long healthy lives; elders are expected to impart wisdom. Both groups respond accordingly.
- Recent declines in health due to outside influences.
- Age exaggeration. Old age brings increased social status.

AGE EXAGGERATION

In 1973, world attention focused on these longevity centers with reports of healthy individuals living well past age 100. The subsequent discovery of age exaggeration (made worse by scientific and tourist visits) was used to discredit the findings and refute the whole idea of life extension.

Typical Longevity Elder	
Claimed Age	100–120
Actual Age	90–100
Biological Age	65–75

There are two ways of interpreting this:

- Look only at the gap between claimed age and actual age. Reject everything these people may have to teach us.
- Look only at the gap between actual age and biological age. (I take this approach.)

"It was the fitness of many of the elderly rather than their extreme ages that impressed me."[59]
—Alexander Leaf, M.D.

"It's an exaggeration to say they live to be 150 but there's no need to gild the lily. The average age is 90 when they die."[60]

—Betty Morales, past president
American Cancer Society
after two visits to the Hunza Valley

A 1969 study, adjusted for age exaggeration, measured low blood pressure and low cholesterol levels among the Vilcabamba elders.[61]

INFLUENCE OF CIVILIZATION

Contact with the outside world has been a mixed blessing. All three regions show declines in health due to outside influences.

Vilcabamba

New roads into this region allowed the introduction of processed chemical-laden foods.[62] Pesticides used on tomato crops polluted the drinking water.[63] Several centenarians died of dysentery after taking antibiotics prescribed by newly arrived doctors.[64]

Numerous Vilcabamba elders apparently died after 1970, when extensive contact with the outside world became common.[65]

Hunza

Non-iodized white salt replaced the traditional brown salt with its naturally occurring minerals. White sugar replaced dried apricot puree. Other newly imported items include white flour, cigarettes, chewing tobacco, processed food, oil, meat and dairy products.[66] These changes contributed to tooth decay, goiters and several other diseases.[67]

Health-care centers reduced TB and dysentery, the principle causes of death in Hunza during the 1970s.[68] The recent introduction of iodized salt has eliminated goiters in children under age 12, but other illnesses remain.

"In old times the only diseases were diarrhea and fever. But now we have many diseases."[69]

—Hunza historian

Before contact with the outside world, at least 50 centenarians were living in the Hunza Valley. By 1972, only six centenarians out of a population of 40,000 remained.[70]

> *"It was a thousand and one times more healthy in the past. I've been to America, and your life didn't seem very healthy. You spray the food with artificial chemicals. The fruits in your country are big and they look very good, but they have no taste."*[71]
>
> —Mir Ghazanfar Ali Khan

Republic of Georgia

By 1972, the Georgians were eating comparatively large amounts of animal products, but this was not always so.[72]

> *"Things are much better now. In Turkey, and when we first came here, we had only beans and vegetables to eat, but now we have meat and wine everyday."*[73]
>
> —local Armenian

The modern Georgian diet derives 30% of its calories from animal products (mostly cheese, buttermilk and yogurt, rather than meat). The Georgian elders were found to have "all kinds of cardiovascular diseases" as a consequence of these foods.[74] Their diet is presented as a lesson in what **not** to do.

LONGEVITY DIETS

> *"The taste for white flour, polished white rice and white sugar shows the failure of man's [and woman's] instinct to serve as a safe guide in the selection of foods."*
>
> *—The Amazing Hunza Diet*

> *"A factor in the long average life spans of the Hunzas may be their drinking of 'glacial milk,' essentially an aqueous extract of rocks. The moving glacier grinds up rocks in its bed and percolates its melting waters through the mineral-rich mush."*[75]
>
> —Roy Walford, M.D.
> *The 120 Year Diet*

Fortunately a record still exists of the traditional Hunza, Georgian and Vilcabamba diets before the outside influences of the past two decades. All three diets included small amounts of meat and cooked food. Consequently no one can advocate a strict vegetarian or 100% raw food diet based on these cultures.

The Hunzas are descendants from the soldiers of Alexander the Great.[76] Vilcabamba was settled by Augustine missionaries during the 17th century.[77] The Hunza and Vilcabamba diets were similar although the Hunza diet had more variety. Both groups have long track records of exceptional health over several hundred years. Both diets have stood the test of time.

Diet	Calories From Animal Products
Hunza[78]	1%
Vilcabamba[79]	1%
Georgian[80]	30%
U.S.A.[81]	44%

	Calories	Fats	Proteins
Hunza[82]	1923	15%	10%
Vilcabamba[83]	1200	12%	12%
Georgian[84]	1800	25%	18%

The Hunzas need more fats and calories than the Vilcabambas because the climate is colder. The Hunza Valley ranges in elevation from 3,500–7,000 feet and is completely enclosed by 20,000 foot Himalayan peaks. The bitter Hunza winters contrast with the 70 degree year-round temperature of Vilcabamba.[85]

Cold temperature and strenuous exercise increase the need for both calories and fats: calories by a large amount; fats by a small amount.

Exercise Level	Temperature	Ideal Fat Intake
Moderate	Warm	10%
Strenuous	Warm	10–12%
Moderate	Cold	10–12%
Strenuous	Cold	10–15%

THE HUNZA DIET[86]

- **Grains:** buckwheat, millet, rice, corn, wheat, barley, rye.
- **Fruits:** apricots, mulberries, grapes, oranges, apples, pears, peaches, cherries, melons, tomatoes.
- **Vegetables:** leafy greens, potatoes, carrots, squash, turnips, onions, cabbage, sprouts.
- **Misc:** dried beans, peas, nuts, seeds, garlic.
- **Local specialty:** fresh ground buckwheat pancakes (chapatis).
- **Cooking:** 80% of vegetables were eaten raw with their skins; 20% were lightly steamed.
- **Apricot seed oil:** all oil extracted from seeds is vulnerable to rancidity. For this reason, the traditional Hunza apricot oil was made fresh and discarded after only 2 days. (Commercial vegetable oils are not recommended.)
- **Animal products:** accounted for only 1% of total calories. Milk, butter and cheese (from goats, sheep and yaks) were consumed sparingly. Small amounts of meat (3 oz. per month) were eaten on special occasions.

Current evidence suggests this diet is near optimum for adult human needs. The goal of the next chapter is to resurrect these principles and apply them to the modern world. The Food Pyramid and Core Recipes are based on the Hunza Diet. (This has been my basic diet for the past 7 years.)

This program is not an all-or-nothing choice. It requires no purity pledge. As with all healthy diets, the more you do, the more benefits you receive. Life has a way of finding those who have little regard for what they eat.

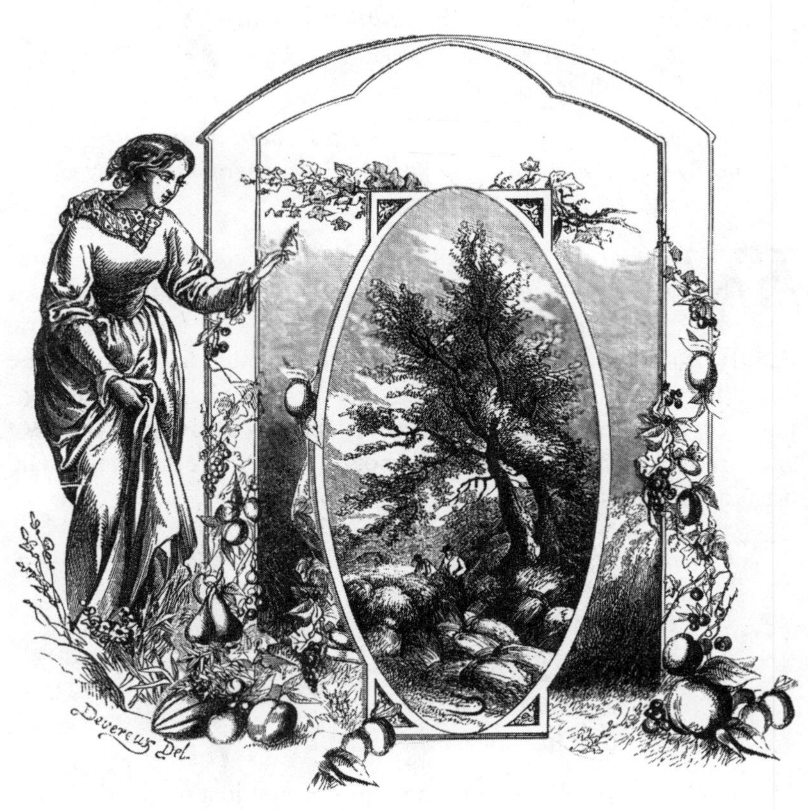
Devereux Del.

CHAPTER 4

Personal Application

"In the arena of human life, the honors and rewards fall to those who show their good qualities in action."
—Aristotle
4th century B.C.

"The consequences of our actions take hold of us quite indifferent to our claim that meanwhile we have 'improved.'"
—Nietzsche, 1886

What we eat is an exquisitely personal choice. The preparation and consumption of food are sacramental rituals for joy, communication and meaning in a depersonalized era. Family, traditions and emotions all revolve around food. To change one's diet is to challenge a lifetime of social and physical conditioning. New habits begin as tiny threads, eventually forming steel cables anchored in concrete. Humans are bound to their lifetime habits and breaking them is not easy.

"I missed most a bottle of good wine and a steak."[1]
—hostage Terry Anderson
after his release

"A Big Mac and a Coke would be nice."[2]
—hostage Edward Tracy
after his release

The goal is to eat for the enjoyment of life, not just to avoid disease or slow the aging process. This will happen rather quickly as your taste buds change. Processed foods rely heavily on spices and fats to provide flavors and stimulation. Unrefined whole foods taste bland by comparison...initially. The life span of a taste bud is about 10 days.

Most of us have grown accustomed to certain types of food. At least 25 brain chemicals (neuropeptides) control food cravings.[3]

Food preference (chemosensory sensitivity) affects the taste buds, liver, fatty tissues, stomach, intestines and neurological pathways.[4] By switching to a plant-centered diet, new flavors are enhanced as the body reprograms itself. Salt, sugar and fats suppress sensitivity.

- To change salt preference may take 2 weeks.
- To change sugar preference may take 6 weeks.
- To change fat preference may take 8–12 weeks.[5]

THREE STEP PROGRAM

1) Decide which health habits are most likely to kill you.
2) Set a goal.
3) Have a master plan.

CONTRASTING GOALS

Average American Goal

"I'm very careful about eating right and carefully trim all visible fat. Heart-healthy choices include low-salt margarine, olive oil and skinless chicken. I've lowered my cholesterol all the way down to 200 by following the government guidelines."

Long Life Now Goal

"I no longer need to be careful when eating because I've developed habits. Foods high in fat, salt or sugar leave a bad taste and discipline is no longer needed. My cholesterol is under 150 by following the longevity guidelines."

Those who fail to set goals are often at the mercy of those who do.

TWO MASTER PLANS

Step-By-Step Plan

- Keep a food record for 1 week. List everything that needs changing, including all substitutes. Set priorities. Modify your old recipes. Clear out the refrigerator.
- Change one food at a time, allowing yourself up to 3 months for each change.
- Cement each habit before moving on.

Cold-Turkey Plan

- Keep a food record for 1 week. List everything that needs changing, including all substitutes. Modify your old recipes. Clear out the refrigerator.
- Change everything in one fell swoop.

You may wish to combine both plans, starting with Step-By-Step and switching to Cold-Turkey at the appropriate time. (This was my personal approach.) Persistent small changes produce great shifts over time, as in water cutting the Grand Canyon.

> *"Choose what is best, habit will soon render it agreeable and easy."*
>
> —Pythagoras (582–500 B.C.)

FIBER

Fiber is the Drano of digestion, the critical missing element in American diets. The Chinese consume 40–60 grams of fiber daily; Americans consume 11 grams. There are two types of fiber, and both are essential for normal function:

Water-Soluble Fiber (Lowers cholesterol)	Water-Insoluble Fiber (Lowers cancer risk)
• oat bran	• wheat bran
• apple pulp	• apple peels
• citrus fruit	• strawberries
• carrots	• whole grains
• sea vegetables	• leafy vegetables
• beans	• beans

Without fiber, the body reabsorbs estrogen and testosterone, thus contributing to breast and prostate cancer. Without fiber, the body reabsorbs bile acids, thus contributing to elevated cholesterol and heart disease.

It's not necessary to count grams of fiber as long as most foods eaten are complex carbohydrates. The more fiber and fluids taken in, the faster food moves through the intestine. The slower food moves, the greater the risk of colon cancer.

Food Transit Time	
Rural Third World	1 day
Average American	2 days
Constipated American	3 days
Elderly American	up to 7 days

Lack of fiber leads to constipation, chronic pancreatitis, colitis, Crohn's disease, cancer and straining. Straining leads to varicose veins, hemorrhoids, diverticulosis and hiatal hernias. The same pattern repeats in countries throughout the world: big stools, little hospitals—little stools, big hospitals. Animal products contain no fiber.

> *"Beef is highly digestible—more digestible, in fact, than vegetables."*
>
> —National Cattlemen's Association
> *12 Myths About Beef*

While in Vietnam, I noticed there were no toilet seats anywhere in the country, except in international hotels and American military bases. At the time, it seemed strange that the Vietnamese culture evolved in such an "unnatural" way.

The problem is anatomical. The typical Western sitting position closes off part of the colon, making full evacuation nearly impossible without straining. The oriental squatting position allows full evacuation without straining. When the unfortunate Western sitting position combines with constipation, problems quickly manifest.

The average human small intestine has an absorptive area equal in size to a football field. About 3 pounds of bacteria grow in the small and large intestines, forming 30–50% of the stool. Humans have more intestinal bacteria than the total number of cells in their body. Even small changes in the intestinal flora can profoundly affect digestion, absorption and overall health. Dietary changes alter the intestinal bacteria.

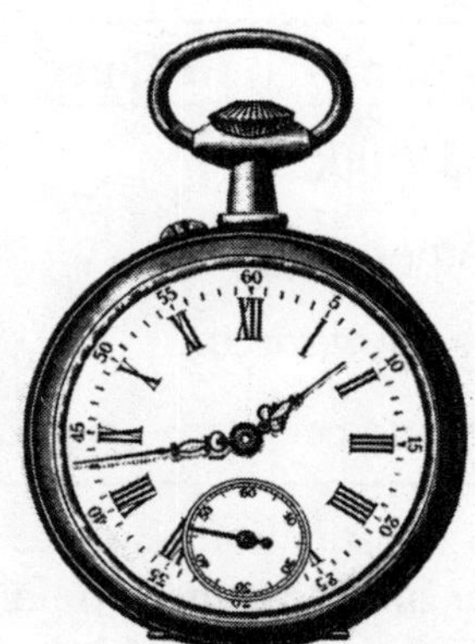

Speed Cooking

> *"Everyone I know is now very, very busy. In our hearts we still love to eat this way, but we've forsaken it because we don't know how to fit it into our lives."*[6]
>
> —Mollie Katzen, author
> *The Moosewood Cookbook*

> *". . . I felt the best I've ever felt in my life. But it took* ***sooo loong*** *to prepare all the food that it just about killed my social life, and with it my career."*[7]
>
> —Casandra Peterson
> a.k.a. "Elvira"

Few problems in modern nutrition are more vexing than the lack of time. There are those who still cling to traditions believing that Americans have ample time to cook from scratch. But philosophy which ignores the persuasion of circumstance is doomed to failure. Cooking meals from scratch is fine for retirees but it doesn't fly with the two-income family. Nutritional programs endure only by their survival in the real world.

THE REAL WORLD

- 6% of American households have two children at home and only one income producer.[8]
- 70% of mothers have outside jobs.[9]
- 75% of women reported their sex lives were affected by lack of time.[10]

- 82% of women lowered their housekeeping standards due to lack of time.[11]
- 50% of adults rely on frozen, packaged, or take-out meals for dinner.[12]
- Average time spent on housework and child care per week: working man—7 hours; working woman—23 hours.[13]
- 25% of commuters eat breakfast while driving to work.[14]

Coming to terms with new realities is never easy. Many Americans learned to cook from their mother or grandmother, who cooked full time. Try that after coming home from a full day at work and you'll quickly run out of life.

> *"In the middle of cooking, you may suddenly slump over, unable to continue. For this reason, it's good to have some late-night backup restaurants that serve bacon cheeseburgers and Chinese food."*
>
> —Bruce Friedman
> *The Lonely Guy's Cooking Tips*

Convenience foods are the direct result of having less time and more cash to spend. What's needed is a viable alternative to fast foods and TV dinners: the 100-year diet prepared in less than 10 minutes, optimal nutrition applied to the real world. Current speed cooking approaches have definite disadvantages.

Option #1: Toss Some Meat On The Grill

Two minutes to prepare it, 10 minutes to cook it, and 5 minutes to clean up the grease. For speed and convenience, it's hard to beat.

> *"For quick snacks, take small wieners, cut long ways in the middle but not to the end. Tuck a small piece of cheese in the cut and wrap a slice of bacon around it. Broil this and you have a delicious serving."*
>
> —Clarence Meyer
> *Old Ways Rediscovered*

Option #2: Throw Something Together

- Steamed vegetables and sautéed onions over instant rice.
- Canned black bean chili and rice burritos, nachos and salad.
- Ready-made soy pizza, sliced tomatoes and chopped onions.
- Ramen noodles, tofu, pilaf mix, vegetables and instant soup.
- Soy tempeh burger on toasted English muffin.
- Spaghetti, canned tomato sauce and soy meatballs.

Busy people often over-utilize these types of meals. Disadvantages: highly processed, low nutritional value, excess fat and sodium.

Option #3: *Long Life Now* Speed Cooking

This approach uses two core recipes: Ten Bean Stew and Seven Grains (see page 114). Cook a large batch from each recipe on the weekend and not cook again for several days (1 week if cooking for 2; 2 weeks if cooking for 1). Place both batches in glass storage jars with screw-on lids. Refrigerate or freeze. For variety, individual meals can be seasoned to taste and prepared differently each day:

- Each batch can be stuffed into burritos, enchiladas, pita pockets, artichokes, eggplants, grape leaves, green peppers, or sandwiches to create grab-and-go foods.
- The Ten Bean Stew can be cut with tomato sauce and turned into soup, talbouli, stroganoff, or falafels.
- Each batch can be combined with "throw something together" meals. The Seven Grains can supplement hot or cold cereals.
- Side dishes can include fruit salads, green salads and steamed vegetables.

Advantages: short preparation and cooking time, fast cleanup, whole unprocessed foods, 25 ingredients per day.

> *". . . against necessity, against its strength, no one can fight and win."*
>
> —Aeschylus (525–456 B.C.)
> *Prometheus Bound*

Food Pyramid

"Foods in one group can't replace those in another. No one food group is more important than another; for good health, you need them all."

—USDA Food Pyramid

Optimal adult nutrition is near 80% carbohydrate, 10% fat and 10% protein. The Food Pyramid, based on the Hunza Diet, provides a visual guide by dividing foods into six groups, each with its ideal percentage of total calories.

FOOD GROUPS

- **B12** – Animal products supply 1% of calories, the only reliable source of vitamin B12. (See Vitamin Wars section.) The Hunzas consume 3 ounces of meat per month, equivalent to 2 square inches or the size of a card deck.
- **High Fats** – Vegetable fats provide 4% of calories, thus raising total fats to near 10%. (Core recipes average 6% fat.)
- **Beans** – Beans are high in protein and should be limited to 1 cup per day or 10% of total calories.
- **Fruits** – Fruits comprise 15% of calories, thus lowering total proteins to near 10%. (Core recipes average 17.5% protein.)
- **Vegetables** – Vegetables supply 30% of calories. The ideal vegetable to fruit ratio is 2:1.
- **Whole Grains** – Whole grains provide 40% of calories. Whole grains contain more fiber, more nutrients and fewer absorbable calories than flour products.

VARIATIONS

- **To Maintain Weight:** Eat 45% grains, high fats and B12 foods; eat 45% fruits and vegetables, and 10% beans.
- **To Lose Weight:** Eat fewer fruits, high fats and flour products, and more vegetables.
- **To Gain Weight:** Eat more fruits, high fats and flour products, and fewer vegetables.

LONG LIFE NOW PYRAMID

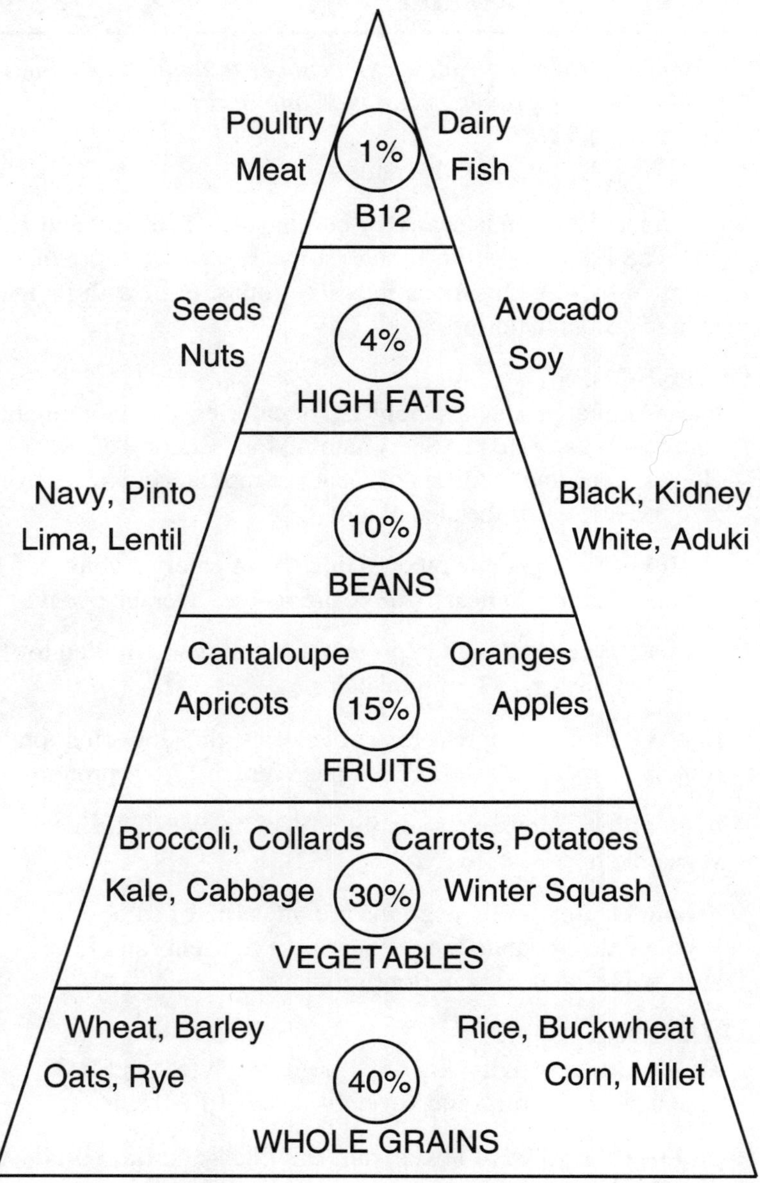

AVERAGE AMERICAN DIET PYRAMID[15]

Canned
3%
Frozen
FRUITS
Canned
4%
Frozen
VEGETABLES
Oil
10%
Margarine
VEGETABLE FATS
Sugar
39%
White Flour
REFINED CARBOHYDRATES
Meat, Poultry
Fish, Eggs
44%
Milk, Cream
Butter, Lard
ANIMAL PRODUCTS

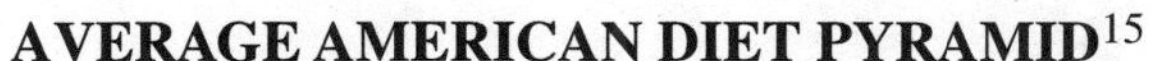

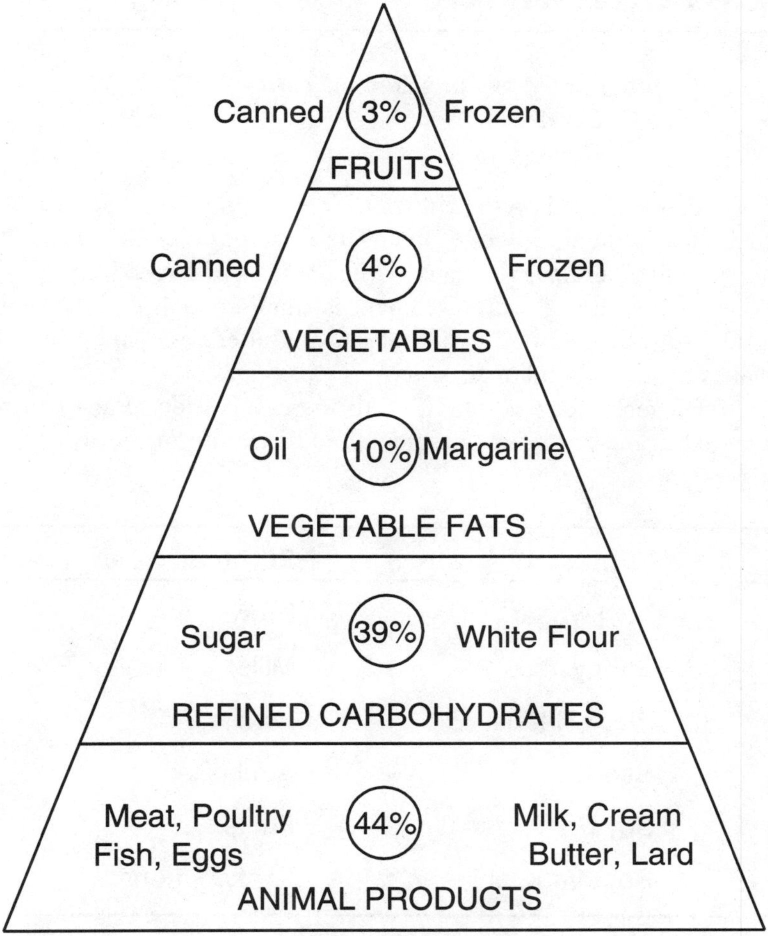

Although the U.S. is one of the most health conscious nations on earth, these pyramids demonstrate a gaping chasm between what we say (perception) and what we do (reality). The average American diet contains 37% fat, 18% protein and 45% carbohydrates. The choices, benefits and consequences are yours alone.

Core Recipes

"The proof of the pudding is in the eating."
—Cervantes
Don Quixote

Core recipes, based on the Hunza Diet, contain no oil, butter, eggs, cheese, salt, sugar, or white flour. These recipes include at least 25 ingredients: 7 grains, 10 beans, 7 vegetables and 1 seed.

The quantity of each ingredient is small enough that the same foods can be eaten daily without causing allergies. This principle makes food rotation unnecessary.

Each recipe can be modified to increase variety. Each can be adapted to the changing seasons by adding more of the following ingredients:

Winter	Summer
Buckwheat	Brown Rice
Barley	Millet
Black Beans	Lentils
Seeds	Aduki Beans
Soy Products	Fruits
Root Vegetables	Leafy Greens

SEVEN GRAINS RECIPE

8 cups total	whole wheat (berries, hard red winter) whole oat (groats) whole barley whole rye brown rice (short grain) buckwheat (groats, untoasted) millet
1½ cups	green lentils
½ cup	flaxseeds
1 cup	currants or raisins (organic)
½ cup	sea vegetables (if available)
15 cups	filtered water
Optional:	cinnamon, nutmeg, grated orange or lemon peel

Batch size: 24 cups
Cooking time: 35 minutes
Fat: 7%
Protein: 14%
Carbohydrate: 79%

To a 10-quart cooking pot, add lentils, flaxseeds and 15 cups of filtered water. Bring to a boil. Add currents or raisins. Stir to prevent clumping. Measure 4 cups of slow-cooking grains (wheat, oats, rye, barley) and rinse. Measure 3 cups of fast-cooking grains (buckwheat, rice, millet) and rinse.

Add slow-cooking grains to the pot and reduce heat to medium. Begin cooking time. Cover and stir as needed. After 15 minutes, add fast-cooking grains and reduce heat to low. Cook for an additional 20 minutes. When grains are done, add sea vegetables.

When Cooking Time Is Up:

- Transfer the batch to glass storage jars and pack tightly.
- Loosely cap the jars and let cool for 30 minutes.
- Before refrigerating, wipe the condensation from inside the lids and cap tightly.

TEN BEAN STEW RECIPE

4 cups total	kidney beans navy beans baby lima beans black beans black-eyed peas garbonzo beans aduki beans red beans great northern beans anasazi or pinto beans
½ cup	green lentils
1 cup	flaxseeds
½ cup	garlic (crushed)
3 pounds	yellow onions (chopped)
4 pounds	red or green cabbage (chopped)
1 cup	scallions or green onions (chopped)
1 cup	green beans (chopped)
1 cup	turnips or rutabaga (chopped)
1 cup	sea vegetables (if available)
12 cups	filtered water

Batch size: 32 cups
Cooking time: 60 minutes
Fat: 5%
Protein: 21%
Carbohydrate: 74%

Optional ingredients: carrots, potatoes, squash, mushrooms, eggplant, peppers, leeks
Optional seasonings: coriander, ginger, turmeric, lemon juice, cumin, mustard seeds, cayenne
Optional thickeners: corn starch, potato starch, rice flour, arrowroot, guar gum, kudzu, agar-agar
Optional thinners: fresh tomatoes, tomato sauce, rice or soy milk

Measure 4 cups of beans and rinse thoroughly. Soak the beans in cold water for 24 hours, changing the water at least once. Use a large pot as beans expand 2½ times their size. Discard any bad beans or floaters.

Stir and drain the soaking water. Add filtered water and bring to a boil. After foam rises to the surface, drain completely. Add 12 cups of filtered water and bring to a simmer. Begin cooking time. Cover and stir as needed.

After 30 minutes, add lentils, flaxseeds and vegetables. When beans are tender, add sea vegetables (optional). When cooking time is up, follow the Seven Grains procedure.

Core Tips

"Knowledge is indeed better than blind practice."
—Bhagavad Gita
2nd century B.C.

With most projects, the often overlooked little things are infinitely the most important.

TEN BEAN STEW TIPS

Bean Cooking Times	
Short	**Long**
Black-eyed peas (cowpeas)	Soybeans
Green peas (whole or split)	Garbonzo (chickpeas)
Lentils	Great Northern
Aduki	Kidney (large red)
Baby lima (butter beans)	Windsor (fava)
Small red	Black (turtle)
Navy (small white)	Pinto

Pre-Soaking Beans

Beans absorb water and expand 2½ times their size after only 4 hours of soaking. The longer you soak them, the shorter the cooking time. If beans are cooked after only 4 hours of soaking, the cooking time will need to be increased. Beans can be safely soaked up to 48 hours if the water is changed. During hot weather, refrigerate the soaking beans to prevent fermentation.

Storage Containers

Uncooked beans and grains are best stored in a cool, dark place in tightly sealed glass jars. I strongly recommend glass containers with screw-on lids. Glass is inert and the lids have an airtight seal.

To avoid tasting plastic, never transfer hot food into plastic containers. After cooking, transfer hot food into storage jars using a 4-cup glass measuring cup as a scoop.

Freezing

Both recipes can be frozen up to 6 months. Glass jars with screw-on lids can be used for freezing Seven Grains, but not Ten Bean Stew. (The high water content may crack the glass.) To freeze Ten Bean Stew, use Pyrex trays with snap-on lids designed for freezing.

- Optional: before freezing, refrigerate for 12 hours and remove condensation from inside the lid.
- Optional: freeze individual servings stuffed into pita pockets using zip-lock bags.

Reducing Gas (Flatulence)

Beans are the nutritional equivalent of nuclear power—a good idea if you can keep them under control. The human nose can detect noxious gas in amounts as small as 1 part in 10 billion (equivalent to 1 postage stamp in a roll stretching 5 times around the earth).

Beans produce gas by containing undigestible sugars (raffinose, stachyose, verbascose) which end up in the colon. Following the recipe (soaking, draining, removing foam) will help reduce these undigestible sugars. Other tips:

- Anasazi beans contain only 20% of the undigestible sugars as pinto beans. (Anasazi in Navajo means "the ancient ones.")
- Lentils, lima beans and aduki beans are also easy to digest.
- Soak the beans for 12 hours and sprout them for the next 12 hours by spreading them on moist paper towels.
- Use boiling water for soaking.
- Use charcoal tablets, Beano enzyme drops, or BeSure enzyme capsules.

Tomatoes

Tomatoes will make the vegetables spoil quickly and should not be used in Ten Bean Stew unless you plan to finish the batch soon. Tomatoes (and salt) will stop the beans from cooking and should be added last.

GRAIN TIPS

Exotic Whole Grains (origin)

- Amaranth (Mexico, Aztec)
- Quinoa (Bolivia/Peru, Inca)
- Teff (Ethiopia)
- Kamut (Egypt)
- Spelt (Northern Europe)
- Brown Basmati Rice (India/Pakistan)
- Wehani Rice (Basmati hybrid)
- Wild Rice (Minnesota)
- Brown Jasmine Rice (Thailand)
- Blue Corn (Native American)

Gluten Content

- High: Wheat, Rye, Oats, Barley
- Trace: Amaranth, Quinoa
- None: Rice, Millet, Buckwheat, Corn

Storing Whole Grains

As long as the outer husk (bran) remains unbroken, most whole grains will last for years without decay. There are two exceptions:

- Maximum storage life for oats is 1 year with refrigeration and 6 months without refrigeration because of its high oil content (16% fat).

- Maximum storage life for brown rice is 6 months with refrigeration and 3 months without refrigeration because of rancid-causing enzymes.

Whole grains are best stored in a cool, dry, dark place in tightly sealed glass jars. Freezing for 3 days will kill any mealworm eggs. Bay leaves also discourage bugs. All processed grains (flour, corn meal, rolled oats, cracked wheat) should be refrigerated and quickly used. Try to turnover all grains and beans within 3 months.

IRON

Excess iron contributes to heart disease and colon cancer; too little iron contributes to iron deficiency anemia. The absorption of iron from plants is enhanced by vitamin C, and inhibited by tannin.

Iron from meats (heme iron) is more absorbable than iron from plants (nonheme iron). Chinese blood levels of iron were found to be higher than American levels despite their plant-based diet and high fiber intake (34g/day vs. 11g/day).

COMPARISONS

- **High Fats:** Seeds are 70% fat and high in zinc; nuts are 90% fat and low in zinc; oils are 100% fat and devoid of zinc. (Seeds are nutritionally superior to nuts, which are nutritionally superior to oils.)

- **Soybeans:** Soybeans and tempeh are 38% fat and high in fiber; tofu is 53% fat and low in fiber. (Soybeans and tempeh are nutritionally superior to tofu.)

- **Brown Rice:** Short grain rice is stickier and higher in fiber; long grain rice is higher in protein. (No significant difference.)

- **Cabbage:** Green cabbage is higher in chlorophyll and vitamin C; red cabbage is higher in vitamin A. (No significant difference.)

ACID-ALKALINE

- Animal products are more acid-forming than beans; beans are more acid-forming than grains; grains are more acid-forming than fruits and vegetables.

- Wheat is the most acidic of the grains; millet is the most alkaline.

- Cranberries are the most acidic of the fruits; prunes are the most alkaline.

- Alkaline-forming minerals: calcium, potassium, magnesium, iron, zinc.

- Acid-forming minerals: phosphorus, sulfur, silicon, boron.

- Sodium chloride salt is neutral.

EATING OUT

- Never eat in a restaurant with a plastic cow on the roof.
- Never eat in a restaurant if the menu pictures the Heinleick maneuver or warns, "Remember what's on your plate in case you need to describe it to a doctor."
- Never eat in a restaurant if the restrooms are marked Steers and Heifers, or (God help us) Pointers and Setters.

PESTICIDES

Processed foods contain more pesticide residues than whole foods. Six ounces of apple juice has more pesticides than 6 ounces of applesauce, which has more pesticides than 6 ounces of apples. When Alar-sprayed apples are processed into apple juice, Alar converts to the carcinogen UDMH (unsymmetrical dimethylhydrazine). Personal pesticide avoidance involves a four-step strategy:

- Reduce animal product consumption to 1% of total calories. Animal products supply 90–95% of the pesticides and PCBs in most American diets.
- Reduce fat intake to 10% of total calories. Most pesticides are fat-soluble.
- Eliminate products containing cottonseed oil. Cotton is the most heavily sprayed agricultural product.
- Buy locally-grown whole foods in season. Switch to organic or unsprayed produce whenever possible.

WATER

Pure water does not exist in nature since water dissolves everything it touches. The human body needs minerals: water is a poor source; food is a rich source. The body does well on either distilled or mineralized water. Distilled water does not deplete the body of minerals, and mineralized water does not contribute to calcium deposits. Water contamination is a far greater concern.

WATER TREATMENT

From a health standpoint, the most important kitchen gadget is a water treatment system tailored to the water in your area. Numerous options exist, each having advantages and disadvantages:

- Ceramic filters contain silver which can leach into water. They do not remove chlorine or lead.
- Reverse-osmosis wastes an average of 6,667 gallons of water each year, requires membrane replacement, and doesn't remove bacteria or viruses. Many have plastic holding tanks.
- Distillation is expensive, noisy, slow, requires cleaning, and doesn't remove volatile organics.
- Loose granular carbon filters allow water to channel and bacteria growth.
- Solid carbon filters are effective for most water supplies although they will not remove fluoride, nitrates, or viruses. Certain carbon filters will remove dissolved lead chloride. (One pound of carbon has the surface area of 6 football fields.)
- Water softeners turn hard water into salt water. (Anion types replace sulfates, nitrates, bicarbonates and chlorides with sodium. Cation types replace calcium, magnesium, iron and manganese with sodium.) Both types increase lead levels. (Sodium leeches lead from faucets and soldered copper pipes.)

KITCHEN SETUP

From a timesaving standpoint, the most important kitchen gadget is a food processor—the bigger, the better.

Other Useful Tools:

- Two 4-cup measuring cups (glass)
- ½-cup measuring cup (non-glass)
- Three large mixing bowls
- Long handle wooden spoon
- Vegetable knives (8 inch)
- Timer
- Wooden cutting board
- Plastic cutting board (for onions)

Stainless Steel Cookware

- 16-quart stock pot (for cooking the Ten Bean Stew)
- 10-quart stock pot (for cooking the Seven Grains)
- Large sauce pan or double boiler (for steaming vegetables)

Glass Storage Jars

- Seven 8-cup storage jars with wide-mouth screw-on lids

  (4 jars for storing the Ten Bean Stew, 32 cups per batch)

  (3 jars for storing the Seven Grains, 24 cups per batch)

> *"The bitterness of poor quality is remembered long after the sweetness of low cost has been forgotten."*
>
> —Michael Hackleman
> *Waterworks*

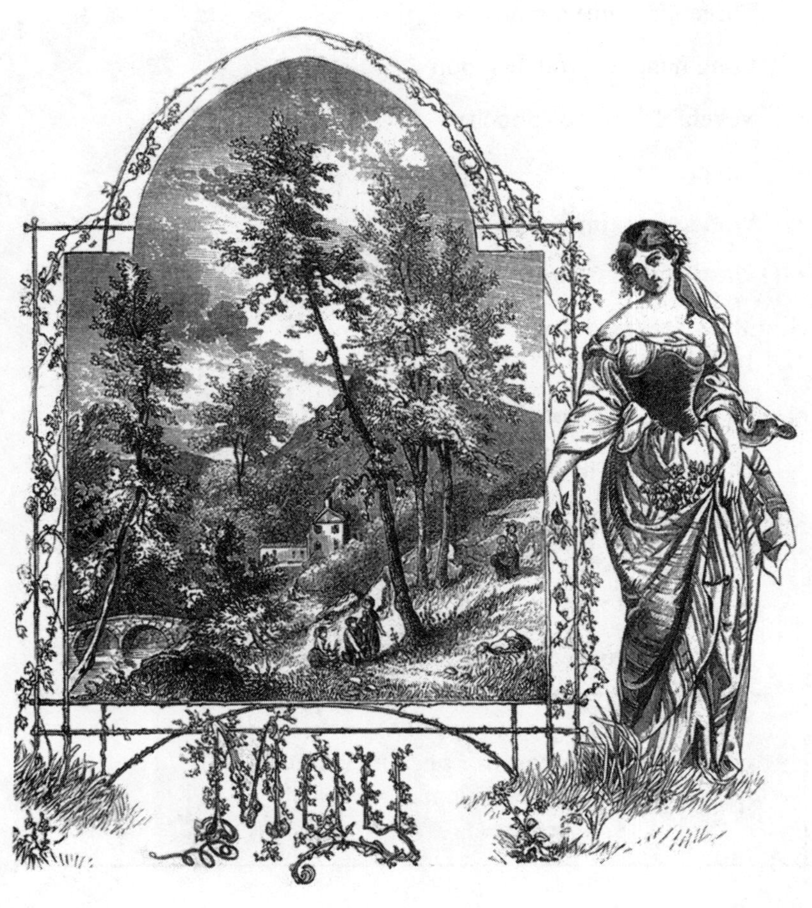

CHAPTER 5
The Human Body

"The doctor of the future will give no medicine, but will interest his patients in the care of the human frame, in diet, and in the cause and prevention of disease."
—Thomas Edison

". . . all diseases may by sure means be prevented or cured, not excepting that of old age, and our lives lengthened at pleasure even beyond the antediluvian standard."
—Benjamin Franklin
letter to an English chemist

Humans are the only species that defy the natural order of things by living decades beyond their peak reproductive years and maximum physical strength. In outliving our biological usefulness, however, the incidence of disease rises with each passing year.

Great scholars probing the depths of medical knowledge, have pondered the age-old question of genetics vs. environment (nature vs. nurture) in the cause of disease. Does the answer lie lurking within the mysterious convolutions of cells, genes and DNA, or within the alchemist miracle of converting plant and animal matter into flesh and blood? Recent research sheds light on this standing scientific challenge.

The Pima Indians of Arizona and the Nauru islanders of the South Pacific share two common traits: obesity and the world's highest incidence of diabetes. During their evolution, both cultures endured times of severe starvation in which the leaner members died off. Those who survived were well adapted to periods of starvation by their ability to conserve fats. When these cultures abandoned their traditional diets in favor of processed high-fat cuisine, obesity and diabetes became rampant.

This selection-by-starvation principle was clearly demonstrated during the Falkland War when Argentina sunk a British supply ship, forcing British troops to live on "short rations." The leaner athletic soldiers had difficulty performing their jobs while the fatter soldiers remained unhindered. Had this situation continued, the athletic soldiers would have starved to death.

Natural selection is one of nature's many tests for insuring the survival of a species. But nature's incessant testing sometimes gets in the way of what we call progress. Obesity, diabetes and cancer are each examples of attempted adaptation to a changing environment. Humans are part of an ongoing experiment and the whole world is the evolutionary laboratory.

Those genetically predisposed to diabetes or cancer will not develop these conditions unless they expose their bodies to the wrong lifestyle. In the absence of promoting factors, genetic proclivity does not manifest. Diabetes rarely occurs among Pima Indians living in the mountains of Mexico—unlike their Arizona relatives. Chronic disease in America develops primarily from the way we live.

According to a recent study, 200,000 native Hawaiians living in Hawaii may be extinct by the year 2044. Native Hawaiians have a cardiovascular disease rate twice that of the general population, 42% are overweight, 33% smoke, and 22% have high blood pressure.

The average American diet constitutes a deviation so extreme that we exhibit afflictions not seen in other cultures: the diseases of civilization. And medicine's armamentarium of surgical and drug intervention offers no shield.

> *"You can drive out nature with a pitchfork, yet she still will hurry back."*
>
> —Quintus Horatius Flaccus
> Roman philosopher (65–8 B.C.)

During the last century, fever and swelling were considered diagnoses rather than symptoms; 50 years from now, diabetes and cancer may be considered symptoms rather than diagnoses. The hard-wired circuitry of genetic programming cannot be altered, but diseases can be mitigated by understanding how the human body works. You can have anything you want once you know what you're doing.

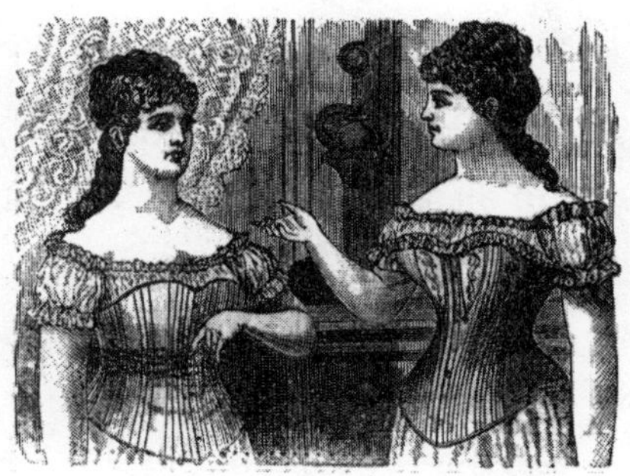

Weight Control

"Never, it seems, have so many worked so hard to lose so little weight."

—Gerald Walker
Time, 1959

"Fat is a real friend. It's a cushion, very comforting at times."[1]

—Roseanne Arnold

"One day I got out of my tub and saw my entire self in a mirror. I was obese."[2]

—Elizabeth Taylor

"I'm not terribly decorative on a beach."[3]

—Peter Ustinov

Does the ice cream call to you from the freezer? Do potato chips and chocolate fudge bars beckon you late at night? When you enter an elevator, do others glance at the capacity sign? You're not alone… America has a weight problem.

When Yankee Stadium was renovated in 1976, the seats needed to be widened by 4 inches to accommodate the larger size of the American fanny. The stadium then held 9,000 fewer seats.[4]

Imagine standing on a bathroom scale holding a 10-pound turkey. That's the amount of weight most Americans gain between Thanksgiving and New Year's Eve. In 1993, Americans collectively gained 155 million pounds through diet,[5] and lost 235,000 pounds through liposuction. Gallup surveys reveal that 90% of Americans want to be thinner.

The U.S. has more obese adults (58 million) than any other nation. America has over 30,000 diets on public record, mostly weight-loss programs. Losing weight is relatively easy compared to keeping it off: 95% of dieters gain their weight back within 2 years, and 99% gain it back within 5 years.[6]

	Average American Female	**Average[7] American Male**
Daily Calorie Intake	1,497	2,154
Daily Fat Intake	61 grams	91 grams
Overweight By 20%	35%	31%
Dieting	50%	25%
Age 25 Body Fat	25%	18%
Age 65 Body Fat	43%	38%
	Height	**Weight**
Average American Female	5'4"	144 pounds
Average Female Model	5'9"	123 pounds

"[Drink] whole milk most of the time, skim milk part of the time, if you need to lose weight."[8]
—National Dairy Council

It's difficult to change while harboring illusions that vested interests would have you believe. Over the past 70 years, Americans cut their calorie intake by 3%, yet the average person weighs more today.[9] About 33% of Americans were overweight in 1995, compared to 25% in 1980.

More than 4 billion people on this earth eat a starch-centered diet (wheat, rice, corn, potatoes) and never become fat. The Chinese eat 20% more calories than Americans, yet Americans are 25% fatter.[10] Not all calories are created equal. Chinese calories are mostly complex carbohydrates (whole grains, vegetables, beans) averaging 15% fat. American calories are mostly animal products, oils, sugars and white flour averaging 37% fat.

The percentage of calories from fat influences body weight more than total calories.[11] Even Carl Lewis, the fastest human alive, was unable to keep his weight down despite his strenuous exercise schedule—until he switched to a low-fat diet.[12]

The body handles fats and nonfats differently. Under normal conditions, carbohydrate, alcohol and protein calories are not converted to fat.[13] Dietary fats convert to body fat so efficiently the molecular structure remains unchanged.[14] Body fat examined under a microscope will reveal the type of fat consumed.

If You Eat	You Carry
Animal fat	Saturated fats
Margarine	Trans fats
Corn oil	Polyunsaturated fats
Olive oil	Monounsaturated fats
Fish oil	Omega-3 fats

Excess carbohydrates are mostly burned as heat. Carbohydrates satisfy the hunger drive; fats do not.[15] Fats may contain up to 11 calories per gram instead of 9.[16] (Carbohydrates and proteins contain only 4 calories per gram.)

Fats are the enemy, not calories. Cut the fats and eat all you want. Replace fats with complex carbohydrates and eat 2½ times more food. You never have to be hungry again.

900 Calories:

6 oz. Potato Chips (60% fat)	OR	5 Baked Potatoes with sour cream (11% Fat)

97 Grams of Fat:

1 Fettuccini Alfredo (1,498 cal.)	OR	485 Baked Potatoes (106,700 cal.)

Most dieters have two strikes against them: they restrict their calories while eating high-fat foods. Examples:

Food	Fat Content[17]
Jenny Craig	20%
Lean Cuisine	25%
Diet Center	19–28%
Nutri/Systems	20–30%
Weight Watchers	27–30%
Extra-lean ground beef	54%

A NEW YOU . . . AGAIN

Extreme calorie restriction produces initial weight loss but it comes at a high price: equal amounts of fat and muscle tissue are lost. Metabolism (calorie burning rate) is forced lower. When the crash dieter gives up and starts eating, more fat is gained back than muscle and the dieter is even worse off. The cycle then begins all over again.

THE YO-YO CYCLE

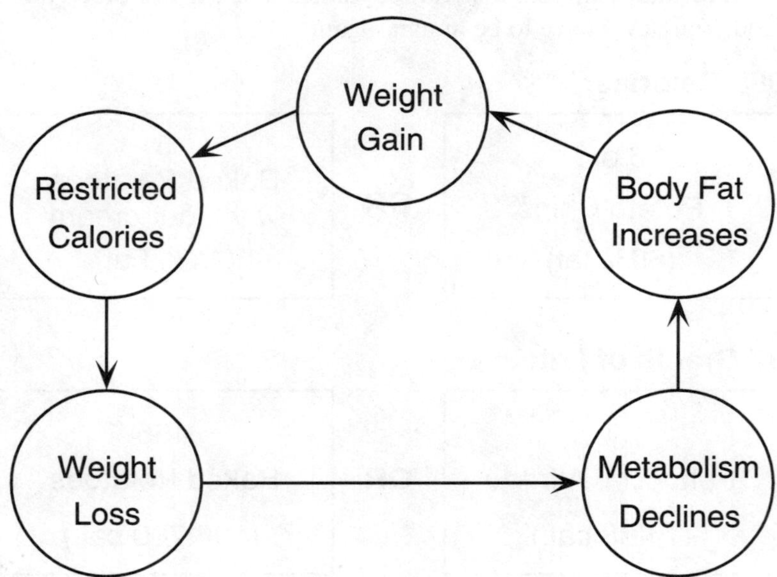

Like Sisyphus pushing the boulder uphill only to have it roll back down, crash dieters are never done with the task. Several yo-yo cycles can condemn the dieter to a lifetime of obesity by causing the following physical changes:[18]

- Higher percentage of body fat (famine mode).
- Lower metabolism (fat burns fewer calories than muscle).
- Activation of the body's fat storage enzyme (lipoprotein lipase) which resists the shedding of fat.

"That's bad news for the well-upholstered of the world. But for American businesses, it represents the marketing opportunity of the century: the chance to sell the same programs to the same people over and over again."[19]
—*Newsweek*

Program	Cost Per Pound Lost[20]
Jenny Craig	$9.32
Optifast	8.64
Nutri/Systems	7.50
Medifast	5.45
Diet Center	3.64
Weight Watchers	0.91

"The frozen foods train the eye to accept small portions."[21]
—Jenny Craig

Small portions cause quick weight loss which leads to quick weight gain. Yo-yo dieters can't keep their weight off no matter how hard they try because they're fighting biology. This tactic is self-defeating since the body is programmed to place survival over appearance. The body will only do what its programmed to do. Starving and bingeing on cardboard food is **not** the answer. Restricting calories to lose weight is one of the great fallacies of our time.

BODY WEIGHT VS. BODY FAT

Another fallacy is the use of body weight to monitor progress. The bathroom scale cannot distinguish between water weight, fat weight and muscle weight. Initial weight loss on a low-calorie diet is almost entirely water. When someone claims to have lost 10 pounds you might ask, "Ten pounds of what?" Accurate monitoring requires the measurement of body fat, not body weight.

> *"In the Middle Ages, they had guillotines, stretch racks, whips and chains. Nowadays, we have a much more effective torture device called the bathroom scale."*[22]
>
> —Stephen Phillips

Each human fat cell can expand 110 times its normal size. Female fat cells can increase both in size and number, especially during puberty, pregnancy and menopause. High-fat diets elevate estrogen levels which accelerates this process.

Top American Food Cravings

Female	Male
1. Chocolate	1. Meat
2. Ice Cream	2. Eggs
3. Candy	3. Potatoes
4. Bread	4. Pizza

Different organs excrete metabolic waste products in different amounts: skin 40%, lungs 40%, kidneys 18%, and colon 2%. This explains why water is critical during times of weight loss.

- Water is needed to flush out the fats that are shed.
- Water helps prevent sagging skin and fluid buildup.
- Water decreases fat storage and increases carbohydrate storage. Lack of water does the opposite.

Carbohydrate is the only nutrient which includes water (hydrate) as part of the word itself. Water is needed for carbohydrate metabolism. A permanent weight control program requires a permanent lifestyle change.

LONG LIFE NOW WEIGHT CONTROL

1) Measure your percentage of body fat:[23]

- Most accurate method: underwater (hydrostatic)
- Medium accurate methods: calipers and electrical resistance (bioimpedance)
- Least accurate methods: infrared and ultrasound

2) Monitor your progress using:

- Repeat body fat measurements (same method)
- Blood pressure and cholesterol levels
- Body measurements and clothing fit
- Cellulite disappearance and energy level
- Appearance in a full-length mirror

3) Eat 10% fat and unlimited complex carbohydrates. Cut back on fruits, juices, salt and flour products. Increase your intake of salads, steamed vegetables and water.

4) Regulate food intake using your appetite only, without counting calories. Never go hungry.

5) Calorie restriction has no place on a long-term weight control program. The body has a natural craving for carbohydrates that cannot be denied.

THE REAL HEAVYWEIGHTS

- Jon Brower Minnoch weighed 1,400 pounds before slimming down to 476 on a crash diet. He then regained 200 pounds in one week.[24]

- Robert Earl Hughes weighed 1,019 pounds before dying of kidney failure at age 32. His coffin (a converted piano crate) had to be lowered by a crane.[25]

Weight control goes far beyond ultimatums from the mirror, tape measure and bathroom scale. At stake is the quality of life. Exercise is the next critical component.

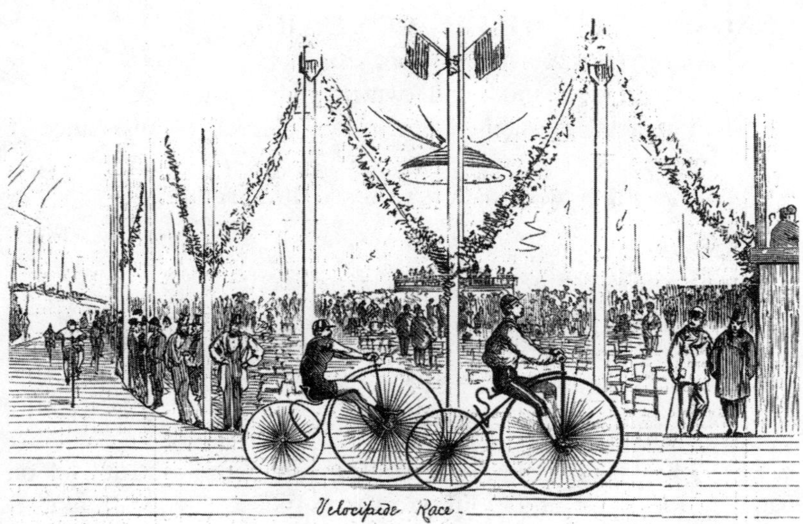

Exercise

"We sit at breakfast, we sit on the train on the way to work, we sit at work, we sit at lunch, we sit all afternoon…a hodge-podge of sagging livers, sinking gallbladders, drooping stomachs, compressed intestines and squashed pelvic organs."[26]
—Dr. John Button Jr.

"A ship in harbor is safe, but that is not what ships are built for."
—John Shedd
Salt from My Attic

Surveys estimate that only 8–20% of Americans exercise at levels sufficient for cardiovascular benefit, and 40–58% of the population is completely sedentary.[27] Most of those who buy fitness equipment stop using it within 6 months. The U.S. would save $4.3 billion annually if sedentary Americans began walking regularly.[28]

By age 74, 25% of American men and 66% of American women cannot lift objects heavier than 10 pounds.[29] You can find marathon runners with arms so weak they can't carry their own luggage, and bodybuilders out of breath after one flight of stairs. To understand the confusing world of exercise, divide everyone into four groups:

1) **Inactives:** completely sedentary.

2) **Moderates:** walkers who seldom raise their heart rates.

3) **Actives:** fitness buffs who raise their heart rates to 60–80% of maximum.

4) **Athletes:** those who push themselves to their physical limits.

Inactive people have the shortest life spans. Athletes and actives have:

- Lower blood pressure
- Lower heart rates
- Higher metabolisms
- Longer life spans
- Stronger immune systems
- Greater cardiovascular fitness

Cardiovascular fitness is measured in terms of:

- Heart muscle strength
- Maximum heart rate
- Recovery time
- Collateral blood flow
- Oxygen utilization
- Lung capacity

EXERCISE AND HEART DISEASE

Jim Fixx, author of *The Complete Book of Running,* was a world-class athlete with elevated cholesterol. He claimed that strenuous exercise protected him from his high-fat diet—until a heart attack killed him during a 10-mile run. Actor Martin Sheen had a heart attack while filming *Apocalypse Now* despite his excellent physical condition.[30]

Olympic gold metal figure skater Sergei Grinkov died of a heart attack at age 28 while skating. Athletes Hank Gathers and Reggie Lewis died of heart attacks on the basketball court. The Masai warriors of Africa and the Soviet Georgians developed heart disease despite their cardiovascular fitness—as did young combat soldiers in Vietnam and Korea. Strenuous exercise offers no escape from a high-fat diet.

The arteries of one adult average 60,000 miles in total length; the surface area of all blood vessels averages half an acre. It's the health of these blood vessels and their ability to transport blood that determines heart attack risk, **not cardiovascular fitness.** Blood vessel health is controlled by diet, not exercise.

EXERCISE AND AGING

In our society, it's normal for muscle mass and metabolism to both decline with age due to decreasing physical activity. It's also normal for calorie needs to drop while nutrition needs stay constant. As a consequence, most middle-aged Americans gain weight. It really comes down to three choices:

- Eat enough calories to avoid nutrition deficiencies and end up gaining weight.
- Eat only enough calories to maintain weight and end up with nutrition deficiencies.
- Eat a low-fat diet and exercise.

Diet is critical because, with age, people develop less tolerance for fats and empty calories. Exercise is critical because the need for calories is determined by muscle mass and metabolism. Exercise maintains both; without exercise, both decline.

SEDENTARY LOOP

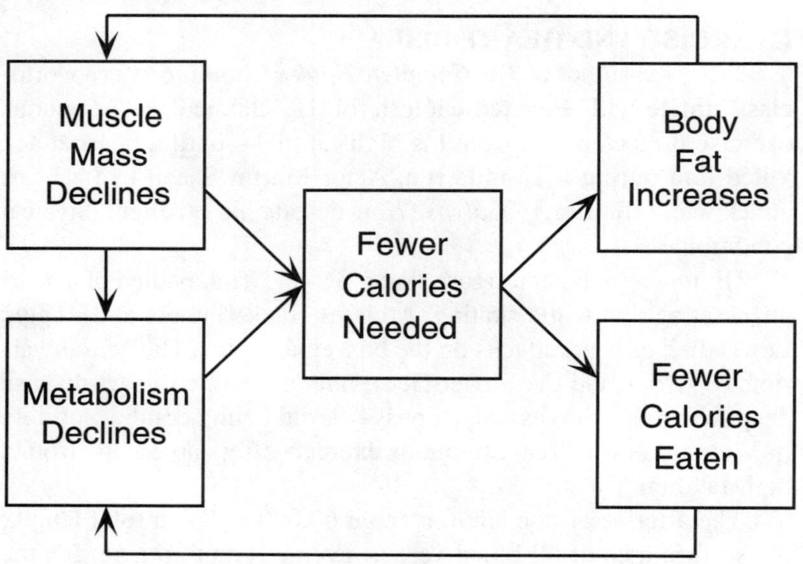

> *"If, in fact, we can maintain or even increase muscle mass, many of these things we called biomarkers of aging might actually be biomarkers of inactivity."*[31]
>
> —Dr. William Evans
> Human Nutrition Research Center on Aging

Exercise reverses everything in the loop, however, not all exercise is effective. Non-aerobic exercise, such as regular walking, maintains neither muscle mass nor metabolism. Physical training enhances the uptake of fats by contracting muscles.[32] Athletes tend to burn fats and conserve carbohydrates; sedentary people burn carbohydrates and conserve fats.

FUNCTIONAL LOSS

The most common reason for seniors entering nursing homes is the loss of ability to perform essential personal care tasks without assistance.[33] In our society, functional ability declines with age. When muscles can no longer lift the body from a chair or bed, when lung capacity declines to the point where simple activity causes fatigue, independent living is irretrievably lost. The process robs seniors of their dignity and savings. Surveys reveal that typical seniors face 11 years of partial or total dependency before they die.[34]

By maintaining lung capacity, muscle strength and the other biomarkers of aging, independent living need never be lost. The minimum oxygen uptake required to maintain independence is estimated to be 12–14 ml/min/kg of body weight.[35] Most sedentary adults lose their independence between ages 75–85. Moderate exercisers (walkers) lose it 10–20 years later.[36] Both decline at the same rate:

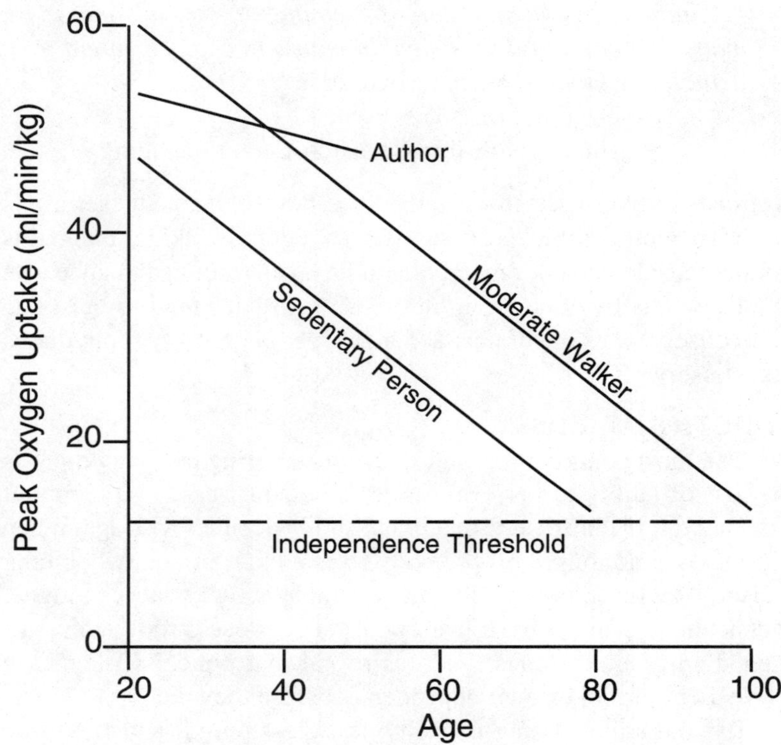

Walking delays but doesn't change the course of old age. Walking is a great exercise if you're happy growing old at the same rate as everyone else. However, if your goal is to avoid institutionalization by maintaining independence for life, you'll need to slow the rate of decline. You'll need to do more than just walk.

VIGOROUS EXERCISE VS. WALKING

Older persons engaged in vigorous aerobic activities were found to have less risk of dying and less disability than average Americans.[37] Middle-aged men assigned to intense workouts experienced enhanced sexual performance compared with those assigned to 1-hour walks.[38] Aerobic exercise improves oxygen uptake more than walking.[39] Vigorous exercise slows the biomarkers of aging; walking confers no such benefit.

Low-intensity workouts do not "maximize fat burning" as claimed by certain promoters. Such assertions are misleading. High-intensity workouts burn more fats and calories than low-intensity workouts for the same time period.[40] If you are able to carry on a conversation during exercise, you receive limited aerobic benefit. The ideal exercise program includes three types of training:

- **Aerobic Exercise:** elevates HDL (good cholesterol), oxygen uptake, cardiovascular fitness and metabolism.
- **Weight Training:** increases muscle mass, strength and metabolism.
- **Stretching:** improves flexibility and helps prevent injury.

Exercise does not lower total cholesterol and plays only a limited role in reducing the risk of heart disease, diabetes and certain cancers.[41] Seniors who avoid chronic disease may still be admitted to a nursing home if they fail to preserve their biological age. Seniors who slow their aging process may still die prematurely of degenerative disease. Diet mitigates disease; strenuous exercise preserves biological age. Doing both offers the surest route to extreme longevity.

Nearly all 100-year-old Americans now languish in nursing homes, but future centenarians can expect more out of life. Many will be running marathons. Where you'll be is largely determined by the actions you take today. The choices, benefits and consequences are yours alone.

Mind and body are one. Only through physical training may we reach our full potential. Only through biological age may we breach the barrier of time.

> *"Afoot and light-hearted I take to the road, healthy, free, the world before me, the long brown path before me leading wherever I choose."*
>
> —Walt Whitman

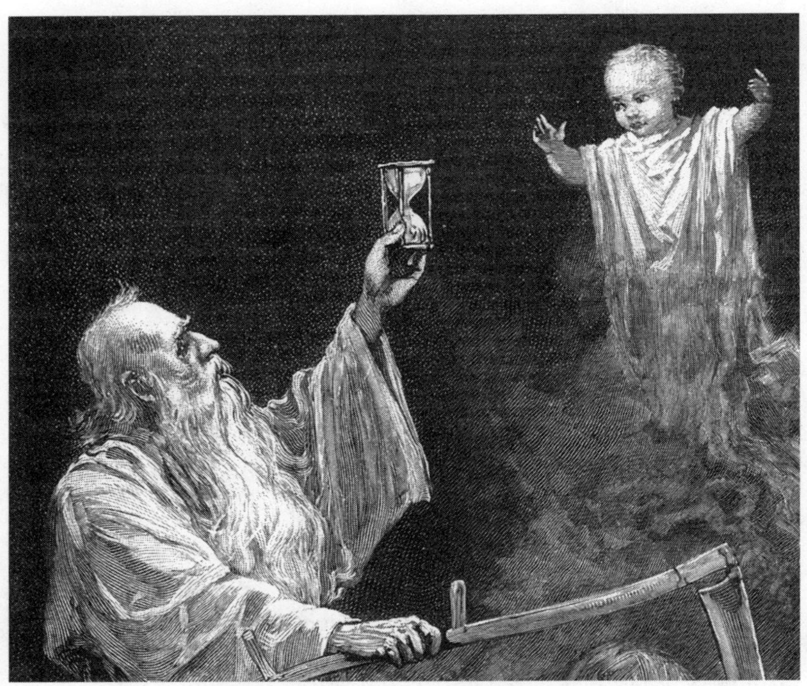

Biological Age

"If it is natural to die, then to hell with nature."
—F.M. Esfandiary
Optimism One

"Some people want to achieve immortality through their works or their descendants. I prefer to achieve immortality by not dying."
—Woody Allen
Woody Allen and His Comedy

"I don't believe in dying. It's been done. . ."
—George Burns
Wisdom of the 90's

"By the time we've made it, we've had it."
—Malcolm Forbes
The Capitalist Handbook

THE REAL CROWN JEWELS

The essence of life comes from playing the cards you've been dealt. But what if you had the power to change those cards, to stay the hands of fate? What if you were given a map leading to fabulous buried treasure? In reality, the most fabulous treasure of all is your biological age. This alone determines how long you'll live and how much fun you'll be physically able to get out of life.

No lifetime accumulation of wealth can compensate for the loss of health. Time is all any of us really have on this earth and we only have two choices: enjoy it while we can or act to preserve it.

Life's real winners are measured by biological age, not by appearance or the trappings of wealth. Howard Hughes died at age 71, not another minute would his fortune buy. All the money and cosmetic surgery in the world makes no difference. Biological age is not for sale—it must be earned.

Normally you don't get much younger as you get older. It's a cold fact of life that the body undergoes predictable changes with advancing age. Biomarkers are the measurements of those changes.

BIOMARKERS THAT DECLINE WITH AGE

- Muscle strength, mass, tone, flexibility
- Vision, hearing, taste, smell
- Reflexes, balance, coordination, reaction time
- Digestion, absorption, metabolic rate, circulation
- Maximum heart rate, cardiac output, endurance
- Immune function, lung capacity, skin elasticity
- Glucose and salt tolerance
- Bone density, kidney filtration rate

> *"At 60 you'll begin to see part of the crowd leaving for the parking lot."*
>
> —Jonathan Winters

People age at different rates. While in college, I volunteered at a methadone clinic for heroin addicts and alcoholics. The long-term users, ravaged by multiple drugs, appeared old before their time.

If we can accelerate the aging process using alcohol, cigarettes, heroin, diabetes and chemotherapy, then we can also slow it down using diet and lifestyle.

By actively slowing the aging process, the gap between chronological age and biological age will widen with time. A fit person of 70 can have greater endurance and athletic prowess than an unfit person of 30. A 65-year-old can have the body of a 45-year-old, and vice versa.[42]

The surface area of adult human lungs is equivalent in size to a tennis court. Lung disease is the third leading cause of disability among Americans. Lung capacity, which declines with age, is the single most accurate indicator of biological age. Most Americans show significant functional decline with age. Examples:

	Age 20	Age 80[43]
Nerve Conduction	100%	85%
Heart Capacity	100%	70%
Kidney Function	100%	70%
Muscle Strength	100%	50%
Lung Capacity	100%	43%
Blood Circulation	100%	40%
Resistance to Infection	100%	25%

The ultimate irony is that the brain remains relatively untouched by the ravages of time…all the better to witness the deterioration of everything else. Contrary to popular belief, Alzheimer's is a disease, not an aging process.

BIOMARKERS THAT RISE WITH AGE

- Resting heart rate
- Blood pressure
- Blood cholesterol
- Blood fats (triglycerides)
- Body weight
- Body fat
- Blood sugar
- Blood insulin

In traditional cultures around the world, where heart disease and cancer are rare, these indicators remain constant throughout life starting at age 20. This represents a challenge that what we consider normal may not be normal at all.

In the grand scheme of things, the human body ages gradually—the lights and machinery shut down one by one. The sequence is genetically programmed; the speed of deterioration is largely up to us. Genetic predisposition determines our time clock; diet and lifestyle move the hands. By slowing the clock, disease inevitability need not manifest.

	American Profile	**Author Profile**
Actual Age	48	48
Sex	M	M
Blood Pressure (mm Hg)	140/90	106/65
Blood Triglycerides (mg/dl)	250	73
Blood Cholesterol (mg/dl)	200	119
Cholesterol:HDL Ratio[44]	4.5:1	3.2:1
LDL:HDL Ratio[45]	4.0:1	1.8:1
Body Fat[46]	23%	6.9%
Weight Gain Since Age 20[47]	23 lb	0 lb
Flexibility (Sit-and-reach test)[48]	11–16"	25"
Lung Capacity (liters)[49]	4.6	5.7
Peak Oxygen Uptake (ml/min/kg)[50]	35.7	48.8
Blood Glucose (mg/dl)[51]	105	71
2 hr. Glucose Tolerance (mg/dl)[52]	127	89
Lifetime Heart Attack Risk[53]	50%	0%
Lifetime Cancer Risk	50%	Near 0%
Biological Age	48	?

"Death does not take the old but the ripe."
—Russian proverb

HEALTH-CARE COST CONTAINMENT

U.S. companies face a major financial challenge:

- General Motors, Ford and Crysler spend about $600 in health-care costs for every vehicle they build.
- Safeway spends four times more on health-care than it earns in after-tax profits.
- In 1993, U.S. companies spent an average of $3,800 per employee for health-care. This cost may climb to $20,000 by the year 2000.[54]

Health-care costs place U.S. companies at a competitive disadvantage in the global marketplace. It's bad business to pay $40 billion each year for heart bypass surgery and angioplasty while the underlying cause is overlooked. Roughly 70–80% of chronic diseases are preventable.[55] The solution is straightforward: financial incentives for diet and lifestyle changes.

People who reported good health habits had medical insurance claims averaging $190 per year. Those with poor habits had claims averaging $1,550 per year.[56] Yet under the current system, obese sedentary smokers pay the same health-care costs as vegetarian athletes. This is wrong. Healthy individuals should not be forced to subsidize the bad habits of others. The system needs reforming and several companies have taken the lead:

- Life insurance companies (including those owned by tobacco companies) charge smokers more for term insurance.
- National Home Life Assurance gives a physical exam that measures aerobic fitness, blood cholesterol and percentage of body fat. Those who qualify receive a discount on their life insurance.[57]
- Baker Hughes (a Houston oil field supplier) gives a physical exam that measures blood pressure, cholesterol, triglycerides and height-weight. Employees who qualify receive an annual cash bonus.[58]

- Hershey Foods and Adolph Coors offer discounts to healthy employees on their medical insurance.[59]

As these programs begin to pay off in terms of lower medical costs, we can expect to see major changes in the workplace. Implications for the future:

- Health insurance premiums based on biological age.
- Biological age pre-employment screening exams.
- Retirement of airline pilots, fire fighters and police officers based on biological age.
- Replacement of age-discrimination with biological age-discrimination.
- Financial penalties for high-risk employees (sedentary obese alcoholic smokers).

Companies can reward healthy employees with paid time off, prizes, bonuses and recognition of achievements. Employees who don't spend their medical deductibles could have that money credited to their retirement. These measures would lower costs, increase profits, extend life and ultimately save the nation billions.

Not all preventive measures offer good value for the resources invested. Reducing blood cholesterol using drugs or 30% fat diets has been shown to cost more than it saves.[60] Reducing cholesterol using a 10% fat diet is cost-effective.[61]

Rising health-care costs are forcing these changes and a spin-off benefit will be longer life for everyone. Scientists are working to perfect the measurements of biological age, and that knowledge will help push life expectancies upward.

Birthdays don't count; biological age is everything.

> *"A switch is not thrown in your nervous system when you reach 65. That age was only an arbitrary invention of the Iron Chancellor, Otto von Bismarck, to coax some recalcitrant generals into retirement."*[62]
>
> —Hugh Drummond, M.D.

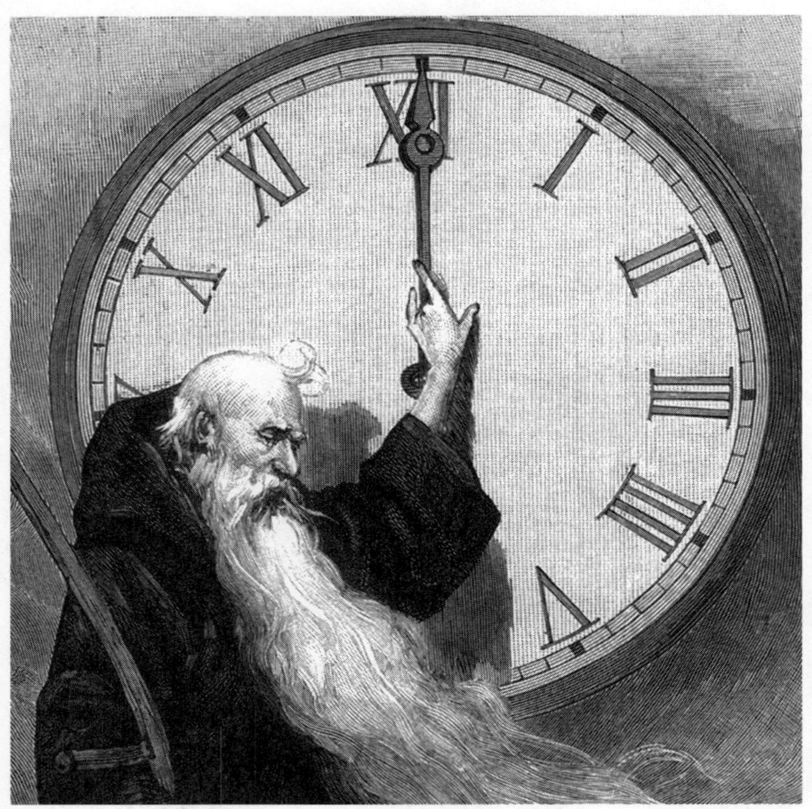

Slowing the Clock

"Youth, large, lusty, loving, youth full of grace, force, fascination. Do you know that old Age may come after you with equal grace, force, fascination?"

—Walt Whitman
Leaves of Grass

"The universe that suckled us is a monster that does not care if we live or die—does not care if it itself grinds to a halt. It is fixed and blind, a robot programmed to kill. We are free and seeing; we can only try to outwit it at every turn to save our skins."

—Annie Dillard
Pilgrim at Tinker Creek

"What is of supreme importance in war is to attack the enemy's strategy...To subdue the enemy without fighting is the acme of skill."

—Sun-Tzu, 300 B.C.
The Art of War

The search for the secret to eternal youth has eluded humanity since time immemorial. Lady Coventry of England painted her face with white lead; Isabeau of Bavaria applied a facial emollient of boar brains, wolf blood and crocodile glands; Mary, Queen of Scots bathed in red wine; ancient Syrians bathed in the blood of children; Romans drank the blood of fallen gladiators; Pope Innocent VIII transfused the blood of young men into his veins.[63]

All in an effort to stem the ravages of time and all to no avail. From ginseng extracts to implanted ape testes, the elusive quest continues today. Dubious and novel procedures abound throughout the world, each promising refuge from fate's icy grasp.

Rejuvenation Injections

- Live cell therapy (fetal sheep cells) – La Prairie Clinic, Montreux, Switzerland; Cost: $10,000
(Clients: Winston Churchill, Dwight Eisenhower, Charlie Chaplin, Henry Kissinger, Charles De Gaulle, Gloria Swanson, Barbara Streisand, Bob Hope, Elizabeth Taylor, George Hamilton, Pope Pius XII)[64]

- Gerovital GH3 (procaine) – L'Aqualigne Clinic, Saint Martin, Caribbean; Geriatric Institute of Romania; Cost: $2,600
(Clients: John F. Kennedy, Marlene Dietrich, Elizabeth Taylor, Imelda Marcos)[65]

- Human growth hormone – Baxamed Medical Center, Basel, Switzerland; El Dorado Rejuvenation and Longevity Institute, Playa del Carmen, Mexico; Cost: up to $25,000

- Human placenta – Wiedemann Clinic, Munich, Germany; Cost: $5,000

- Cattle, goat and shark embryos – Tijuana, Mexico; Cost: $4,000

Cryonic Suspension

- Freeze your body in liquid nitrogen – Trans Time Inc., Oakland, CA; Life Extension Foundation, Ft. Lauderdale, FL; Alcor Life Extension Foundation, Riverside, CA; Cost: $120–$140,000 (substantial discount for frozen brain)

Mummification

- Preserve your body as a New Age mummy – Summum, Salt Lake City, UT; Cost: $8,000 for funeral in pyramid, $26,000 for sealed bronze sarcophagus (additional cost for mausoleum and Plexiglas display case)

Make no mistake, the causes of aging are legion—an assault on all fronts by an army of petty thieves stealing from us in the night. Youth and vitality are the spoils of plunder. No single assassin the cause, no armor a shield, and no fortress a sanctuary from the great equalizer and ultimate unwelcomed guest.

To even the strongest, aging eventually draws near. Pop vitamin pills and the foe snickers cynically…it's unimpressed. In time, chronic disease comes calling and to slow the onslaught requires an organized counterattack. The laws of nature are simple but enforced without mercy. Ignore the laws and grow old before your time. In this arena, you play for keeps.

THE LAWS OF NATURE

Law #1: You are fully responsible for your own actions. Although this law is an alien concept in our society, nature is an exquisitely ruthless enforcer. In nature, there are no excuses, rewards or punishments…there are only consequences. Nature is neutral.

Law #2: A double-edged sword cuts both ways. Disease risk cannot be lowered without slowing the aging process; disease risk cannot be raised without accelerating the aging process. This is the double-edged sword of metabolism, a sword over which you have control.

The unrelenting and predatory laws of nature can be your closest ally or your bitterest foe. As humanity's oldest adversary, this thief of time brings our species to its knees. We can defy the process only by understanding how the process works.

"During each day the average adult produces and sheds more than 500 billion cells and synthesizes 300 grams of protein—an amount of protein produced and destroyed annually which is greater than the mass of the average human body. The outward appearance of stability is an illusion... Without constant self-construction, life would long ago have disappeared into the crust of the earth from which it arose."[66]

—Dr. Richard W. Young

We age from things that happen within our assemblage of 60–100 trillion cells. All living organisms engage in constant battle against the forces of decay and hostile environmental insults. Evolution arms us with elaborate intracellular backup systems, upon which survival depends. When hostile forces deplete our reserves, cellular damage occurs.

DNA (deoxyribonucleic acid) contains the genetic blueprint passed from one cell to the next. When DNA is damaged, new cells become less efficient and eventually die. Premature cell death leads to premature aging. DHEA (dehydroepiandrosterone) is the second most common steroid in the human body (after cholesterol). DHEA declines between ages 20–30 more than any other known substance. Aging is a more complex biological phenomena than cancer.

FREE RADICALS

Free radicals are strange unstable molecules which damage cells, proteins, fats and DNA. They come in several models, each having an abnormal number of electrons:

- Oxygen with one electron – superoxide radical
- Oxygen with two electrons – hydrogen peroxide radical
- Oxygen with two electrons (opposite spin, higher energy) – singlet oxygen radical
- Oxygen with three electrons – hydroxyl radical

Free radicals steal electrons from other molecules. (Oxygen with four electrons is water.) They rust out cars, eat holes in the ozone layer, turn pages yellow and sliced apples brown, and wreak havoc on the human body—all while lasting only a few thousandths of a second. Every disease process involves free radicals.

The immune system destroys bacteria, viruses and toxins using free radicals as weapons. Problems arise when invading organisms overwhelm the defenses, turning free radicals against the host. If free radicals aren't controlled, more cells are destroyed than regenerated. When cell damage exceeds cell repair, we age. Free radicals are agents of both life and death.

Rancid fats generate free radical chain reactions (lipid peroxides). Every cell is vulnerable to this process since every cell has a fatty membrane. Free radicals react with any fat they contact, and the bodies of most Americans provide ample fuel:

- High cholesterol level
- High body weight
- High triglyceride level
- High body fat

The liver removes fats from the bloodstream but fat clearance becomes less efficient with age. Each process takes a cumulative toll, eventually breaking down the immune system. Premature aging occurs when several factors combine.

COLLAGEN

Pinch older skin and it stays up like a ridge of putty. The same sun that gives a healthy glowing tan at age 20 makes skin look like crepe paper at age 50. The difference is collagen.

Collagen protein supports every cell in the body: skin, bones, muscles and organs. When free radicals damage collagen, the fibers undergo the classical signs of advanced age:

- Skin collagen – wrinkled
- Muscle collagen – reduced flexibility
- Lens crystalline collagen – cataract
- Artery collagen – reduced blood supply
- Kidney collagen – decreased kidney filtration
- Lung collagen – decreased lung capacity

AGING LOOP

Damaged collagen at the cellular level leads to the vicious cycle of organ malfunction and accelerated aging.

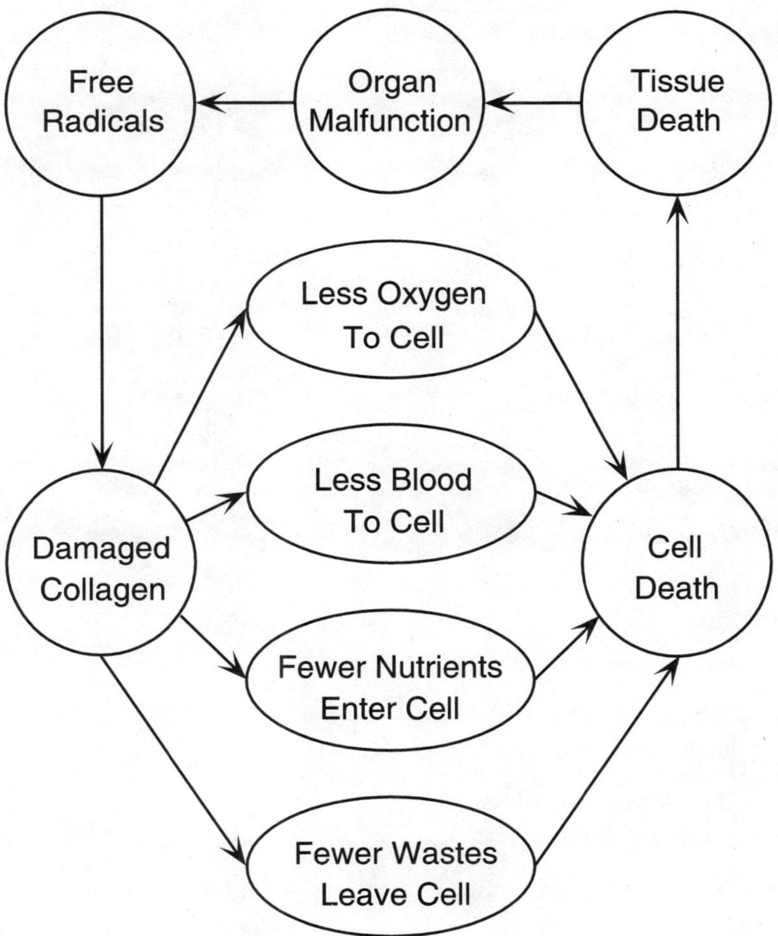

Young collagen: soft, flexible and permeable.

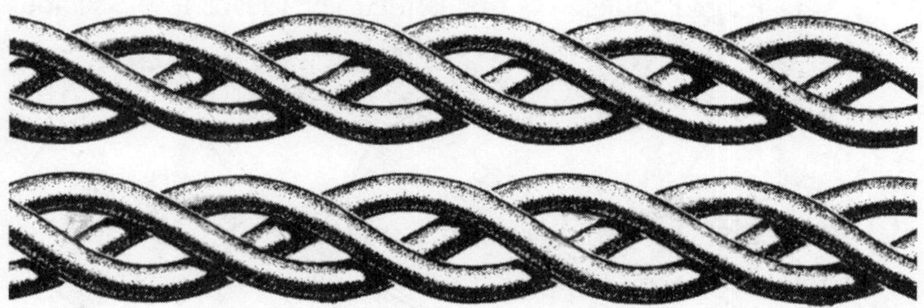

Old collagen: tough, rigid and less permeable.

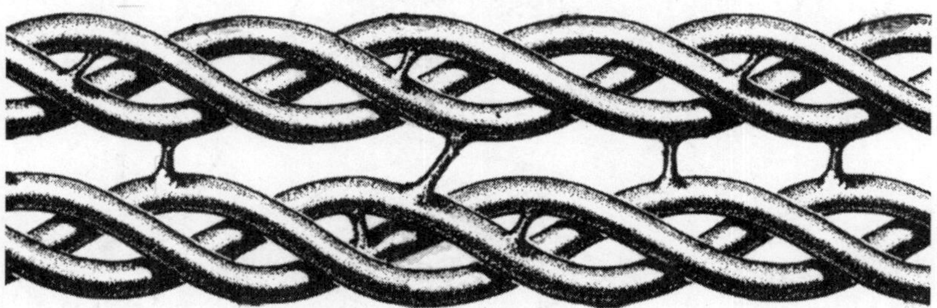

There are four basic strategies for protecting yourself from damage caused by free radicals:

- **The Easy Way:** antioxidants from pills (vitamins C, E and beta-carotene).
- **The Moderate Way:** antioxidants from foods (vegetables, fruits and whole grains).
- **The Hard Way:** source control (reduce fat, protein and sugar intake).
- **The Long Life Now Way:** do all the above.

Belief: You'd need to eat 20,000 calories' worth of food a day to get the same nutrients that will slow down age-dependent disease.[67]

Reality: Age-dependent disease is due primarily to dietary excess, not deficiency.

Belief: Strenuous exercise causes free radical damage.

Reality: Free radical damage manifests only when the immune system deteriorates, as with a sedentary lifestyle. Free radicals are essential for life itself, generating energy within each cell.

Belief: Free radicals cause premature aging.

Reality: Free radical damage is a symptom of premature aging, not the cause. Free radicals behave like any other opportunistic bacteria, virus, fungi or disease. All are held in check by the immune system; all are unleashed when the immune system fails. Free radicals, like fire, can warm your hearth or burn down your house.

THE IMMUNE SYSTEM

From the beginning, molds, fungi and bacteria have competed for living space within us. Molds have a track record of developing poisons against bacteria. Bacteria have a track record of developing resistance against poisons. Long-term human survival depends more on immune system strength than on finding the right antibiotic.

The primary purpose of the yeast candida albicans is to turn the human body into topsoil after it dies—a recycling program you may not want working on your body while its still alive.

Human skin is host to a whole array of microscopic organisms. If the body were to suddenly disappear leaving these critters in place, the bacteria layer would form a perfect image. A healthy immune system is essential for survival on this planet and ultimately determines our capacity to thrive.

Over millennia, humans have developed elaborate defenses for dealing with rogue cells, noxious agents and microscopic invaders setting up shop inside us. Examples:

- Defense enzymes which destroy toxins using free radicals.
- Antioxidant enzymes which neutralize free radicals (catalase, superoxide dismutase, glutathione peroxidase).
- DNA repair system which guards against mutated cell growth and damaged collagen.
- Killer T cells which attack bacteria, viruses and cancer cells.[68]

As each arsenal deteriorates, illness quickly takes hold. It's normal in our society for cancers and infections to rise dramatically with age, thereby accelerating aging. For the average 30-year-old, disease risk doubles every 8 years for life. Fortunately, each of us has the means to challenge this human condition. Diet intimately determines immune system strength.

> *"Many years ago, I showed that with age the level of cholesterol increased not only in the blood but in the T lymphocytes of the immune system. There, it directly interferes with the ability of these cells to fight off disease."*[69]
>
> —Vladimir Dilman, M.D.
> Petrov Research Institute of Oncology
> St. Petersburg, Russia

Immune system strength intimately determines biological age. The key to longevity requires holding in check the "normal" changes in metabolism:

- **Fat Metabolism –** elevated blood cholesterol, triglycerides, body fat and body weight.
- **Carbohydrate Metabolism –** decreased glucose tolerance; increased blood glucose and insulin resistance.
- **Protein Metabolism –** decreased kidney function and bone density; increased uric acid level.

Metabolism has many masters: genetics in the backseat, environment in the frontseat, and the average American diet in the driver's seat. Attempting to slow the aging process by taking vitamins is consistent with treating symptoms while ignoring the cause. Knowing how the process works is the true free radical shield.

To master the aging process is to live the oldest of dreams. To preserve youth is to walk serene in the shadow cast by the beast…your medical destiny. An extra 40–50 years is like a whole new lifetime. By living that unlived life in each of us, by changing the face of what it means to grow old, you become the future of humanity.

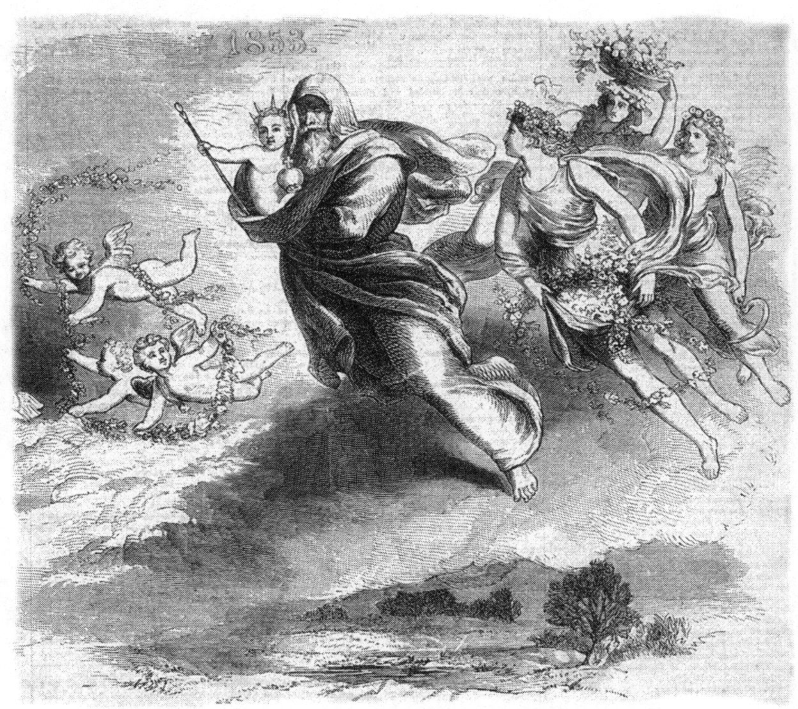

American Seniors

"The society which fosters research to save human life cannot escape responsibility for the life thus extended."[70]
—Walter Bortz, M.D.

As the dawn of a new millennium approaches, no issue presents a greater challenge of our national resolve than how we accommodate our seniors. Health is fleeting for most Americans over age 75. Each passing year brings yet another reminder of mortality and another nudge towards institutionalization.

Anyone who's placed a loved one in a nursing home remembers their heartache and guilt. And anyone who sees what goes on inside remembers the unmitigated doom—physical, mental, social—of growing old in America. That's not the way it has to be.

Today an entire generation has vowed not to allow their bodies to deteriorate the way their parents have. This is the first generation in history to make such a vow and the first generation with the knowledge to pull it off. By altering diet and lifestyle to extend life, you exercise the most fundamental of birthrights: control over your medical destiny.

THE NATION GROWS OLDER

Year	Americans Over 65[71]
1970	1 in 10
1990	1 in 8
2040	1 in 5

As of 1994, the oldest verified age anyone survived was just over 120; more people are expected to reach this age in the coming decades.[72] Our senior population will rise dramatically starting in 2011 when the baby boom generation begins reaching age 65. The government is making preparations by pushing Social Security back to age 70, eventually to age 75.

Job security is now an obsolete vestige from a bygone era. Mid-life career changes, continuing education and two-income families are now the norm. The high costs of housing, raising children and caring for aging parents will challenge the resources of the sandwich generation. For boomers and all succeeding generations, the years beyond age 65 will be the most productive in history—out of sheer economic necessity. Slowing the aging process is no longer a luxury. Personal fitness throughout life now determines financial survival.

QUALITY OF LIFE

For too many seniors, the passage of time inevitably leads to disability and the catastrophic costs of long-term nursing home care. Loss of independence is a senior's greatest fear.

- Of all Americans who turned 65 in 1990, nearly half will enter nursing homes.[73]
- Of those that enter, one-third will die within their first year, half will be sedated with psychotrophic drugs, 19% will be physically restrained, and 50% will develop Alzheimer's.[74]
- The nation would save $3 billion per month if the institutionalization of elderly Americans could be postponed.[75]

Our nation has traded the acute infections from earlier this century for the chronic wasting diseases of affluence. Medical life-saving technology has outstripped prevention with seniors living longer in abject misery.

> *"Death is a refuge from the real fear of aging: Chronic Illness."*[76]
>
> —Hugh Drummond, M.D.

CHRONIC HEALTH PROBLEMS

Diabetes:	26% by age 85
Heart disease:	31% by age 65
Arthritis:	50% over age 65
Kidney function loss:	33–50% by age 80
Hearing impairment:	39% by age 70
High blood pressure:	50% by age 65
Cataracts:	46% by age 70
Dentures:	66% by age 75
Hemorrhoids:	50% by age 50
Diverticulosis:	75% by age 75
Urinary incontinence:	50% by age 80
Gallstones:	40% by age 65
Require assistance:	33% by age 85

Female Problems

Breast cancer:	11% by age 85
Varicose veins:	40% by age 65
Osteoporosis:	90% over age 75
Spinal fractures:	40% by age 80
Hip fractures:	32% by age 90

Male Problems

Colon polyps:	67% by age 65
Prostate enlargement:	50–75% over age 50
Prostate operations:	25% by age 80
Impotence:	25% by age 65
Osteoporosis:	50% over age 75

> *"Health consists of having the same diseases as one's neighbors."*
>
> —Quentin Crisp

LIFE AT ANY COST

To avert the coming demographic disaster—a pileup of frail and helpless untouchables—this nation can no longer afford the luxury of ignoring the cause. In 1988, 27% of all Medicare costs were spent on patients during their last year of life, and half those costs were spent on patients during their last 60 days.[77]

Squandering our resources to maintain people in poor health is not the answer…nor is the marriage of cost-containment to death-with-dignity. The only real long-term solution is the prevention of premature aging.

Surveys show that typical sedentary seniors face 10 years of partial dependency and 1 year of total dependency before they die.[78] This age-related functional loss is not seen in other societies with radically different diets. What we consider normal is not normal at all. What we call old age is actually the cumulative damage from the way we live. Premature aging is, to a great extent, preventable.

Two recent studies reported that American seniors are increasing in number but decreasing in disability.[79] The goal of *Long Life Now* is to accelerate this trend. History suggests our national institutions—government, science, medicine—have done little to protect us from degenerative disease. We must learn to protect ourselves.

The time has come to start building a new American society where nursing homes and besetting infirmities are relics of the past, where immunity from medical disfigurement is taken for granted, where the final years are savored without physical constraints.

THE FUTURE

Senior Olympic athletes today, at age 65, would have qualified for the 1904 Olympics. Senior athletes are living examples of what lies ahead.

- James Ward, age 74, is the oldest finisher of the Ironman Triathlon (2.4 mile swim, 112 mile bike ride, 26 mile run).
- Paul Spangler, age 94, is the oldest marathon runner and plans to be the first human to run a 26-mile race at age 100.

Such feats will become the new standard by which we as a people measure our progress. Senior athletes defy the boundaries of human limits and help dispel society's current perception of old age.

What used to be age 50 is now considered age 60–65. This emerging phenomena (down aging) will accelerate as the population ages.[80] The future will bring an ever widening gap between those who slow down and those who accelerate their biological aging process. With human potential pushed to its limit, the lines between young and old will blur.

> *"No question: In the 21st century, people will live 30 to 40% longer, to about 150. This will be done by extending the periods of youth and mid-life, not old age."*[81]
>
> —Roy Walford, M.D.

The fastest growing group of Americans are those over age 85. By the year 2040, there will be 1 million Americans over age 100 (up from 45,000 in 1992).[82] But unlike today's centenarians, many will be competing in athletic events.

We're here on this earth for only three reasons: to learn, to grow and to have fun. Lying in a hospital bed with tubes in each orifice can make the enjoyment of life more difficult. Taking control over the final stage of life, making it livable and worth attaining, is a highly spiritual act.

Taking control requires information.

ENDGAME

It's a sad commentary on our society that the residents of Sun City, Florida (a retirement community) were upset by the buzzards circling overhead.[83] It's sadder still that the suicide rate increased among American seniors while a book on committing suicide became a national bestseller (*Final Exit* by Derek Humphry).[84]

Terminal illness is relentlessly corrosive to the human spirit while "rational suicide" offers the ultimate escape from intolerable pain and pointless suffering. There is another option—a legacy no one can take away and no amount of money can buy—the gift of long life and freedom from disease.

This most precious gift comes from a true understanding of things at the point of cause, an understanding that lasts a lifetime. It is my highest hope that you'll gain this gift, master those things necessary to pull it off, and embark on the most compelling frontier of our time: the grand adventure of extending your life.

"[Future generations will be given the knowledge but not the questions. Past generations had the questions but not the knowledge.]
"In all of the four-billion-year history of life on our planet, in all of the four-million-year history of the human family, there is only one generation privileged to live through that unique transitional moment: that generation is ours."

—Carl Sagan
Broca's Brain

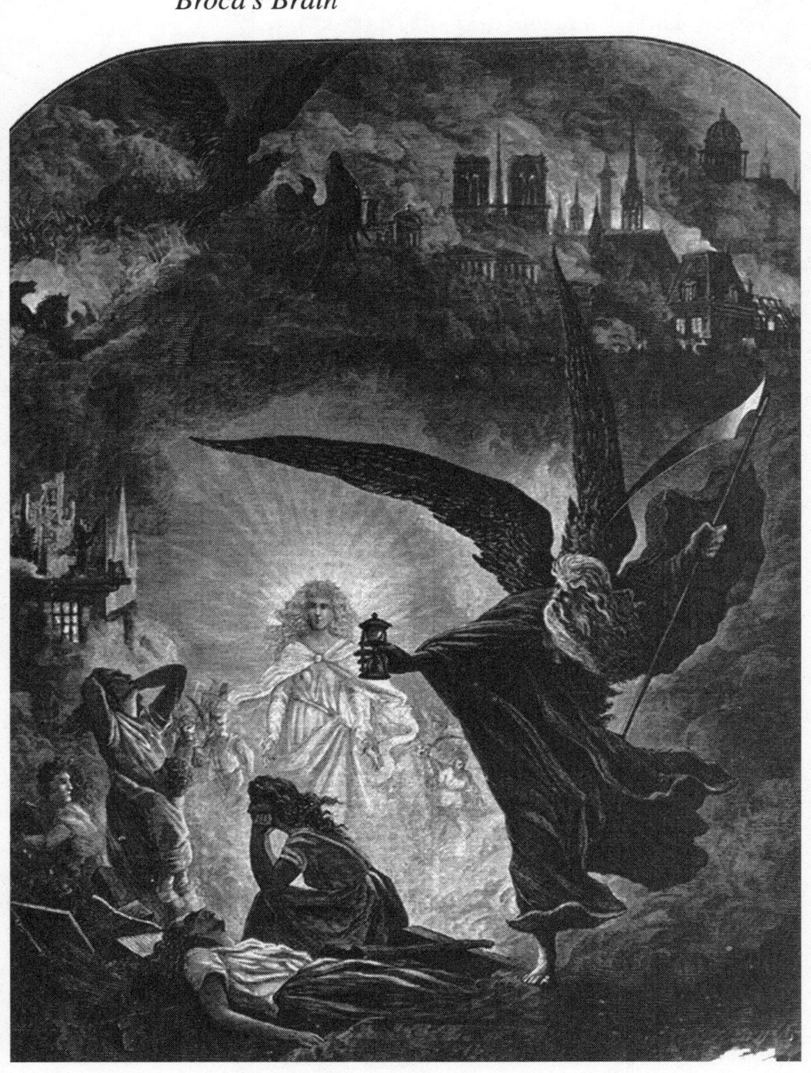

CHAPTER 6
Survival Skills

"When health is absent, wisdom cannot reveal itself, art cannot manifest, strength cannot fight, wealth becomes useless and reason becomes powerless."

—Herophilies, 300 B.C.
physician to Alexander the Great

"I have a right to decide what happens to my own body, not because I know more than anyone else, but simply because it is my body. And I have a right to acquire the information that can help me make those crucial decisions."

—Audre Lorde
A Burst of Light

"Rule of survival: Pack your own parachute."

—T.L. Hakala

Humans have recognized the link between food and disease since the dawn of civilization, but only recently has nutritional consensus been touched by the specter of corporate influence. During the 1950s, vegetable oil companies launched a publicity campaign claiming that cholesterol was the main culprit leading to heart disease. Although unanimous scientific agreement was lacking, heavy promotion lead to the campaign's acceptance.

During the 1960s, the National Live Stock and Meat Board funded studies of the Masai tribes in Kenya and Tanzania.[1] The Masai subsisted on meat, milk and blood, yet they appeared immune from heart disease despite their 73% fat diet.[2] Early studies reported heart disease to be a consequence of inactivity, rather than diet. This conclusion was later modified when Masai autopsies revealed extensive cardiovascular damage.[3]

In 1987, the National Dairy Board recommended that American teen-agers eat double cheeseburgers, milkshakes, lasagna, cheese-topped potatoes and pizza.[4] Current evidence suggests these recommendations may be less than exemplary.

Every culture harbors its own plague. The Masai suffer from diseases of poverty (malaria, parasites, malnutrition and water-borne dysenteries); Americans have diseases of affluence (degenerative, autoimmune and environmental). To battle the top killers, one must first be aware of what the killers are.

10 Leading Causes of Death: United States, 1993[5]

Rank	Cause of Death	Number	Percent
1	Heart Disease	738,860	32.6%
2	Cancer	530,870	23.4%
3	Stroke	149,740	6.6%
4	Lung Disease	101,090	4.5%
5	Accident	88,630	3.9%
6	Pneumonia, Influenza	81,730	3.6%
7	Diabetes Mellitus	55,110	2.4%
8	HIV Infection	38,500	1.7%
9	Suicide	31,230	1.4%
10	Homicide	25,470	1.1%

According to the Surgeon General, diet-related diseases account for 68% of U.S. deaths.[6] Conventional medicine offers early detection and treatment at the expense of prevention. However, few degenerative conditions are due to medication, X-ray or laboratory test deficiencies.

Popular tests for liver function and intestinal permeability have their place, but not as a substitute for changing the diet. Procedures which fail to address the underlying cause fall short of prevention. True prevention means avoiding the medical system altogether through an understanding of disease processes.

Heart Disease

"The role of the artery must be absolute, universal and unobstructed, or disease will be the result."[7]

—Andrew Taylor Still, D.O.
founder of osteopathy, 1897

"I am so healthy that I expect to live on and on."[8]

—J.I. Rodale
founder of *Prevention* magazine
moments before his death from a heart attack

Heart disease kills four times as many American women each year as breast cancer. Cardiovascular diseases kill nearly twice as many American women each year as all forms of cancer combined.[9] For 300,000 people each year, the first and only symptom of heart disease is sudden death.

According to the Centers for Disease Control, only 18% of Americans over age 18 are free of heart disease risk factors: high blood cholesterol, smoking, overweight, diabetes, hypertension and inactivity.[10]

The heart is a magnificent organ that gets noticed mainly when it stops working. Each heart attack costs our health-care system at least $40,000. Heart disease is a $40 billion dollar industry with bypass surgery and angioplasty among the most lucrative medical procedures. Heart surgeons generate more revenue per in-patient hospital admission than any other specialty.

During my senior year of chiropractic school, a classmate sitting next to me suffered a heart attack. It seemed remarkable that such a thing could happen in an institution dedicated to prevention. One of my grandfathers died of a heart attack at age 56; the other took nitroglycerine tablets for angina. The key to avoiding heart disease is understanding how the process works.

In our society, it's normal for atherosclerosis to begin in early childhood. Several studies showed fatty streaks in the arteries of American children by age 10.[11] It's common in the U.S. for blood cholesterol to rise with age. What we consider normal is not normal at all.

National Cholesterol Levels (mg/dl)[12]			
	Range	Average	Borderline High
U.S.A.	155–274	206	200–240
China	88–165	127	150

About 80% of the human race have cholesterol levels below 150 and will never have a heart attack.[13] The Tarahumara Indians of Mexico and the Yanamomes of Brazil have average cholesterol levels from 133–137.[14]

Blood cholesterol below 150 offers immunity from heart attack independent of "good" HDL (high density lipoproteins) and "bad" LDL (low density lipoproteins).[15] Total cholesterol divided by HDL should ideally be under four. The higher the cholesterol above 150, the greater the heart disease risk and the more this ratio matters.[16] Low HDL (35 or less) is a risk factor only when total cholesterol is above 150.

A cholesterol level of 206 may be normal for most Americans who die in their 70s, but it's not normal for those planning to live past 100. Life extension is difficult when arteries are clogged with yellow wax-like substances.

Belief: *"There's no physiological benefit from cholesterol levels under 180. Don't strive for ultra-low numbers unless you are under special medical treatment."*[17]

—George Blackburn, M.D.
Harvard Medical School

Reality: Most of the human race would respectfully disagree.

Belief: Low blood cholesterol is associated with stroke.[18]

Reality: There are two types of stroke and neither is caused by low blood cholesterol.[19] Blood clot stroke (cerebral embolus) is caused by high blood cholesterol. Bleeding stroke (cerebral hemorrhage) is caused by high blood pressure.

Belief: Low blood cholesterol is associated with cancer.[20]

Reality: When cancer patients have low blood cholesterol, it's the disease (often undetected) that causes the drop.[21]

Belief: Low blood cholesterol is associated with suicide.[22]

Reality: A higher suicide rate was observed among users of cholesterol-lowering drugs.[23] Other studies found no association between cholesterol and suicides.[24]

Belief: Eating less butter and more vegetable oil will help prevent heart disease.

Reality: Only if you feel comfortable substituting cancer for heart disease while the overall death rate remains unchanged.[25]

Belief: Aspirin tablets help prevent heart attacks.

Reality: Only if you feel comfortable substituting hemorrhagic stroke and intestinal bleeding for heart attacks.[26] The most common intestinal irritants are aspirin and alcohol.

Belief: Margarine with "zero cholesterol" helps prevent heart attacks.

Reality: Margarine contains trans fats (hydrogenated fats) which elevate cholesterol more than other types of fat. Cancer and heart disease deaths are highest among users of trans fats.[27]

Belief: Beef, chicken, fish and cheese all have the same effect on the body.

Reality: All have essentially the same level of cholesterol but different levels of saturated fat. In a 4-ounce serving of each, the saturated fat ranges from 0.1 grams in fish to over 20 grams in cheese.

Saturated fat raises blood cholesterol far more than dietary cholesterol. Countries with the highest intake of saturated fat reported the highest mortality from heart disease.[28] Dairy protein and excess vitamin D are additional risk factors for atherosclerosis.[29]

Oxidized cholesterol is especially damaging to the artery walls.[30] The metabolism of refried lard, powered milk and eggs, fluoride, chlorine, chlorinated pesticides, and polyunsaturated oils generates oxidized cholesterol.[31] Chlorinated pesticides elevate blood fats and interfere with carbohydrate metabolism, thereby contributing to atherosclerosis and diabetes.[32]

Blood cholesterol is normally converted into bile salts by the liver, excreted into the intestine, and carried away by fiber. Without fiber, bile salts are reabsorbed and converted back into cholesterol. Animal products contain no fiber.

Sugar is another risk factor for atherosclerosis since it elevates the insulin level. Dietary fats and simple sugars convert to acetate, from which blood cholesterol is derived.

Blood cholesterol can be effectively lowered by reducing fats to 10% and animal products to 1% of total calories.[33] Secondary measures include garlic, onions, oat bran, psyllium, green tea, activated charcoal, niacin (non-time-release), gugulipid (Indian herb), vitamin C (2,000 mg), and vitamin E (200 IU dry form).

Atherosclerosis is not stopped by following the American Heart Association guidelines (30% fat, 300 mg of daily cholesterol, and 4 eggs per week).[34]

THE POLITICS OF HEART DISEASE

The risk of heart disease from meat, poultry, eggs and dairy is far greater than what these industries would have you believe. Numerous studies funded by the Egg Board,[35] the Missouri Egg Merchandising Council,[36] the Egg Industry Research Council,[37] the Poultry Research Council,[38] and the National Dairy Council[39] reported that eggs have no significant effect on blood cholesterol.

However, these studies may be flawed since people with high baseline cholesterol intake show little change when additional cholesterol is given.[40] In contrast, vegetarians fed cholesterol show a much greater response.[41]

Calcium lowers blood cholesterol according to studies funded by the dairy industry,[42] the pharmaceutical industry,[43] and Procter & Gamble.[44] Beef lowers blood cholesterol according to studies funded by the meat industry.[45] However, most current evidence suggests that heart disease is a consequence of excess fats—not calcium or beef deficiency.

Heart disease patients may be placed on "cholesterol reduction" diets (30% fat) under the guise of nutritional intervention.[46] Such diets seem guaranteed to fail. When symptoms worsen, physicians recommend invasive procedures:

- Heart bypass patients have a 4–79% risk of permanent brain damage from the heart-lung machine during surgery.[47]
- Heart bypass patients have a 25% risk of developing cardiac arrythmias (abnormal heart rhythm).[48]
- Following heart bypass surgery, 50% of bypassed arteries clog up within 5 years.[49]
- Following balloon angioplasty, 33% of dilated arteries clog up within 4–6 months.[50]

In most cases, these procedures relieve chest pain but fail to improve survival.[51] In contrast, a 10% fat diet and exercise program reduces chest pain by 91% within 24 days while reversing heart disease.[52] Others advocate a different approach:

> *"Findings in the Journal of the AMA show that lean meat not only fits in a general heart-healthy diet but also plays an important role in therapeutic low-fat diets for high-risk populations."*[53]
>
> —National Live Stock and Meat Board

The AMA released a nutritional videoclinic to help doctors lower cholesterol in their patients. The videoclinic teaches "Choice, rather than avoidance" and was "Made possible by an educational grant by the National Live Stock and Meat Board, the Beef Board, and the Pork Board."[54]

> *"Of course, the human body NEEDS cholesterol—some 1,000 milligrams a day. . ."*
>
> —National Cattlemen's Association
> *12 Myths About Beef*

Cancer

"There are no odes to cancer. Chronic disease is an unsung presence which hovers, fluttering, like an uncertain bird of prey...Health becomes less a memory, more of a mirage, like the voice of a dead lover—thin, unreal, longed for, elusive."[55]

—Hugh Drummond, M.D.

"I lost my hair, I lost my job, I lost my health, I lost my breast, I lost my boyfriend. There's not a day that goes by that I don't miss all those things."[56]

—Pam Onder

"The best armor is to keep out of range."

—Italian proverb

Envision a 3-mile-long black granite wall etched with over 4 million names, the names of all Americans who died in war from 1964–72. This would be the memorial to the war on cancer. Each year breast cancer kills nearly as many American women as all Americans lost during the Vietnam war.

Cancer was a rarity during centuries past. The 1909 edition of the standard U.S. textbook, *Principles and Practice of Medicine*,[57] devoted only 15 pages to cancer. (Breast and prostate cancers received no mention; colon cancer received 2 lines.)[58] In contrast, the 1994 edition of *Principles of Internal Medicine*[59] devoted 174 pages to this affliction. Cancer is the most feared, most complex group of diseases known: an elusive, multi-faceted adversary growing anywhere in the body in hundreds of forms.

Hopes were high when President Nixon signed the Conquest of Cancer Act in 1971, initiating the war on cancer. But despite the estimated $1 trillion spent on research and treatment during the past two decades, cancer deaths continue unabated.

Cause of Death (Ages 55–84)	**Percent Change[60] (1973–1987)**
Cardiovascular Disease	– 33%
Cancer	+ 12%

Only rarely does an industrialized nation change its No. 1 cause of death, an event soon to occur in the U.S. Cancer is the only major disease for which age-adjusted deaths are still increasing.[61] For Americans aged 35–53, cancer has now overtaken heart disease as the leading cause of death.[62] The American Hospital Association predicts cancer will pass heart disease by the year 2000 and become the "dominant specialty of American medicine."[63]

CANCER INCIDENCE

Americans born during the 1940s have a 50–100% higher risk of nonsmoking-related cancers than their grandparents.[64] Experts often blame the victims by pointing to lifestyle factors such as high-fat diets, smoking, drinking and sunbathing.[65] But that doesn't explain the 25% increase in brain cancers or the 73% increase in non-Hodgkin's lymphoma.[66] Nor can experts explain why cancer is the leading cause of death in children ages 1–14,[67] an increase that cannot be attributed to better detection alone.

Studies suggest that pesticides promote cancers of the breast, prostate, brain, kidney, liver, central nervous system, blood cells and skin.[68] Non-Hodgkin's lymphoma (the cancer that killed Jacqueline Kennedy Onassis) is commonly diagnosed among Vietnam veterans and farmers. Dioxins have been linked to its onset.[69] American fat tissues contain dioxin levels so high that if the tissues were soil, the Dutch government would ban cattle from grazing on it.[70]

Pesticides and dioxins are factors that didn't exist in generations past. One in three Americans will be diagnosed with cancer. New cancer cases increased 22% over the past 18 years,[71] and may reach 50% by the year 2007.[72] It would then be considered "normal" for Americans to develop cancer. The war on cancer is not going well.

RISK FACTORS

Japanese men smoke more cigarettes than American men, yet have fewer lung cancers. The high-fat American diet is a major contributing factor. Cancer begins when several factors are brought to bear on a single cell:

- Elevated insulin has been shown to be an independent risk factor for breast cancer.[73] Insulin accelerates breast cancer cell growth up to 12-fold and increases the bioavailability of estrogen and testosterone.[74]

- Fats increase hormone production, activity and bioavailability.[75] Estrogen and testosterone stimulate cell proliferation in the breast and prostate.
- Estrogen and testosterone are normally removed from the blood by the liver, excreted into the small intestine, and carried away by fiber. Without fiber, these hormones are reabsorbed.[76] Animal products contain no fiber.
- Colon cancer is linked to excess cholesterol, iron, bile acids and fatty acids in the colon. Meat increases all four. Fats suppress the immune system.
- Fats alter the intestinal bacteria (clostridia) which transforms bile acids (deoxycholic acid) into carcinogenic steroids. This has a local effect on the colon and a systemic effect on the breast and prostate.
- Ammonia (a by-product of protein metabolism) kills cells, stimulates cell division, alters DNA and promotes tumors. Protein metabolism generates ammonia.
- Americans consume about 150 mcg of pesticides and PCBs each day.[77] Animal products account for 90–95%. Pesticides can mimic hormones and suppress immune function.
- Most pesticides are fat-soluble. High-fat diets increase pesticide intake; obesity increases pesticide storage capacity.

Cancer is the local expression of a systemic disorder. Tumors can be either benign or lethal. Tumor grade (divergence from normal) and cell doubling time determine lethality. The strength of the cancer and of the immune system it faces determine the eventual outcome more than the therapy chosen.

- Cancer patients have been successfully treated with standard medicine (surgery, radiation, chemotherapy, hormone therapy) but many more have died.
- Cancer patients have been successfully treated with alternative therapies (Macrobiotics, Gerson, Hoxsey) but many more have died.

- Some cancer patients die after exhausting all conventional and alternative therapies. Others have spontaneous remission with no treatment at all. Still others are "cured" only to have the cancer return with a vengeance.
- Most cancers can be **prevented** with nutrition alone. Few cancers can be **cured** with nutrition alone.

BREAST CANCER

Breast cancer is the most common cancer in American women and the second leading cause of cancer death.[78]

Year	Breast Cancer Incidence[79]
1960	1 in 20 (85-year lifespan)
1996	1 in 9 (85-year lifespan) 1 in 8 (95-year lifespan)

Breast Cancer Luminaries:

- Betty Ford
- Happy Rockefeller
- Nancy Reagan
- Shirley Temple Black
- Olivia Newton-John
- Bella Abzug
- Rachel Carson
- Ingrid Bergman
- Julia Child
- Gloria Steinem
- Ann Jillian
- Lorraine Day

Breast cancer is a systemic disease with microscopic spread even in its early stages.[80]

Test	Average Age of Tumor[81] When Detected
Self-Examination	10 Years
Mammography	8 Years

The ability of early detection to improve survival is controversial.[82] One reason is overdiagnosis. Autopsy studies reveal that 39% of women ages 40–50 have breast tumors, most of which never progress into metastatic cancer.[83] About 23% of breast cancers diagnosed by mammography are ductal carcinoma in situ, many of which never become invasive cancer.[84]

The overdiagnosis of breast cancer increases incidence, the 5-year survival rate and the number of cancer survivors, but does not increase actual survival. Metastatic breast cancer patients live no longer today than patients 80 years ago.[85] Modern women just live with the knowledge longer due to earlier detection. The early diagnosis of breast cancer improves the cosmetic outcome but does not increase survival.[86]

Roughly half of pre-menopausal breast cancer patients are still alive after 14 years. Among women with invasive breast disease, 20-year survival is less than 10-year survival, and 30-year survival is lower still. Most women diagnosed with metastatic breast cancer will eventually die of breast cancer if followed long enough.[87] It therefore seems disingenuous to pronounce patients "cured" after only 5 years.

> *"We can no longer ignore the possibility that screening may not reduce mortality in women of any age, however disappointing this may be."*[88]
>
> —M. Maureen Roberts, M.D., former director
> Edinburgh Breast Screening Project, Scotland
> shortly before her death from breast cancer

The hallowed triad of mastectomy, chemotherapy and radiation confers no survival benefit over lumpectomy alone.[89] Lymph node removal offers no survival advantage.[90] Breast cancer can spread to distant body sites bypassing the nodes. Radiation therapy decreases local recurrence but increases recurrence in the opposite breast, and may lower survival by suppressing immune function.[91] Radiation therapy may cause lung scarring and rib fractures.

Chemotherapy increases the risk of leukemia, bladder cancer, brain tumors and fatal infections.[92] Terminal breast cancer patients may be treated with chemotherapy until death even when doctors know it's not effective.[93]

The well informed patient or family member will ask whether the treatment has been shown to save lives—before submitting to aggressive procedures. As with all medical decisions, it's prudent to consider the current weight of evidence. Clinical studies provide our truest bearing in a turbulent sea of siren songs.

The cell doubling time of breast cancer averages 100 days (range 23–940 days). Most invasive breast cancers turn lethal after 40 cell doublings, spreading faster in premenopausal women. According to the American Cancer Society, breast cancer cannot be prevented since most patients have no known risk factors. This position fails to consider two facts:

- In our culture, a 30% fat diet is not considered a risk factor even though it greatly increases breast cancer risk compared to 10% fat.
- During the past 30 years, researchers have largely ignored the connection between toxic chemicals and cancer.

Most breast cancers can be prevented by addressing these underlying factors. Breast cancer patients on low-fat diets live longer than those on high-fat diets.[94] The survivability of breast cancer depends more on a woman's immune system than on medical intervention at her chest wall. All the surgery and chemotherapy in the world pales compared to her own fork and spoon.

MAMMOGRAPHY

In 1972, the National Cancer Institute (NCI) and the American Cancer Society (ACS) were warned of the radiation hazard posed by mammography to women under age 50. These warnings came from the National Academy of Sciences and NCI's scientific staff. The ACS and NCI ignored these warnings and went ahead with mass mammography screening to gain favorable publicity and more research funds.[95]

Several studies reveal higher breast cancer mortality among pre-menopausal women undergoing mammograms compared to those who avoided mammograms.[96] Early detection leads to early treatment and chemotherapy, which may shorten survival in some patients.[97] The pre-menopausal breast is 50 times more sensitive to radiation than the post-menopausal breast. Mammography radiation may contribute to breast cancer either directly or by activating the pesticides contained in breast tissue.[98] Breast compression during mammography may increase the risk of spreading cancer cells.[99]

The ACS is nearly alone in promoting mammograms to women under age 50, despite the lack of patient benefit. Mammography is a high-profit enterprise. The ACS receives support from G.E. (maker of mammography machines), DuPont (maker of X-ray film), and self-interested radiologists.[100]

About 5% of women screened by mammography have a suspicious abnormality, of which 80–93% are false positives leading to unnecessary procedures including surgery. Several recent studies showed no significant benefit of mammography to women of any age.[101] Current evidence fails to justify screening mammography as a publicly funded health measure.

PROSTATE CANCER

Prostate cancer is the most common cancer in American men and the second leading cause of cancer death.

Prostate Cancer Luminaries:

- Francois Mitterrand
- John Paul Stevens
- Harry Blackmun
- Alan Cranston
- Robert Dole
- Jesse Helms
- Linus Pauling
- Norman Schwarzkopf
- Don Ameche
- Telly Savalas
- Frank Zappa
- Michael Milken

Autopsy studies reveal that 80% of Western men in their 80s (and practically all men over 100) harbor prostate cancers, up to 90% of which never become clinically significant.[102] Current screening cannot distinguish between latent and aggressive prostate tumors. The overdiagnosis of prostate cancer increases incidence but does not improve survival.

The early detection and treatment of prostate cancer confers no survival advantage.[103] The 10-year survival of patients who undergo treatment (radical prostatectomy or radiation therapy) is lower than for those who avoid treatment.[104] Prostate cancer treatment may result in castration, urinary obstruction, incontinence, impotence, rectal injury, cardiopulmonary complications, pain, cost and early death. External beam radiation therapy is especially damaging in suppressing immune function.

Virtually all men undergoing screening tests for prostate cancer believe that early detection saves lives, a belief not supported by clinical evidence. Until such time as prostate cancer treatment has been shown to increase either the quality or length of life, all screening tests for prostate cancer must be considered fraudulent.

Most tumors detected by digital rectal exam are 10 years old.[105] Transrectal ultrasound and the PSA blood test (prostate specific antigen) yield variable results. The cell doubling time of prostate cancer averages 5 years, spreading more slowly in men over 55.[106] This is why most men die with prostate cancer, rather than from it.

Patients with metastatic prostate cancer on low-fat diets outlived by 13 years those who made no dietary change.[107] A 10% fat diet corrects the biochemical risk factors leading to cell proliferation; medical treatments do not. Patients warned against falling prey to the specter of "doing nothing" may wish to keep this difference in mind. The survivability of prostate cancer depends more on a man's immune system than on medical intervention inside his pelvic cavity.

COLON CANCER

Colon cancer is the second leading cause of cancer-related death among Americans.

Colon Cancer Luminaries:

- Audrey Hepburn
- Mary Martin
- Elizabeth Montgomery
- Vince Lombardi
- Ronald Reagan
- Tip O'Neil
- Steve Allen
- Robert Reed
- Jackie Gleason
- Joe Carcione
- John Tower
- Willy Brandt

Studies suggest that fats, proteins, carcinogens, and lack of fiber each play a role in the cause of colon cancer. Irritation to the colon's lining results in cell proliferation from which polyps arise. Fiber reduces polyp formation.[108] Approximately 5–10% of Americans over age 40 have polyps. Colon cancer develops after polyps have been present for 10–35 years.[109] The larger the polyp, the greater the risk. Treatment has little effect on long-term survival once the disease reaches an advanced stage.

Screening for colon cancer remains controversial. Fecal occult blood tests confer no benefit.[110] Flexible sigmoidoscopy at age 55 has been shown to reduce colon cancer mortality despite half of all polyps located above its reach (60 cm).[111] The discovery of polyps warrants colonoscopy (130–170 cm). However, the early detection and removal of polyps fails to address the underlying cause. Those who rely on such procedures while ignoring diet play a most dangerous game.

CANCER RESEARCH

The National Dairy Council, the American Cancer Society and the National Cancer Institute co-sponsored two studies indicating that calcium prevents colon cancer.[112] Other studies reported that aspirin prevents colon cancer.[113] The Dairy Bureau of Canada funded two studies showing that calcium prevents breast cancer.[114]

Population studies strongly suggest these cancers are due to fats and animal protein, not calcium or aspirin deficiency. Breast, prostate and colon cancers rarely occur in populations consuming a plant-based diet. Asian countries with lower cancer rates do not have better medicines—they have better diets.

AMERICAN CANCER SOCIETY

The ACS is not without conflict-of-interest. Several of the 300 ACS board members have close ties to petrochemical and pharmaceutical industries.[115] Many of the carcinogens downplayed by the ACS are by-products of profitable industries in which its directors have financial interests.[116] The ACS rebutted Bill Moyer's PBS documentary on pesticide risk.[117]

Neither the ACS nor the NCI supported the Toxic Substances Control Act, the Clean Water Act, the Clean Air Act, or efforts to reduce chemical pollution. The ACS has yet to emphasize the role of toxic chemicals in cancer causation.

- Cancers caused by diet: up to 60%[118]
- Cancers caused by environmental factors: up to 90%[119]

Each year, the ACS solicits approximately $350 million from the public, nearly all of which supports cancer treatment, rather than prevention. While treatments have become more toxic, expensive and profitable over the years, their success in prolonging life has largely remained unrealized. Many believe prevention offers our only real hope of eventually controlling this disease.

> *"Don't quit on us now. We're already half way there."*[120]
> *"Fight cancer with a checkup and a check."*
> *"We want to cure cancer in your lifetime."*
> —American Cancer Society slogans

NATIONAL CANCER INSTITUTE

Following its founding in 1937, the NCI devoted one-third of its research budget to the dietary causes of cancer. Then something happened:

> *"After World War II along came chemotherapy, which represented a more profitable and fashionable area of investigation."*[121]
>
> —Dr. Dean Burk
> founder of NCI

As far back as 1968, researchers reported a link between elevated pesticide levels in fatty tissues and cancer incidence. But the NCI has yet to undertake large epidemiological studies of toxic chemicals which are known dietary contaminants. There are two primary reasons:

- The National Cancer Advisory Board lacks expertise on environmental carcinogens.[122]
- Close financial ties between the NCI and the pesticide–pharmaceutical companies.[123]

The President's Cancer Panel (which determines NCI policy) was recently chaired by Armand Hammer, head of Occidental Petroleum and the Hooker Chemical Company. Past chairman, Benno Schmidt, was an investment banker with close ties to oil, drug and chemical industries. Samuel Broder, director of the NCI, left his position to join a chemotherapy company (Ivax Inc.).[124]

Less than 5% of NCI's budget addresses chemical pollution and occupational exposures as causes of cancer.[125] The NCI and the Olin Chemical Company co-sponsored a curious study which found no relation between DDT levels and cancer.[126]

The NCI downplays the risk of toxic chemicals. When a recent Harvard study found an increase in bladder and rectal cancers from chlorine in drinking water,[127] the NCI responded with a press release which began:

> *"Chlorinated drinking water offers immense health benefits."*[128]

THE POLITICS OF CANCER

- Companies producing both pesticides and drugs: Abbott Labs, American Cyanamid, BASF, Bayer, Ciba-Geigy, Dow, DuPont, Hoechst, ICI-Zeneca, Eli Lilly, Marion, Merck, Miles, Monsanto, Pfizer, Rhone-Poulec, Sandoz, Schering-Plough, and Upjohn.

- ICI-Zeneca, maker of tamoxifen (an anti-estrogen drug), sponsors Breast Cancer Awareness Month (October). Their educational materials stress early detection but exclude prevention and carcinogens.[129] The more women diagnosed, the more money they make.

- Schering-Plough, maker of flutamide (an anti-testosterone drug), sponsored Prostate Cancer Awareness Week (September 20).[130] Prevention was again excluded.

- Harvard University Medical School received funding from Monsanto.[131]

- Memorial Sloan-Kettering Cancer Center received funding from Dow Chemical, DuPont and Union Carbide. Several Sloan-Kettering board members have close ties to pesticide, chlorine and drug companies.[132]

"With us, you'll never be a routine cancer patient."[133]
—Sloan-Kettering advertisement

National cancer policies—under the guise of concern for public welfare—promote early detection and treatment over prevention. The pesticide and drug industries oppose changing national cancer policies because prevention would be bad for business. Prevention would negatively impact pesticide and chemotherapy drug sales.

By producing pesticides and treating the results, profits are maximized. National cancer policies are a true gift to the petrochemical, pharmaceutical and cancer treatment industries.

PREVENTIVE MEDICINE

True prevention is unprofitable since it cannot be patented or prescribed. In the medical arena, cancer prevention often denotes "chemoprevention." The NCI's Breast Cancer Prevention Trial involves 16,000 healthy women testing the drug tamoxifen to prevent breast cancer. Concerns have been raised that tamoxifen may increase the risk of uterine cancer, liver cancer, colon cancer, eye damage and blood clots.[134] The industries involved are not held accountable for the unintended consequences of their actions.

The NCI's Prostate Cancer Prevention Trial involves 18,000 healthy men testing the drug Proscar (finasteride) to prevent prostate cancer. The side effects of Proscar include impotence and decreased libido.[135]

More than 150,000 women will participate in the Women's Health Initiative Study testing 20% fat diets and hormone replacement therapy. Drug companies are testing Sulindac and DFMO (difluoromethylornithine) to prevent colon cancer. Female hormone manipulation is also being investigated.[136] The long-term health consequences of chemoprevention are unknown.

Preventive medicine includes finding the gene responsible for familial breast cancer. Women who test positive would have the option of protecting themselves by having their breasts removed. This approach, however, makes two rather troubling assumptions:

- Women are genetically defective.
- Familial breast cancer risk is unrelated to mother/daughter eating patterns.

The NCI has yet to investigate 10% fat diets.

CANCER EPILOGUE

Many people avoid thinking about cancer. I never thought about it until my wife was diagnosed with breast cancer (ductal adenocarcinoma) at age 44. She passed away less than 6 months later. During that time, we fought this disease with two mastectomies, radiation treatments, macrobiotics and herbal remedies. Nothing stopped the spread. We then drove to the Gerson Clinic in Tijuana and joined other desperate patients drawn from around the world by the promise of hope.

This was not a passive program. The regimen combined coffee enemas, carrot juices, castor oil drinks, B12–laetrile injections, thyroid pills, ozone therapy, liver-gallbladder purges and "healing reactions." Patients and their partners had little time to ponder the things and events that brought them to this place.

Another young couple arrived at the clinic after the husband was diagnosed with inoperable brain cancer (astrocytoma). Paul was a Mormon minister and had always led a clean Mormon lifestyle. He had no family history of disease. But Paul grew up on a farm and one of his childhood chores was to fill the hopper behind his father's tractor with pesticides. He wore no mask and, 30 years later, developed brain cancer. His low-fat diet offered no apparent protection.

The four of us talked of going backpacking together someday. But as things became progressively worse, it became clear that someday would never come. The agony that followed completed my awakening to the totality of cancer, an awakening only partly tempered by memories of the good times.

After the memorial service, I thought of her father who died of lung cancer, her mother who wears a colostomy bag from colon cancer, her uncle who died of prostate cancer, and my grandfather who died of colon cancer. To live in a society where the diagnosis of cancer is considered normal is not acceptable. This epidemic must be stopped.

Our private lives offer no shield from angry DNA. For cancer victims and their families, the grim specter of terminal illness carries a harsh lesson in the consequences of despoiling the human body. That's not the way it has to be. No one need suffer the ravages of a pestilent scourge, nor live in fear of a painful and premature death. Each of us is free to heed the warning and to seek a safer path.

In our society, the early detection of breast, prostate and colon cancer is considered preventive medicine. But in other cultures around the world, such tests are avoided and cancer rates are low. They don't practice early detection to the exclusion of prevention. They don't live in fear of cancer because they're not at the mercy of cancer. Freedom from fear is your birthright.

> *"Women agonize...over cancer; we take as a personal threat the lump in every friend's breast."*[137]
>
> —Martha Weinman Lear

Proposed Cancer Policy Reform

- Amend the National Cancer Act to remove the NCI from direct Presidential authority, placing it within NIH. Eliminate the President's Cancer Panel.
- Appoint members to the National Cancer Advisory Board with expertise on carcinogens and alternative medicine. Require full financial disclosure.
- Dedicate at least half of NCI's budget to primary prevention.

What You Can Do

- Withhold contributions to the American Cancer Society.
- Advocate an NCI mandate that gives top priority to the role of diet and chemicals in the cause of cancer.
- Embrace the dietary practices of those successful in preventing cancer.

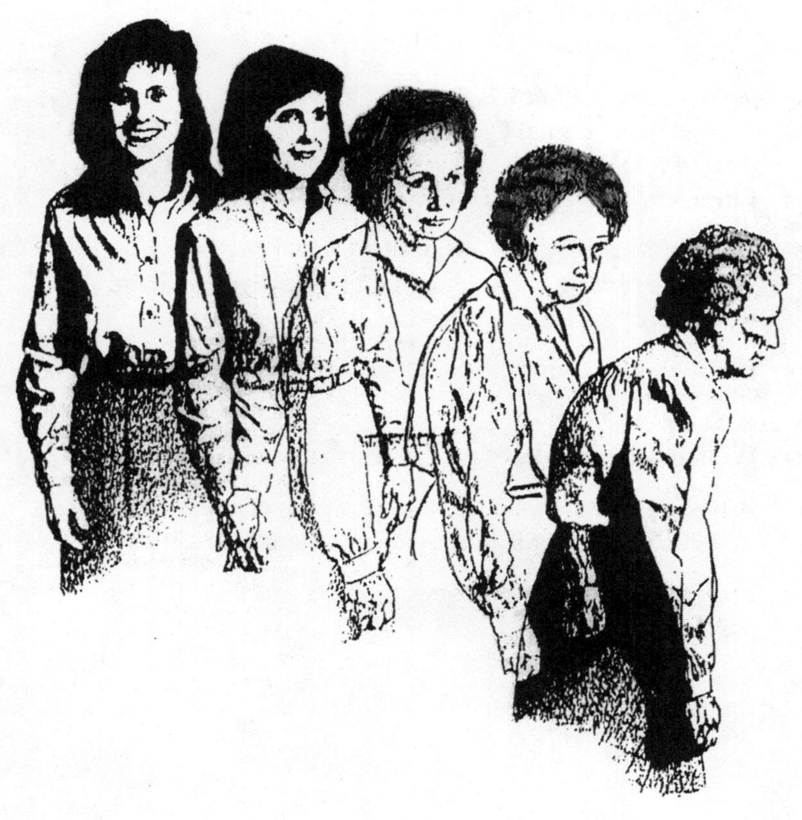

Osteoporosis

"If we knew more about osteoporosis and developed ways to prevent its onset, we could simultaneously enrich life for elderly women, reduce hospital visits and stays in nursing homes, and save billions of dollars a year."[138]
—Hillary Rodham Clinton

"Adult Americans don't get enough dairy products in general and enough skim milk in particular."[139]
—George Blackburn, M.D.
Harvard Medical School

"Beware of little expenses; a small leak will sink a great ship."
—Benjamin Franklin

Ask any American woman what disease she fears most and she'll probably say breast cancer. Yet hip fractures kill more women than cancers of the breast, cervix and uterus combined.[140] Each year, more than 280,000 Americans suffer hip fractures; half are unable to walk again unassisted, 25% end up in nursing homes, and 25% die within 3 months of surgery. (Eva Gabor died of complications following a hip fracture.)

Osteoporosis literally means "porous bones," a crippling and disfiguring disease marked by the progressive loss of bone tissue, loss of height and fractures. One third of American women over age 65 will suffer a spinal fracture and half will lose 50% of their bone density. Osteoporosis is a major health problem in industrialized nations but relatively rare in developing countries.

Few health issues generate greater controversy and few battles within scientific circles rage more bitterly than the role of calcium in preventing osteoporosis. Prestigious medical journals and airwaves are besieged by conflicting calcium studies. What exactly is the optimal calcium intake needed to maintain bone health?

In 1984, the National Institutes of Health convened a Consensus Development Conference on Osteoporosis which recommended 1,000–1,500 mg/day of calcium for all women. The National Osteoporosis Foundation concurred with these recommendations. The sales of dairy products and calcium supplements have since reached record levels.

In 1993, the NIH and the National Osteoporosis Foundation convened a new Consensus Conference which urged 1,000 mg/day of calcium for premenopausal women and 1,500 mg/day for postmenopausal women. This reinforced the earlier recommendations.

Each Conference reached this position after considering all evidence presented, and most medical studies support calcium in maintaining bone density.[141] However, the experts may have overlooked the elusive and often confounding variable of who paid for the research—a signal failing inherent in the current system.

SPECIAL INTERESTS

Of all studies published since 1981 supporting calcium in preventing osteoporosis, at least 26 were funded by special interests including the National Dairy Council,[142] the Institute for Dairy Research,[143] Procter & Gamble,[144] the USDA,[145] the pharmaceutical industry,[146] and General Mills.[147]

The National Dairy Council[148] and the National Live Stock and Meat Board[149] sponsored two studies claiming that meat doesn't cause calcium loss. Procter & Gamble sponsored studies showing that calcium citrate-malate is better absorbed than calcium carbonate[150] (blackboard chalk). Calcium citrate-malate is found only in Procter & Gamble products.

Three drug companies (Mead Johnson, Wyeth-Ayerst, Procter & Gamble) fund research grants from the National Osteoporosis Foundation.[151] Pharmaco Pharmaceuticals is conducting a study of 1,000 healthy women taking the drug raloxifene HCl for up to 5 years to prevent osteoporosis.

THE WEIGHT OF EVIDENCE

If enough research is published showing a particular result, national policy will eventually be changed to conform to the weight of evidence. This is the scientific method and it works well most of the time. However, the system breaks down when biased studies, ill-conceived and fraught with mischief, dominate the medical literature. Credibility is further undermined when special interests enlist the same researchers over and over again.

Current government guidelines recommend increasing calcium intake, rather than decreasing protein intake. This seems unfortunate considering that 80% of the human race avoids osteoporosis by consuming foods fundamentally different than those of Americans. The countries with the highest consumption of meats, calcium and dairy products also have the highest rates of hip fractures.[152]

PROTEIN VS. CALCIUM

The key to preventing osteoporosis is understanding how the process works. In ranking priorities, the body places maintenance of blood calcium well above the maintenance of bone strength. The body is programmed to sacrifice its skeleton to maintain blood calcium, and the body will only do what it's programmed to do.

Protein is composed of amino acids which turn the blood slightly acidic. The body neutralizes these acids by dissolving bone calcium leading to urinary calcium loss.[153] The more protein in the diet, the greater the calcium loss.[154] Doubling the protein intake increases urinary calcium by 50%.[155]

The average American consumes 44% of their calories from animal products, 70% of protein from animal products, and 75% of calcium from dairy products.[156] Much evidence suggests that such a diet leads to bone loss despite a high calcium intake.[157]

> *"Osteoporosis is a disease of calcium loss, not calcium deficiency. American women are hemorrhaging calcium."*[158]
>
> —Michael Klaper, M.D.
> Institute of Nutrition Education and Research

There is no evidence to demonstrate that high-calcium intakes help prevent osteoporosis.[159] In fact, the opposite seems to be true.[160]

- In countries where both calcium and protein intakes are low, osteoporosis is rare.
- In countries where both calcium and protein intakes are high, osteoporosis is common.

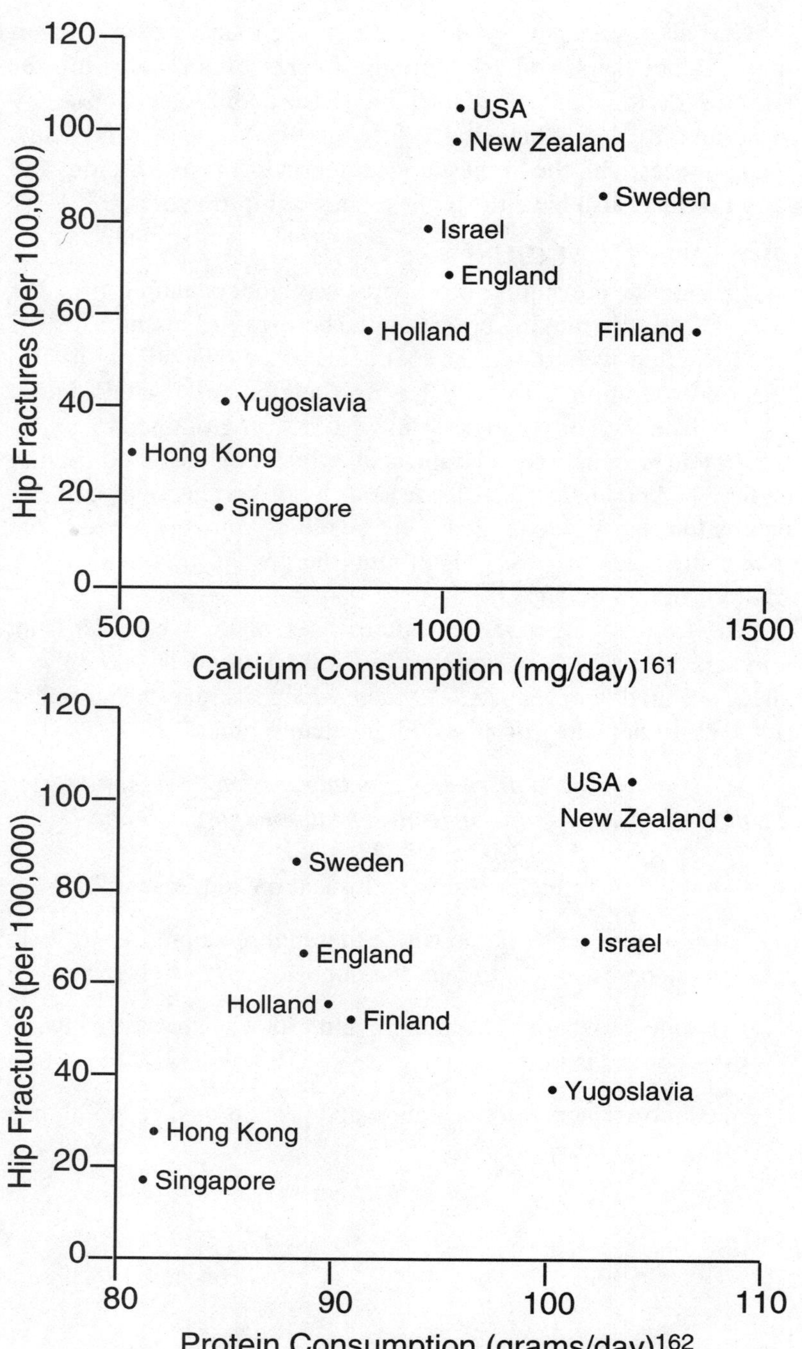
120
100
80
60
40
20
0
Hip Fractures (per 100,000)
USA
New Zealand
Sweden
Israel
England
Holland
Finland
Yugoslavia
Hong Kong
Singapore
500
1000
1500
Calcium Consumption (mg/day)[161]
120
100
80
60
40
20
0
Hip Fractures (per 100,000)
USA
New Zealand
Sweden
England
Israel
Holland
Finland
Yugoslavia
Hong Kong
Singapore
80
90
100
110
Protein Consumption (grams/day)[162]

High-protein diets increase the need for calcium, however when calcium intake rises, absorption efficiency falls.[163] Since the body absorbs protein more efficiently than calcium, a high-calcium intake alone cannot halt protein-induced calcium loss.[164] Most Americans absorb only 20–40% of their calcium intake while losing 320 mg of calcium each day.[165]

When calcium intake rises, the body lowers the blood level of calcitriol, which causes calcium to be inefficiently used. A lifetime of consuming calcium-rich foods (or supplements) will train the body to inefficiently absorb and utilize calcium.[166] When postmenopausal women lose the protection of estrogen, their inability to conserve calcium may contribute to greater bone loss. In other words, high-calcium intakes may actually do more harm than good.

High-fat diets elevate hormone levels. Estrogen levels are 50% higher in premenopausal women consuming high-fat diets compared to premenopausal women on low-fat diets.[167] Postmenopausal women eating high-fats thus experience a sharper drop in their estrogens, which may contribute to bone loss and hot flashes.

Elevated estrogens also contribute to PMS, migraines, uterine fibroids, endometriosis, breast tenderness, fibrocystic breasts, ovarian cysts, cervical dysplasia, fluid retention, weight gain, gall bladder disease, hypertension, blood clots, diabetes, depression, early menarche and late menopause. PMS and hot flashes do not exist in other cultures with lower fat diets.

PLANT VS. ANIMAL FOODS

Vegetarian women have lower calcium intakes, lower estrogen levels and greater bone densities than meat-eating women.[168] There are several possible reasons:

- Calcium from green leafy vegetables is more absorbable than calcium from milk.[169]
- Animal proteins erode bone by forming ammonia and uric acid. High protein diets suppress calcium reabsorption by the kidneys.[170]
- Animal proteins contain twice the sulfur of plant proteins. Sulfur erodes bone by forming sulfuric acid and hydrogen sulfide. When soy protein replaces animal protein, less calcium is lost in the urine.[171]

- Vegetables and beans contain plant estrogens (phytoestrogens) which may reduce bone loss without the negative side-effects of synthetic hormones.[172]
- Meat, poultry and fish contain 15–20 times more phosphorus than calcium.[173] Phosphorus stimulates parathyroid hormone which erodes bone for its calcium.[174]
- Animal products contain no fiber and tend to be high in fat. Both factors increase insulin resistance leading to calcium excretion.[175]
- Plant-based diets are high in magnesium which suppresses parathyroid hormone. Fruits and vegetables generate alkaline compounds (sodium and potassium hydroxide).
- Animal products are low in magnesium which decreases calcium absorption. (Dairy milk has a calcium-magnesium ratio of 8:1.)

POPULATION STUDIES

Traditional Chinese consume plant-centered diets in sharp contrast to those of Americans. The following table is standardized for 143-pound adult males:[176]

	China	USA
Calcium	544 mg	1,143 mg
Calcium From Dairy	0%	75%
Protein	64 g	91 g
Protein from Animals	7%	70%
Calories From Animals	6%	44%

In rural regions of China, osteoporosis is rare despite half the calcium intake of Americans. Animal protein intake overrides calcium in the development of osteoporosis. This suggests the need to shift the American diet from animal-centered to plant-centered.

American Calcium Sources	Oriental Calcium Sources
1. Dairy Products	1. Green Vegetables
2. Fortified Foods	2. Beans
3. Supplements	3. Whole Grains

"Ironically osteoporosis tends to occur in countries where calcium intake is highest and most of it comes from protein-rich dairy products."[177]

—Dr. T. Colin Campbell
China Health Project

Alaskan Eskimos consume up to 2,500 mg of calcium and 200–400 grams of animal protein each day.[178] The Eskimos have one of the world's highest rates of osteoporosis affecting both men and women starting at age 40, despite their heavy weight-bearing exercise. This suggests that diet overrides exercise in maintaining bone health and further suggests the need to shift the American diet.

Osteoporosis is a multi-factorial disease with risk increasing when several factors combine. To prevent osteoporosis, calcium absorption and retention take priority over calcium intake.

Factors That Decrease Calcium Absorption

- High fat intake
- High calcium intake
- Sodium, phosphorus
- Sugar, alcohol, dairy protein
- Oxalates from spinach
- Antacids, low stomach acid
- Low vitamin D
- Low magnesium

Factors That Decrease Calcium Retention

- High protein intake
- Reducing diets
- Elevated insulin
- Sodium, caffeine
- Soft drinks, coffee
- Reduced lung capacity
- Parathyroid hormone
- Diuretics

Soft drinks contain several acids (carbonic, malic, erythorbic, phosphoric) which increase calcium loss. Fluoridation of drinking water contributes to hip fractures.[179] Reduced lung capacity generates excess acid-producing CO_2 molecules (hydrogen ions) which must be neutralized with calcium. Lung capacity is diminished by asthma, emphysema, smoking, air pollution and lack of exercise.

PHOSPHORUS

Phosphorus alters calcium balance in three ways: phosphorus decreases calcium absorption, decreases urinary calcium loss and increases fecal calcium loss.[180] These forces balance each other.

Animal products upset this balance. When animal products are consumed, the net effect decreases calcium absorption, increases urinary calcium loss and increases fecal calcium loss. This places a triple burden on calcium balance. In maintaining bone health, animal protein supersedes calcium and phosphorus.[181]

CALCIUM STUDIES

The actual need for calcium is far less than what the dairy industry would have you believe. All varied plant-based diets contain sufficient calcium. Excess calcium from dairy products and supplements is usually not absorbed, thus protecting the body from calcium toxicity.[182] Several studies show no relationship between calcium intake and bone density, especially during the 5 years following menopause.[183]

In a recent study, postmenopausal women were given 1,000 mg calcium supplements daily for 2 years.[184] The difference in bone density between the calcium and placebo groups diminished with time and there was no significant difference after 2 years. The researchers concluded this was probably due to decreased calcium absorption from the intestine and kidneys which occurs during long-term calcium supplementation.[185] Most calcium studies are less than 2 years in duration and need to be interpreted with caution.

In a National Dairy Council study, women drank an extra 24 ounces of low-fat milk daily for 1 year.[186] Despite the extra 1,471 mg of calcium, the women still lost more calcium than they absorbed after a full year. The researchers concluded:

> *". . . this may have been due to the average 30% increase in protein intake during milk supplementation."*[187]

	Whole Milk	Skim Milk
Fat	51%	4%
Protein	21%	44%

Removing the fat from dairy products concentrates the protein. This places an added burden on bone tissue. Dairy products contribute to, rather than prevent, the development of osteoporosis.

Postmenopausal women who are heavy meat and dairy product consumers are at increased risk and should monitor their bone density using Dual Photon Absorptiometry (DPA) or Dual Energy X-ray Absorptiometry (DXA) of the lumbar spine.

HORMONE REPLACEMENT THERAPY

During menopause, estrogen levels fall but never reach zero. The body still makes estrogen from the ovaries, adrenal glands, fat tissues and other hormones. Estrogen raises HDL (good cholesterol), and enhances magnesium and calcium uptake by the bones. This offers resistance to osteoporosis and heart disease. However, estrogen also increases the risk of breast cancer, uterine cancer and stroke.[188]

The goal should be to prevent all five conditions, not two out of five. All five diseases can be prevented by embracing the dietary practices of those successful in preventing all five. In countries where osteoporosis and heart disease are lowest, hormone replacement therapy is not available.

The most popular estrogen is Premarin (derived from pregnant mares' urine) which contains two types of estrogens: estrone (E1) and estradiol (E2). Both increase breast cancer risk. Estriol (E3), made by the human placenta, may protect against breast cancer.

Estrogens slow bone loss but don't generate new bone formation.[189] Non-prescription natural progesterones (Pro-Gest) generate new bone and help protect against breast cancer.[190] Prescription synthetic progestins (Provera) increase breast cancer risk.

My concern is that hormone pills, creams, drops and patches will be used as a substitute for changing the diet. A price is always paid when symptoms are treated while the cause is ignored.

PREMENOPAUSAL OSTEOPOROSIS

Research with female athletes shows that strenuous exercise can suppress ovulation leading to premenopausal osteoporosis despite normal estrogen levels.[191] Only progesterone builds new bone; only ovulation stimulates progesterone production. Anything which stops ovulation leads to progesterone deficiency and loss of bone.

Studies suggest that significant numbers of premenopausal women are failing to ovulate after age 35 during otherwise normal menstrual cycles.[192] These women will face menopause with osteoporosis already underway. Petrochemicals may be contributing by disrupting normal hormone balance.[193] The dioxin concentration of American fat tissues is at or near levels causing reproductive abnormalities in animals.[194]

PUBLIC HEALTH POLICY

The top priority of public health policy is to first do no harm. American women are told they need 3–5 times more calcium than the amount consumed in other countries. If every women actually required 1,000–1,500 mg of calcium, osteoporosis and hip fractures would be epidemic worldwide.

Much evidence suggests that osteoporosis is caused by excess protein, not calcium deficiency. Something is seriously wrong when such evidence is ignored and when nutritional recommendations possibly do more harm than good. The cost of osteoporosis is over $10 billion. If the current recommendations are incorrect, this expenditure will rise dramatically as the baby boom population loses bone mass. Disastrous consequences of that magnitude will cost us dearly. This nation can no longer afford to look the other way.

THE POLITICS OF OSTEOPOROSIS

Recent articles on preventing osteoporosis appeared in the *Harvard Health Letter*,[195] the *Tufts University Diet & Nutrition Letter,*[196] the *U.C. Berkeley Wellness Letter,*[197] the *John Hopkins Medical Letter*,[198] and the *Center for Science in the Public Interest Nutrition Action Healthletter*.[199] These articles emphasize calcium intake but exclude any mention of protein.

In 1993, the American Dietetic Association and the National Dairy Council held an osteoporosis conference in Washington, D.C. This conference recommended increasing dairy products and calcium, but downplayed the risks of excess protein.[200]

The National Osteoporosis Foundation and Sandoz Pharmaceuticals published a booklet titled *Boning Up on Osteoporosis*. This booklet recommends calcium intake, drug therapy and estrogen replacement therapy. Protein is mentioned only briefly:

> *"More studies are needed in this area to determine if these substances [protein and sodium] actually cause a loss of calcium. . . ."*[201]
>
> —National Osteoporosis Foundation

The first study showing protein-induced calcium loss was published in 1930.[202] Hundreds of similar studies have been published since. The pamphlet, *How Strong Are Your Bones?* by the National Osteoporosis Foundation, lists 14 risk factors for osteoporosis: low calcium is included; excess protein is overlooked.[203]

> *"It's not that Americans get too much protein, it's that they don't get enough calcium."*[204]
>
> —Lori Limberg, spokesperson
> National Osteoporosis Foundation

> *"Usually a diet liberal in calcium is recommended [to treat osteoporosis]. This includes at least 1 quart of milk, hard cheeses and the normal allowance of other foods daily."*[205]
>
> —American Medical Association

> *"There seems to be little increased risk of osteoporosis from eating a high-protein diet."*[206]
>
> —Food and Nutrition Board
> National Academy of Sciences

> *"Meat helps build strong bones."*[207]
>
> —*Prevention* Magazine

> *"If high protein diet is mentioned as cause of osteoporosis, it would be considered misleading information."*[208]
>
> —John Renner, M.D.

John Renner tried to secure $75,000–$100,000 from the National Live Stock and Meat Board to "foster the appropriate patient education."[209] Dr. Renner is a trustee of the National Osteoporosis Foundation (NOF). The treasurer of the NOF represents the AMA.[210]

The eradication of osteoporosis will remain elusive as long as intransigent government agencies overlook the underlying cause and place corporate economic interests above the health and welfare of this nation.

OSTEOPOROSIS EPILOGUE

While writing this chapter, I remembered the circumstances that lead to my father's death. At age 77, his daily calcium intake was over 1,000 mg from meats, dairy products and supplements. While sitting in a chair and coughing, he suffered a spontaneous spinal fracture paralyzing the nerves to both legs. He never walked again. After rushing my father to the hospital and viewing his lumbar compression fracture on X-Ray, it became clear that postmenopausal women have no monopoly on osteoporosis. (George Bernard Shaw died of complications following a hip fracture.)

My father was then transferred to a Medicare-approved skilled nursing home. Most nursing home admissions are considered a prelude to death, and state law required me to make funeral arrangements before gaining admission. During the days that followed, I became familiar with the workings of that facility.

What struck me was the degree of frailty among the residents. Most were elderly women about 4 feet tall, some with spinal deformities so severe they were unable to straighten up and breathe. Those who weren't bedridden or wheelchair-bound, walked with a painfully-slow measured gait. Nearly all required assistance as any sudden movement could cause a fracture. The residents coped with this living hell as best they could, but it was not a fun place to be.

The cafeteria served "balanced" meals representing the four food groups (meat, milk, canned vegetables, white flour). The entire cafeteria was dedicated to smoking and there were no facilities for exercise. The recreation room contained one huge color TV. Lest someone trip and fall, there were no stairs, carpets, or rugs anywhere in the building.

In the physical therapy room, dedicated people struggled in vain to help my father to walk. Less than 2 weeks later, my father passed away from a combination of osteoporosis, stroke, cancer, liver cirrhosis, radiation treatment, end-stage lung disease, and lack of purpose. It never ceases to amaze me what the human body and spirit will endure.

The elderly residents of that nursing home were beyond help, but it's not too late for succeeding generations. Current evidence gives individuals a clear choice:

What You Can Do

- To prevent osteoporosis, follow the diet of people with a track record of preventing osteoporosis.
- To develop osteoporosis, ignore protein intake and follow the guidelines of the National Institutes of Health and the National Osteoporosis Foundation.

Arthritis

"What we do is slow down how fast they get worse."[211]
—Robert Meenan, M.D.
American College of Rheumatology

"When a patient with arthritis walks in the front door, I feel like leaving out the back door."[212]
—Sir William Osler, M.D.
19th century

The scourge of civilization strikes over 37 million Americans[213] leaving untold misery in its wake. Science has no cure for our nation's primary crippler, despite the wealth of conflicting advice. Arthritis accounts for more disability among middle-aged and older adults than any other affliction.[214]

Year	Health-Care Costs	Lost Work Days[215]
1989	$8.6 billion	27 million
1995	$54.6 billion	115 million

As a group of more than 100 diseases, arthritis affects the joints, muscles, tendons, ligaments and coverings of internal organs. The three most common forms are rheumatoid arthritis (RA) which favors younger women, osteoarthritis (OA) which favors older women, and gout, which favors indulgent males as its victim of choice.

Joint diseases have existed since antiquity, as ancient skeletons attest. Remains of Java Ape man, Neanderthal man, Neolithic man, Egyptian mummies and dinosaurs reveal signs of arthritis. Most archeological evidence suggests that RA, of the severity seen today, rarely occurred in centuries past.[216] RA appears to be a disease of modern origin.[217]

RHEUMATOID ARTHRITIS

RA is a systemic, progressive, autoimmune disease in which the body attacks its own tissues. RA usually spreads to several joints, destroying cartilage, bone, surrounding structures and life itself. RA patients historically die 10–15 years earlier than expected.[218]

Uncontrolled inflammation leads to irreversible joint damage during the first 2 years of onset.[219]

Among traditional Asian and African populations, RA rarely occurs.[220] The Pima Indians of Arizona, after abandoning their ancestral diet for processed foods, develop five times the RA as most Americans.[221] Conventional doctrine holds that diet plays no part, but current evidence suggests otherwise. Consider the following:

- RA is linked to food allergens in the blood.[222]
- The most common food allergens are undigested proteins, especially dairy proteins.[223]
- Undigested proteins are absorbed through the intestinal tract on a regular basis.[224]
- Intestinal permeability is increased by aspirin, antibiotics, immunodeficiency and allergies.[225]
- The immune system triggers allergies by attacking undigested proteins as foreign invaders.[226]
- Undigested proteins can migrate into joint tissues, provoking inflammatory reactions.[227]
- Certain polyunsaturated fats (fish oil and evening primrose oil) reduce inflammation by suppressing immune function.[228]
- Saturated animal fats worsen arthritis.[229]

RA commonly develops from an autoimmune reaction to animal products. Patients with RA often have serum antibodies to cow protein in their blood.[230] Autoimmune reactions to animal protein may trigger allergies to wheat gluten, corn and citrus. Controlled studies demonstrate the effectiveness of vegetarian diets (without dairy products) in treating RA.[231]

OSTEOARTHRITIS

Osteoarthritis (OA) develops as cartilage erosion, bony spurs and eventual joint fusion. This disease accounts for more disability among the elderly than any other affliction.[232] Obesity, injury and overuse are accepted contributing factors to OA in the knees, hips and spine. The effects of mechanical stress on these weight-bearing structures is easy to understand. However, mechanical factors alone do not explain the following:

- OA occurs in the hands (Heberden's nodes and Bouchard's nodes).
- Multiple OA joint involvement is more common in women.[233]
- OA occurs more frequently in affluent countries.[234]

Both mechanical and metabolic factors must be considered. Current evidence suggests an autoimmune component in the origin of generalized OA.[235] Autoantibodies against collagen were found in 50% of OA cartilage samples.[236] The synovial cells of joints may be stimulated to release enzymes (proteases) capable of destroying cartilage.[237] Dietary factors likely play a role in the inflammatory reactions of both RA and OA.

GOUT

Gout is among the most illustrious diseases of antiquity. Hippocrates noted its clinical manifestations during the 5th century B.C. Roman physicians Celsus and Galen recognized gout's affinity for the rich, powerful and indulgent.

Diet accounts for nearly 90% of all gout cases, arising from excessive uric acid levels in the blood. Meats are the major uric acid producers; alcohol inhibits uric acid excretion by the kidneys.[238] Elevated uric acid leads to needle-like crystals which deposit in joint tissues. These crystals cause the intense pain characteristic of classical gout attacks.

Gout rarely occurs in populations consuming a low-protein, plant-centered diet.[239] Filipinos living in the U.S. have higher uric acid levels than Filipinos in the Philippines.[240] This suggests that diet affects uric acid levels independent of genetics. Others take a different point of view:

> *"Gout is a special kind of arthritis, caused by an inherited defect in body chemistry, not by high living[241]. . . .If you are on gout medication you probably will not have to change your diet."*[242]
>
> —Arthritis Foundation

THE POLITICS OF ARTHRITIS

"Diet is not a factor in the cause or treatment of arthritis."[243]
—National Institutes of Health

"The simple proven fact is: no food has anything to do with causing arthritis and no food is effective in treating or 'curing' it."[244]
—Arthritis Foundation

These positions are not supported by current evidence. Research solidly indicts diet as the primary cause of inflammatory arthritis. Yet the Arthritis Foundation recommends a 30% fat diet[245] which includes beef, chicken, eggs, milk, cheese, pizza, white bread, sugar, jelly and oil.[246]

"Deciding that meat...or eggs may be responsible for your arthritis and eliminating them from your diet could make you feel weak and without energy."[247]
—Arthritis Foundation

"Animal sources of food such as meat and fish contain 'complete' proteins. This means that the nutrients in animal products more nearly match those of the human body and are more easily used by the body."[248]
—Arthritis Foundation

In the area of treatment, the Arthritis Foundation lists several "unproven remedies of doubtful benefit" including prayer, copper bracelets, vibrators and vegetarian diets.[249] Most rheumatologists favor drug therapy as the treatment of choice.

DRUG THERAPY

Arthritis sufferers fuel the voracious drug market by spending billions on a smorgasbord of dubious palliatives. Doctors write over 70 million prescriptions each year for nonsteroidal anti-inflammatory drugs such as "arthritis strength" aspirin (caffeine or antacid added). Side-effects include 200–300,000 cases of gastrointestinal bleeding leading to 10–20,000 deaths annually.[250]

More powerful drugs have serious side-effects: methotrexate (liver damage), antimalarial agents (eye damage), and cortisone injections (brittle bones). These drugs fail to alter the course of arthritis.[251] In one study, most RA patients were either dead (35%) or severely disabled (19%) after 20 years of drug therapy.[252] The concept of "remission-inducing" drugs appears fallacious. Yet the Arthritis Foundation heavily promotes drugs in its literature. Consider the following ad:[253]

> Introducing New
>
> Arthritis Foundation Pain Relievers
>
> For Relief You Can Count On Until We Find A Cure!

The Arthritis Foundation uses its name to sell Johnson & Johnson aspirin, ibuprofen and acetaminophen.[254] This anti-diet, pro-drug position seems curious in light of current information. Several factors could help explain this:

- The Arthritis Foundation is chaired by Jerry Langley, vice president of international finance for McDonald's Corporation.[255]
- The Arthritis Foundation accepted donations from Procter & Gamble ($100,000)[256] and SmithKline Beecham Pharmaceuticals (over $1 million).[257]
- Wyeth-Ayerst Laboratories funds the Arthritis Foundation's medical bulletin.[258]

What You Can Do

- Be wary of advice from the Arthritis Foundation.
- Follow the diet of people successful in preventing arthritis.
- Advocate an NIH mandate that shifts the National Institute of Arthritis and Musculoskeletal and Skin Diseases (NIAMS) budget from drug research to diet research.

Diabetes

"What gout is to the nobility of England, diabetes is to the aristocracy of India,"[259]

—*British Medical Journal*, 1907

"Candies enjoy an established position in the child's diet."[260]

—*Journal of the AMA* advertisement, 1950s

Each year diabetes kills more than twice as many American women as breast cancer.[261] Diabetic retinopathy is the leading cause of blindness in Americans under age 65.[262] Diabetes flourishes only in those cultures where rich foods prevail. One in 20 Americans has diabetes and nearly half the world's diabetics live in the U.S. About 90% of diabetics have Type II non-insulin-dependent diabetes mellitus.

In industrialized countries such as ours, blood sugar and insulin levels rise progressively with age. This "normal aging process" does not occur in other cultures with different diets. The key to avoiding diabetes is understanding how the process works.

When blood sugar rises, the pancreas secretes insulin which transports glucose into liver and muscle cells. Several factors can disrupt this process. For example, chlorinated pesticides alter hormones, carbohydrate metabolism, insulin secretion, receptors, vitamin C uptake, glucose transport proteins, and blood fats.[263] High-fat diets increase pesticide intake; obesity elevates pesticide storage capacity. Diabetes invariably develops from multiple dietary factors.

The World Health Organization recommends 0–10% of calories from sugar but most Americans consume 23%.[264] Two scientific reports (*The Surgeon General's Report on Nutrition and Health,* and the National Research Council's *Diet and Health*) claim that sugar does not contribute to diabetes. However, mounting evidence suggests that sugar, fiber and fat each play a role.

DIETARY CAUSES OF TYPE II DIABETES[265]

- High fat intake
- Obesity
- Sugar-fiber ratio

At least 80% of type II diabetics are obese. Fat paralyzes insulin response and hinders insulin clearance from the bloodstream by the liver. Both factors elevate insulin levels. High-sugar, low-fiber diets cause blood sugar spiking and elevated insulin, which impairs the insulin receptors.[266] Fiber helps control blood sugar spiking by slowing carbohydrate absorption. [267]

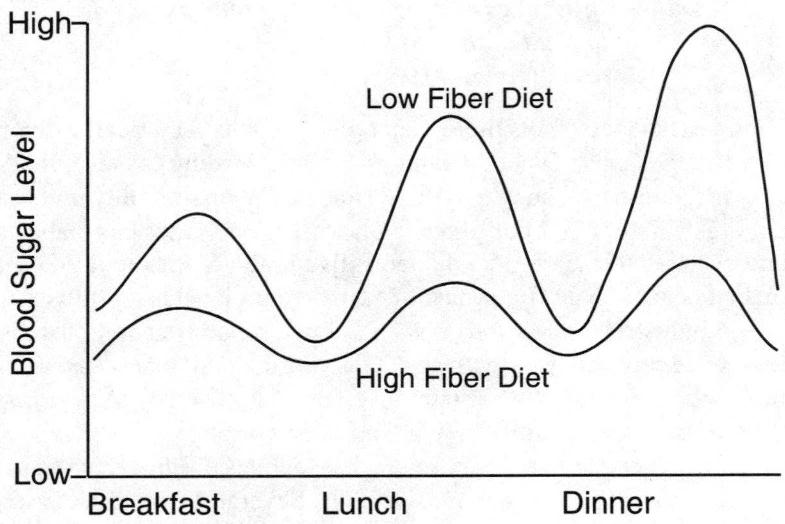

Insulin resistance results from cell receptors becoming less sensitive to insulin.[268] High fat diets, obesity and blood sugar spiking each contribute to insulin resistance and other serious metabolic changes. Researchers at Cornell Medical Center found that obese teenagers secreted large amounts of tumor necrosis factor (TNF) in their blood cells.[269] Heavy TNF secretions are strongly associated with insulin resistance and the development of diabetes.

> *"Do not bite at the bait of pleasure 'til you know there is no hook beneath it."*
>
> —Thomas Jefferson

DIABETES LOOP

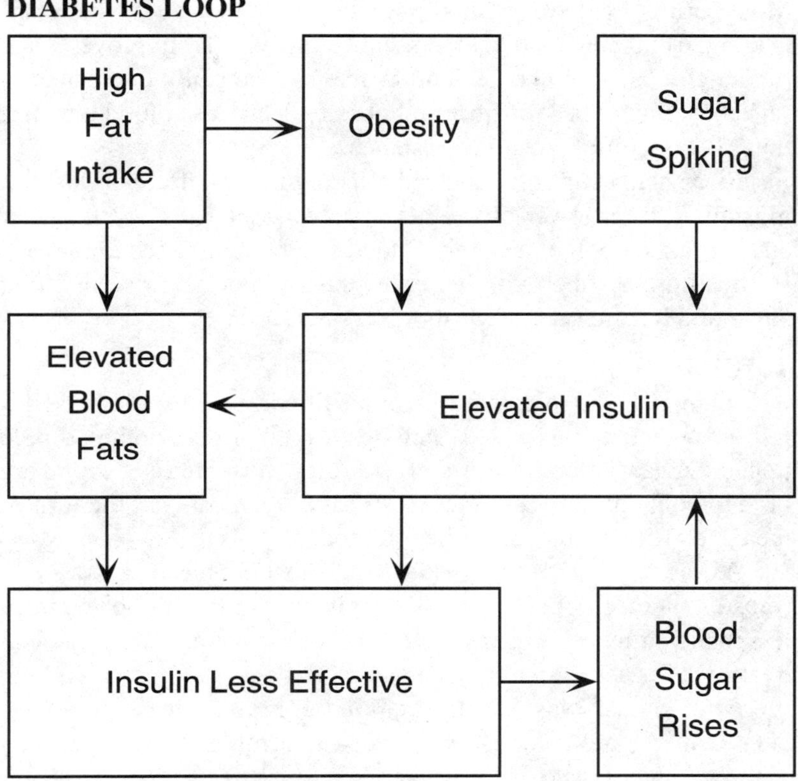

STAGES OF DIABETES

The sequence of events leading to full blown diabetes follows a four-stage process:

- Resistance of the muscle and liver cells to insulin; blood glucose rises.[270]
- Compensatory increase in insulin secretion by the pancreas.[271]
- When blood glucose level reaches 140mg/dl, insulin secretion declines and liver glucose production increases.[272]
- Blood glucose continues to rise while insulin secretion continues to drop.[273]

Most current evidence points to insulin resistance as the hallmark leading to diabetes.[274] Insulin resistance consistently improves when blood glucose is lowered, and worsens when blood glucose is raised.[275] Sugar, lack of fiber and obesity each raise blood glucose, thus contributing to insulin resistance.

Fiber helps control diabetes by its regulatory effect on insulin: high-fiber foods lower blood fats by lowering insulin levels; sugar and refined carbohydrates raise blood fats by raising insulin levels. By maximizing fiber, you help prevent the "normal" rise in blood sugar and insulin seen in most older Americans.[276]

JUICES

Juicing is a poor way to maximize fiber intake. Apple juice has less fiber than applesauce, which has less fiber than apples. Apple juice is sugar water and little else. Fruits on the market today are bred to contain up to 50 times more sugar than fruits at the turn of the century. Fruit juice is no health food.

A 6-ounce glass of orange juice contains 1½ tablespoons of sugar (mostly sucrose) which converts to glucose in the bloodstream in less than 1 minute.[277] Orange juice is used as an emergency medical treatment for acute low blood sugar.

An 8-ounce glass of carrot juice contains the same sugar, beta-carotene and calories as 3 medium carrots but less fiber than 1 carrot. Juices with poor sugar-fiber ratios lead to blood sugar spikes, insulin spikes, insulin resistance and weight gain—especially if consumed on an empty stomach.

Sucrose (white sugar) contains one glucose and one fructose molecule. Glucose elevates insulin; fructose elevates triglycerides; both elevate cholesterol. Juice-sweetened foods offer no advantage over sugar-sweetened foods. All added sugars are best avoided. One can of regular soda contains 9 teaspoons of sugar—equivalent to eating over 30 feet of sugar cane.

Under the guise of nutritional education, the sugar industry exploited the fear that people will switch to higher fat foods if sugar intake is curtailed...a notion proven false.[278]

> *"I didn't say it was good for you, the king replied, I said there was nothing like it."*
>
> —Lewis Carroll
> *Through the Looking Glass*

THE POLITICS OF DIABETES

Four dietary factors (sugar, fiber, dietary fat, body fat) regulate blood sugar control. Unfortunately the American Diabetes Association (ADA) currently recommends the following foods to treat low blood sugar:[279]

- 4 teaspoons of sugar
- 4 ounces of fruit juice
- 4 ounces of soft drink
- 3 hard candies
- 3–10 glucose tablets
- 1 cup of skim milk

These foods contain no fiber. The ADA also recommends a diet up to 30% in fat.[280] *The New Diabetic Cookbook* (endorsed by the ADA) contains recipes using margarine, oil, sugar and white flour.[281]

A recent study in the *Journal of the AMA* reported that ice cream can be safely included in diabetic diets.[282] These recommendations conflict sharply with numerous studies supporting high-fiber, low-fat diets in the control of blood sugar.[283]

Fredrick Stare, founder of Harvard's Department of Nutrition, testified before Congress that cereals containing up to 70% sugar were more nourishing than an old-fashioned breakfast. The Kellogg Company later donated $2 million to his department.[284]

TAKE THE SUGAR TEST

Elementary school children in Hartsdale, New York, were given a nutrition test by their teacher. This test, along with the curious answers, was provided by the Sugar Association.[285]

Questions:

1) Sugar contributes importantly to good nutrition.
   Fact ☐ **Fiction** ☐
   (Children who answered "Fiction" were marked wrong.)

2) Fruits provide a better source of carbohydrates than sugar.
   Fact ☐ **Fiction** ☐
   (Children who answered "Fact" were marked wrong.)

> *"The message in all of our programs and publications is the role sugar can play, in moderation, in a healthful diet."*[286]
> —Sylvia Rowe, public relations
> The Sugar Association

Hypertension

"We're talking about a problem where, if you live long enough, only a minority of Americans escape. All families will be touched by it."

—Jeffrey Cutler
National Heart, Lung and Blood Institute

There are cultures on this planet where low blood pressure is the norm, cultures where 80-year-olds have the same blood pressure as teenagers.[287] We don't live in one of them. Among Western societies such as ours, blood pressure rises progressively with age—creating a time bomb in the brain, eyes, heart and kidneys. For 25% of untreated patients, the first symptom of hypertension is sudden death.[288] Hypertension is the most common reason for Americans seeking medical attention.

Food	Sodium (mg)
Peach	1
Shredded Wheat (1 oz)	3
Green Beans (1 cup)	5
Baked Potato (4 oz)	6
Salt (1 tsp)	2,132
Pizza Hut Super Supreme Pizza	2,200
Denny's Taco Salad	2,628
Hardee's Big Country Ham Breakfast	2,870
House Lo Mein Chinese Dinner	3,460
Shoney's Reuben Sandwich	3,873

The average American consumes 4,000–6,000 mg of sodium daily (75% is hidden in processed foods, 15% comes from the saltshaker, and 10% occurs naturally in foods). The actual human requirement for sodium is far less:

Minimum Sodium Requirements

• New England Journal of Medicine	50 mg[289]
• Food and Nutrition Board	115 mg[290]
• American Heart Association	200 mg[291]
• RDA "safe minimum" amount	500 mg[292]
• RDA "safe and adequate" amount	1,100–3,300 mg[293]

Suggested Maximums

• National Heart, Lung, and Blood Institute	2,300 mg[294]
• Center for Science in the Public Interest	2,400 mg[295]
• National Academy of Sciences	2,400 mg[296]
• American Diabetes Association	3,000 mg[297]
• American Heart Association	3,000 mg[298]

Much attention has been given to the link between blood pressure and sodium. However, sodium by itself does not cause hypertension, nor does sodium restriction always prevent it.[299] Hypertension invariably develops from multiple dietary risk factors.

DIETARY CAUSES OF HYPERTENSION

- Insulin resistance
- Blood flow resistance
- Sodium-potassium ratio

Insulin resistance (caused by blood sugar spiking, fat intake and obesity) is the key to both hypertension and diabetes.[300] Insulin resistance in non-diabetics can vary up to 5-fold.[301] Non-diabetics who are insulin resistant compensate by secreting large amounts of insulin, which raises blood pressure by several mechanisms:[302]

- Elevated insulin alters kidney function leading to sodium retention, fluid retention and calcium loss.
- Elevated insulin stimulates the adrenal glands to produce adrenaline and causes the autonomic nervous system to produce norepinephrine (a neurotransmitter).

- Elevated insulin raises blood cholesterol and blood fats (triglycerides) leading to atherosclerotic plaques.
- Elevated insulin increases fat storage and inhibits fat breakdown leading to obesity.
- Elevated insulin stimulates proliferation of arterial muscle cells which thickens the blood vessels leading to blood flow resistance.

Blood pressure is the product of blood volume times its resistance. Blood flow resistance is increased by blood cell sludging and artery-constricting hormones (prostaglandins) released when platelets clump together following a high-fat meal.[303]

The sodium-potassium ratio influences blood pressure only when sodium intake exceeds potassium intake.[304] Humans evolved eating vast amounts of potassium and little sodium. As a product of that evolution, the human body is designed to excrete potassium while conserving sodium. Whole plant foods have sodium-potassium ratios of 1:100; animal products and processed foods have sodium-potassium ratios of 100:1. Low-potassium foods lead to sodium retention which raises blood volume and pressure.

Blood pressure rises when multiple risk factors combine, as with the average American diet. The largest hypertension study to date—the Intersalt Study of 10,079 people in 52 centers around the world—clearly reveals this effect:[305]

Finding: Chinese in the Tianjin province had low blood pressure despite the highest salt consumption of any group studied.

Interpretation: Low intakes of fat, refined carbohydrates and sugar have a greater combined influence on blood pressure than salt consumption alone. Rural Chinese food is typically high in potassium and fiber.

Finding: American blacks in Chicago had hypertension despite the lowest salt consumption in the industrialized world.

Interpretation: High intakes of fat, refined carbohydrates and sugar have a greater combined influence on blood pressure than salt consumption alone. American food is typically low in potassium and fiber.

Finding: The primitive tribes of Papua New Guinea and the Yanomamo Indians of Brazil had the lowest blood pressure and the lowest salt intakes.

Interpretation: Low-fat, low-sodium, high-potassium, mostly vegetarian diets resulted in the lowest blood pressure.

Populations in Northern Japan and Tianjin China consume up to 15,500 mg of sodium daily. It takes a Yanomamo Indian 3 years to eat the amount of salt a Northern Chinese consumes in 1 day, yet both have low blood pressure. Vegetarians commonly have lower blood pressure than meat-eaters, regardless of their salt intake.[306]

In 1896, it was reported that certain cannibal tribes in Australia would not eat the flesh of Caucasians because it tasted too salty and caused nausea.[307]

THE POLITICS OF HYPERTENSION

The National Dairy Council sponsored at least eight studies suggesting that calcium lowers blood pressure.[308] The drug industry funded studies showing similar results.[309] However, that doesn't explain how populations in developing countries avoid hypertension with half the calcium intake of Americans. Hypertension manifests from dietary excess, not calcium deficiency.

Most current evidence points to insulin resistance as the prime cause of hypertension.[310] Insulin resistance is linked to excess fat, refined carbohydrates and sugar. Hypertension, diabetes, cancer, heart disease, osteoporosis and premature aging develop from dietary excess, not deficiency. Thinking in terms of excess is critical for survival in this society.

One of the most debilitating consequences of hypertension is blindness. No strategy for staying alive would be complete without the protection of eyesight.

> *"Do not stand in a place of danger trusting in miracles."*
> —Arabic proverb

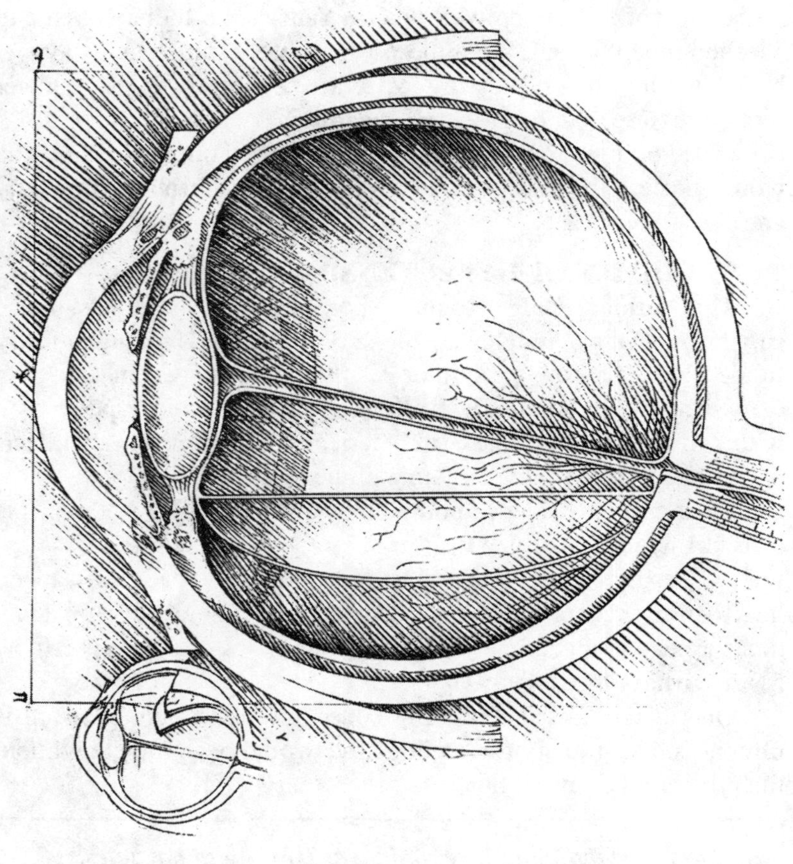

Eye Protection

"Who would believe that so small a space could contain the images of all the universe?"
—Leonardo da Vinci (1452–1519)

"I who am blind can give one hint to those who see...Use your eyes as if tomorrow you would be stricken blind."
—Helen Keller

As you watch a butterfly dance in the sun atop a red rose, your brain watches a movie by way of nerve fibers. Behind every human eye is a dime-size screen called the retina. Thousands of times each second when images hit the screen, 132 million light-sensitive cells convert the pictures into electricity: the language of the brain. Loss of sight is perhaps the most feared disability of life. The preservation of our most precious sense is a gift beyond measure.

The sun nurtures all life on earth. But as the sun gives, it also takes away. Sunlight destroys different things in different ways: plastic lawn furniture turns to dust; skin becomes wind-shredded crepe paper; eyes go blind. Light travels in straight lines at 186,000 miles per second...until it hits something.

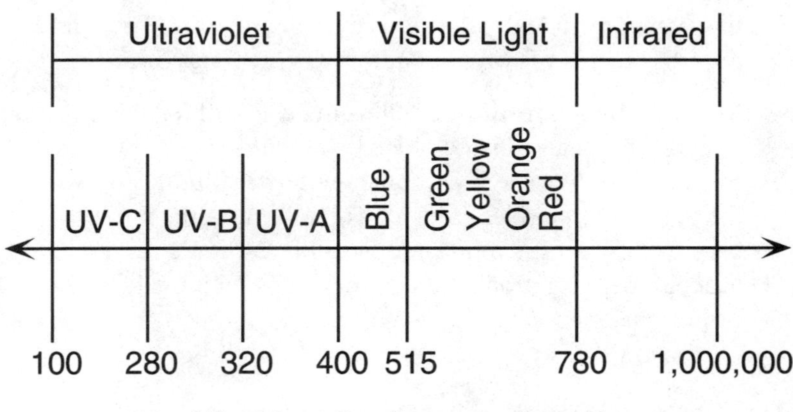

HARMFUL RAYS

- **UVC (Ultraviolet C):** UVC rays are normally filtered out by the ozone layer and do not reach the earth's surface.[311] UVC causes problems only in those exposed to artificial sources (welding arcs).

- **UVB (Far Ultraviolet):** UVB rays are scattered by clouds, blocked by windows and are most intense during clear summer days. UVB causes suntanning, sunburn, blisters, surface wrinkles, snow blindness, skin cancer and vitamin D.

- **UVA (Near Ultraviolet):** UVA rays pass through clouds and windows and are equally intense throughout the year. UVA is 100–500 times more abundant in sunlight than UVB. UVA causes suntanning, deep wrinkles and skin cancer.

- **Infrared:** Infrared rays produce heat and are normally harmless to the eye. Infrared causes problems only in those exposed to artificial sources (lasers).

SUNLIGHT-RELATED EYE DISEASES

- **Cataracts:** The world's leading cause of blindness and the most common major surgical procedure among American seniors.[312] Cataracts are caused by UVB rays striking the lens and turning it cloudy by the process of oxidation.[313] Cumulative damage gradually develops over many years. The lens absorbs most UVB rays but allows UVA to pass through.[314]

- **Macular Degeneration:** The leading cause of legal blindness among Americans 65 and older.[315] Macular degeneration is caused by UVA rays[316] combined with blue light[317] striking the eye's inner surface (retina). The macula is the most sensitive part of the retina and lies directly at it's center. Macular degeneration gradually develops with the loss of central vision.

MACULAR DEGENERATION

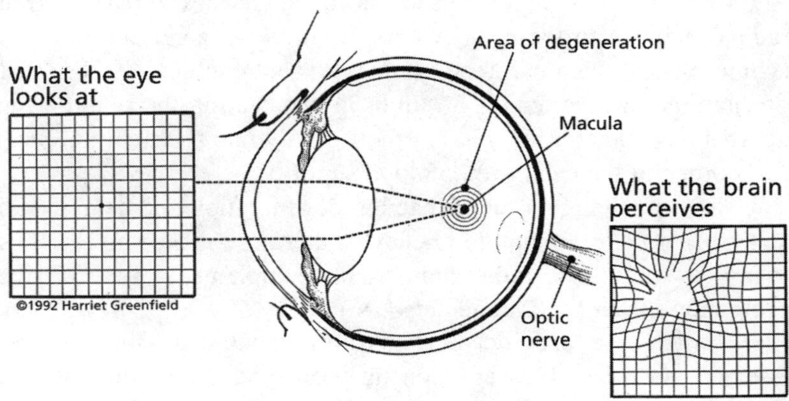

The eye has three built-in defenses which partially protect against macular degeneration:

- Eye pigment – macular degeneration is less common among Orientals, Hispanics and others with deeply pigmented eyes.
- Eye melanin – provides light filtration and antioxidants. Eye melanin decreases with age (50% loss by age 60).[318]
- Pupil constriction – bright light constricts the pupil which limits light entering the eye.

WARNING

- Dark sunglasses cause pupil dilation. Dark wrap-around sunglasses that fail to block blue light (below 515 nm) can leave eyes more vulnerable to macular degeneration than no sunglasses at all.
- Sunglass polarization, color and darkness offer no protection against UV rays.[319]
- Sunglasses labeled "100% UV Protection" block UVB rays only; they block neither UVA nor blue light. For maximum protection, sunglasses should block all three.[320]

ANTIOXIDANTS

Since macular degeneration and cataracts develop from free radical damage to the eye, experts often recommend antioxidants (vitamins C, E, beta-carotene) to help prevent damage.[321] The level of vitamin C in the lens is 36 times higher than in the blood. This approach sounds reasonable but there's only one problem: the lens and cornea of the eye have no blood supply.

The underlying cause of macular degeneration and cataracts is sunlight, not antioxidant deficiency. It therefore makes more sense to rely on sunglasses, rather than vitamin supplements, for effective protection. A hat brim alone cuts UV rays by 50%.

Whole foods provide nutrients not available in supplements. Green leafy vegetables are rich in lutein and zeaxanthin, which form the macula's yellow pigment. Yellow pigment absorbs blue light. Supplements are no substitute for vegetables, which are no substitute for sunglasses.

RATING SUNGLASSES

The FDA and the Sunglass Association of America developed the following rating system. Sunglasses labeled "Meets ANSI Requirements" meet the guidelines of the American National Standards Institute for one of three categories:

Amount of Light Blocked

	UVB	UVA	Visible Light
Cosmetic Lens	70%	20%	60%
General-Purpose Lens	95%	60%	60–92%
Special-Purpose Lens	99%	60%	20–97%

Unfortunately this rating system offers little protection against UVA rays and completely ignores the blue light hazard. And the new FDA rating system (currently under development) also falls short of optimum.

ALTERNATIVE

Blue-blocking lenses are superior to other types because they selectively remove only the harmful rays (UVB, UVA, blue) without blocking the harmless rays (green, yellow, orange, red). The additional visible light entering the eye causes pupil constriction for added protection against **both** cataracts and macular degeneration.

Blue-blocking lenses protect against all sunlight-related eye diseases.[322] Blue-blocking lenses are orange (the opposite of blue) but do not interfere with the red-yellow-green color discrimination needed for traffic lights.

Sunglasses that block all rays below 515 nanometers remove 99% of blue light. Sunglasses that block all rays below 550 nanometers remove 100% of blue light.

Proposed Sunglass Rating System

- The more light blocked below 550 nanometers, the higher the rating.
- The more light allowed in above 550 nanometers, the higher the rating.

What you can do

- Purchase your sunglasses with blue-blocking protection in mind and tell the sales person why.
- Write letters to the other sunglass companies telling them why you didn't buy their products.

Ozone depletion and ultraviolet levels worsen with each passing year. Simultaneously, diets are improving. If this trend continues, we may someday find this nation inhabited by healthy blind people. Don't be one of them. Protect your eyes.

> *"What does it mean to redefine one's relationship to the sky? What will it do to our children's outlook on life if we have to teach them to be afraid to look up?"*[323]
>
> —Al Gore
> *Earth in the Balance*

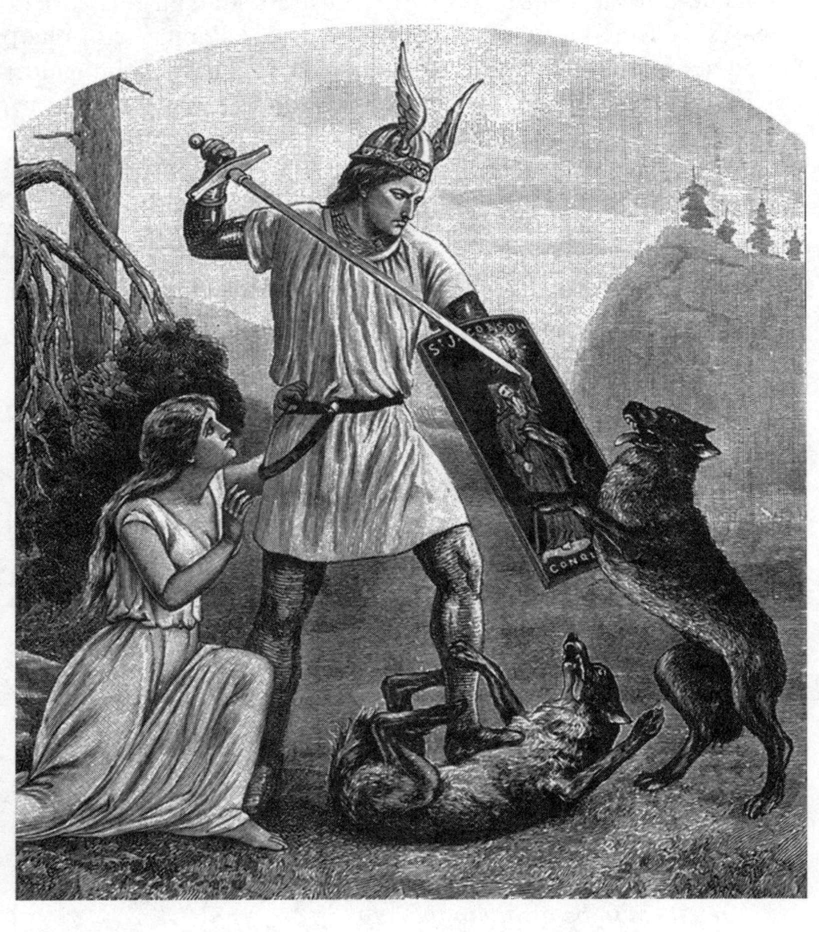

CHAPTER 7
Industry

"Burning hydrocarbons is a way of life."[1]
—U.S. Petroleum Institute

One of the most prominent landmarks of the San Francisco Bay Area never appears in tourist brochures: the Chevron Oil refinery. Amidst throbbing pipes and hissing valves, strange unmentionable chemicals mix and percolate as flames shoot upward from shiny smokestacks. While working in this refinery, I observed that petrochemical pesticide production is not the cleanest of industries.

Two decades ago, the Worldwatch Institute warned that humanity had 40 years to reverse environmental degradation of the planet, or face ruinous social and economic consequences. Since then, all major environmental trends have worsened. The U.S. now faces critical ecological and medical pressures brought on by industrialization. In our search for solutions, much can be learned from history, our most woefully underutilized resource.

During the 1930s, insecticides included lead arsenate, food colors included lead chromate, and patent medicines contained strychnine.[2] Jamaica ginger, an over-the-counter drug, permanently disabled at least 35,000.[3] Clearly new laws were needed to protect the public and, despite industry resistance, Congress eventually passed the Food, Drug and Cosmetic Act of 1938.

This law served its purpose well during the era of World War II but can no longer cope with today's technology. Annual carcinogen production has increased 400-fold since the 1940s.[4] Petrochemical interests now dominate the world's top 10 corporations:

1) Exxon
2) General Motors
3) Royal Dutch Shell
4) Ford
5) Mobil
6) Texaco
7) Royal Iranian
8) Standard Oil
9) British Petroleum
10) Gulf

In 1962, Rachel Carson published *Silent Spring,* her landmark expose on DDT. Industry fought back. The National Agricultural Chemical Association trashed her book using hired experts, front groups, media mailings and scientific misinformation.[5] Rachel Carson died of breast cancer before her book was vindicated. Her warnings have yet to be heeded.

During the 1960s, the new miracle ingredient hexachlorophene was loudly trumpeted in mouthwash, shampoo, Dial and Phisohex soaps, and feminine hygiene sprays. Unfortunately for consumers, hexachlorophene is an industrial waste product containing dioxins. Exposure led to damaged immune function,[6] birth defects[7] and several infant deaths.[8] Hexachlorophene, water fluoridation, food irradiation and mercury dental fillings convert industrial waste products into economic assets.

The double-edged sword of technology generates prosperity and opportunities for life enhancement on a scale not imagined in generations past. Technology's seductive lure allows humans mastery over all that we survey with blind disregard for the web of life. This mode of thinking carries a price: extinction. Petrochemicals have a darker side.

Toxic chemicals now blanket the earth altering the reproductive health of animal species in ways unprecedented in recorded history. It seems we have poisoned all of creation and undermined the biological basis of human existence. The world's gene pool is now at risk. Pesticides steal from generations yet unborn and time is not on our side as we rapidly approach our day of reckoning for poor planetary stewardship.

Clearly new laws are needed to protect the public health. But more urgent than laws, a national consensus is needed between government, science, industry, medicine and the public to safeguard our most treasured inheritance from irreversible harm.

During World War II, German scientists developed poisonous gas for the planned extermination of an entire race. Those same organophosphate chemicals now serve as insecticides. This chapter addresses the petrochemical industry infrastructure, tentacles and all.

Only by fully understanding industry's interconnected pillars can an aroused public bring about reform. Only through reform can we advance with confidence into the future, beckoned by the great wonders and adventures before us.

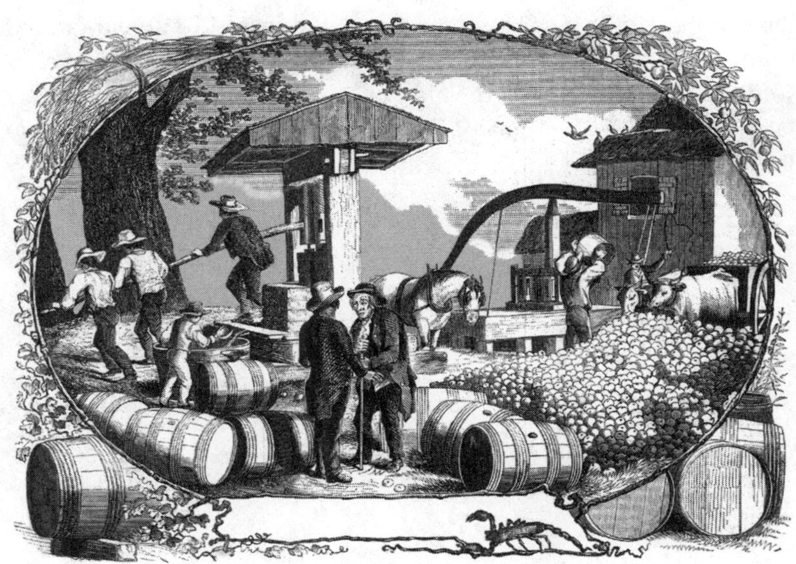

Pesticides

"Without chemicals, life itself would be impossible."
—Monsanto slogan, 1977

"DDT is good for me-e-e!"
—advertisement, 1950s

". . . if you drink much from a bottle marked 'poison,' it is almost certain to disagree with you, sooner or later."
—Lewis Carroll
Alice in Wonderland, 1865

"The Atomic Age began at exactly 5:30 Mountain War Time on the morning of July 15, 1945, on a stretch of semi-desert land about 50 airline miles from Alamogordo, New Mexico.

"And just at that instant there rose from the bowels of the earth a light not of this world, the light of many suns in one."
—William Laurence
New York Times, Sept. 26, 1945

During the 1950s, our nation conducted at least 130 above-ground nuclear explosions at the Nevada Test Site. Low-ranking soldiers were ordered into the blast areas soon after detonation. Years later, many developed cancer. Residents living downwind were told there was no danger.

> *"Fallout levels have been very low, slightly more than the normal radiation which you experience day in and day out where you may live."*[9]
>
> —Atomic Energy Commission
> *Atomic Tests Effects,* 1955

There's a parallel between this statement and the following:

> *"[Agent] Orange is relatively nontoxic to humans and animals."*[10]
>
> —U.S. Army, 1969

> *". . . 2,4,5-T [Agent Orange] is about as toxic as aspirin."*[11]
>
> —Dow Chemical Company

These statements reflected the best science available at the time—the long-term health effects of radiation and Agent Orange were unforeseen. With current medical knowledge doubling every 8 years, our future understanding of pesticides will be far greater than what is known today.

During the Vietnam War, the level of dioxin contamination in Agent Orange varied greatly between different manufacturers (Dow Chemical, Monsanto, Diamond Shamrock). Elevated dioxin levels were allowed because Agent Orange was to be sprayed only on the enemy and would never contact Americans…or so they thought. The U.S. and South Vietnam governments conducted PR campaigns to convince civilians that Agent Orange was safe. Workers were sent to remote villages where they demonstrated the safety of Agent Orange by washing their faces in it.

Following the war, American servicemen and Vietnamese reported sharp increases in birth defects, miscarriages, stillbirths and cancers. This damage included abnormal chromosomes rarely seen in humans. Vietnamese women in Da Nang now have dioxin levels in their breast milk 75% higher than American women.[12] When we use technologies in war and in peace whose consequences are unknown, we are still responsible for each of those consequences.

While traveling the rivers of Vietnam's Mekong Delta, I witnessed vast barren regions totally stripped of life. Viewing these moonscapes, I felt safe from ambush and grateful that Agent Orange was on our side. Thoughts of ecological devastation and long-term health risks simply never occurred to us. We had other concerns.

RISKS

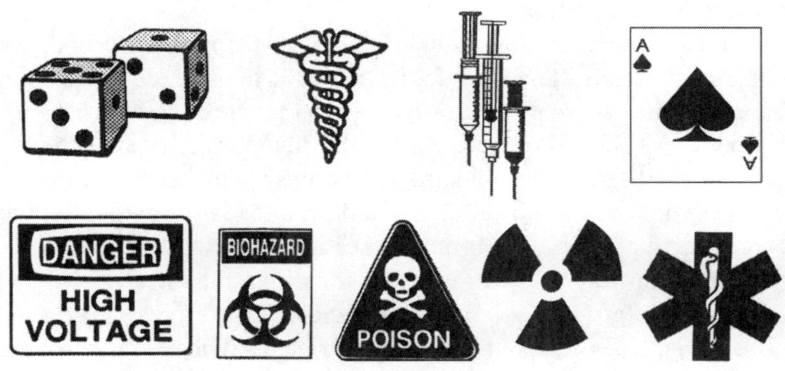

Life is filled with risks. Driving a car and taking a commercial flight both present risks. During a car crash, you have some control over the situation by being in the driver's seat. But during a plane crash, you've placed your life in the hands of someone else and you likely expect the pilot to be competent. Faced with less control, our risk tolerance drops.

It's a modern fact of life that pesticides are present in food and consumers can do little to detect or remove them. In 1992, the USDA analyzed 5,592 samples of washed and peeled fruits and vegetables. Pesticide residues were detected in 61% of the samples.[13] Grapes contained 21 different pesticides; apples had 25. Systemic pesticides cannot be removed. Agent Orange was formerly sprayed on apples to prevent premature fruit drop.[14]

> *"What is the risk of toxic chemicals? I think that there's almost a fear and dread of some of these environmental hazards and, in many cases, it's justified."*[15]
>
> —Dr. James Mason, director
> Centers for Disease Control

The EPA ranks pesticides as the number three cancer risk, after smoking and radon.[16] Ingesting one toxic chemical will increase personal risk only a tiny amount. But the EPA cannot measure the cumulative hazard of multiple pesticides. Chemical companies now produce over 50,000 different pesticide products.[17] Sensitive to image, the National Agricultural Chemical Association changed its name to the American Crop Protection Association.

CIRCLE OF POISON

Banned pesticides, including DDT, may be present in food. We still manufacture illegal pesticides and sell them to countries that have no ban. These countries then ship their produce back to us. Chlordane is banned in the U.S., yet chlordane residues are detected on imported fish, rice, mushrooms, squash and beef.[18] Half our winter produce is imported. Imported produce is twice as likely to carry illegal pesticides as foods domestically grown.[19]

DDT can travel through the air for thousands of miles before falling to the ground in rain or snow. Scientists traced DDT in the Great Lakes to sources in Central America, Africa and Asia, where the pesticide is still used.[20] Windblown DDT has found its way to Antarctica.[21] Eggshell thinning from DDT was recently observed among bald eagles in Washington state.[22] This suggests there are no pesticide-free areas left anywhere on earth.

America is the world's largest producer of pesticides. More than 30% of our exported pesticides are banned or restricted in the U.S.[23] Thousands of Latin American banana workers were made sterile by the pesticide DBCP which was exported by U.S. companies long after its dangers became known.[24] Dow Chemical, Monsanto, Miles and Eli Lilly are among the U.S. companies that produce and export banned pesticides.[25] Powerful industry lobbies defeated past efforts to control pesticide exports.

The U.S. government finances pesticide exports through three agencies: the Export-Import Bank, the Overseas Private Investment Corporation, and the Agency for International Development.[26] These programs helped quadruple U.S. pesticide exports since the late 1960s.

It's difficult for corporations to convince cancer victims that their disease is justified on the basis of cost-benefit analysis, that chemical company interests supersede the right to a clean environment, that shareholder profits supersede life itself.

BITTER LEGACY

Since DDT was banned in 1972, researchers have found no overall decrease in human breast milk.[27] The DDT levels commonly found in breast milk would be banned by the FDA if found in cow's milk. Once DDT is stored in human fat tissue, its breakdown product (DDE) can persist for a lifetime. Pesticides mimic the body's sex hormones (estrogens) and there's growing evidence that exposure may lead to cancer.

Two recent studies found that breast cancer patients have more DDE in their blood than those without cancer.[28] Five other studies detected elevated organochlorine levels in the breasts of cancer patients.[29] Several studies found higher pesticide levels in patients with stomach cancer and lung cancer.[30] The increased cancer risk among farmers is well documented.[31]

Worldwide sperm counts dropped 50% during the last half-century; U.S. testicular cancers increased 50% in the last 20 years.[32] An estimated 20% of American males were considered functionally sterile in 1980; infertile males were found to have more pesticides in their semen.[33] If sperm counts continue dropping at the same rate, most men will be sterile in two generations.

> *"Every man in this room is half the man his grandfather was."*[34]
>
> —Dr. Louis Guillette
> speaking before Congress

Pollution appears to be emasculating wildlife. Studies show permanent changes in the brain, genitals, sperm and sex hormones of wildlife after exposure to estrogenic chemicals.[35] Male alligators in Florida have genitals only 33–50% their normal size. Undescended testicles are becoming more common. Despite growing scientific concerns, current regulations do not consider hormonal disruption in risk assessment to humans. Industry uses estrogenic chemicals with impunity, squandering our biological inheritance and opening the door to large-scale genetic destruction.

Pesticides have made our nation's food production the envy of the world, but that bounty carries a heavy price: the human gene pool. Several clusters of birth defects and childhood cancers have been linked to pesticides.[36] Children of California farmworkers are twice as likely to be born with deformed limbs.[37]

As with nuclear waste disposal, politicians with short political lives are visiting their decisions upon future generations. Politicians are not gods, yet they hold the power to make godlike mistakes when unbridled arrogance overshadows all else.

> *"Sure, it's [Chlordane] going to kill a lot of people, but they may be dying of something else anyway."*[38]
>
> —Othal Brand
> Texas Pesticide Regulatory Board

Decisions to develop, market and apply technologies are often made by corporate and government officials without the burden of public imput or informed consent. Today's technological wonder carries the risk of becoming tomorrow's nightmare.

> *"DDT enjoyed a great popularity as an insecticide partly because it combined high toxicity for insects with low toxicity for people and animals."*[39]
>
> —American Council on Science and Health

Pesticide "inert ingredients" may include DDT.[40] U.S. pesticide policy: Place an infant inside a crib with a pacifier and a hand grenade. Then turn off the lights and say, "Don't worry. Things have always worked out before."

THE POLITICS OF PESTICIDES

Corporations spend millions in campaign contributions to block tougher pesticide regulations. Their investment has paid off:

- In 1958, Congress passed the Delaney Clause which prohibits all food additives shown to cause cancer. But Congress also allowed the continued use of all pesticides approved before 1958.
- In 1970, the EPA assumed responsibility for setting safe pesticide limits. But Congress again permitted the continued use of all pesticides approved before 1970.
- In 1978, more accurate testing procedures were adopted. But all pesticides approved prior to 1978 were again exempted.

Several older sprays, grandfathered into use without adequate testing, persist for years and would not be allowed on the market today.

The National Academy of Sciences estimates that 90% of the cancer risk from pesticides stems from those approved before 1978.[41]

In contrast to other industrialized nations, breast cancer deaths in Israel (which had been rising for 25 years) dropped sharply between 1976–1986. During this same period, known risk factors actually worsened: Israeli alcohol, fat and total calorie consumption increased; fiber, fruit and vegetable intake declined; and childbearing was delayed.

The apparent reason for Israel's declining breast cancer was their program to ban organochlorine pesticides (DDT and lindane) in 1978.[42] The pesticide level in Israeli breast milk and cow's milk has fallen since the ban. Scientists believe organochlorines are "complete" carcinogens, which both initiate and promote cancer growth.

U.S. breast cancers increased sharply in recent years despite a drop in consumption of fat and alcohol. U.S. pesticide exposure worsened during the last decade. Pesticides contribute to breast cancer risk independent of fat intake. Counties with toxic waste sites have elevated breast cancer rates.[43] Our government has failed to curtail dangerous pesticides, not because we lack information, but because we lack political resolve.

The Delaney Clause requires the EPA to deny approval of new pesticides that are less carcinogenic than older pesticides currently in use.[44] Congress inflicted this intolerable situation on the public and only Congress can undo the damage.

Proposed Pesticide Reform

- Immediately revoke the registration of all pre-1978 pesticides not tested under current standards. (Manufacturers could re-apply for registration.)
- Ban the production and export of any pesticide not allowed on American food.
- Regulate and phase out estrogenic chemicals.
- Require manufacturers to list all "inert" pesticide ingredients, including DDT.
- Require growers to disclose which pesticides they use. Require a country-of-origin labeling law.
- Mandate civil and criminal penalties for violators.

There are those who still cling tenaciously to tenets of the past. The chemical industry with its powerful lobbies, legislative cohorts and indentured academic consultants, has relentlessly pursued profits with little regard for biological consequences. While lives are being lost, members of Congress accept campaign contributions from pesticide companies.

The government's pesticide regulatory system is fundamentally compromised by special interests, an approach not compatible with public health. A sustainable society cannot place corporate profits and campaign war chests over cancer risks to the public at large. A sustainable society tempers technology with accountability and gives people a voice.

In 1954, John Wayne, Susan Hayward, Agnes Moorehead and producer Dick Powell filmed *The Conqueror* on the sand dunes outside St. George, Utah—about 150 miles downwind from Atomic bomb testing. For 3 months, the filmmakers breathed dust laced with radioactive fallout.

Of the 220 people in the cast and crew, 91 had contracted cancer by late 1980, and half the cancer victims had died of the disease. These included John Wayne, Susan Hayward, Agnes Moorehead and Dick Powell.[45]

The U.S. government apologized to the citizens of Utah for the lives lost in the name of national security...40 years after the fact. We cannot wait for the same apology with pesticides. The stakes have grown too large in this macabre game of poker. The seeds are sown and nothing short of concerted national action can halt cancer from becoming our nation's leading cause of death.

Every time history repeats itself, the stakes go up.

"Tomorrow is the most important thing in life...It hopes we've learned something from yesterday."[46]

—John Wayne (1907–1979)

Chlorine

"Our massive tampering with the world's interdependent web of life...could trigger widespread adverse effects, including unpredictable collapses of critical biological systems whose interactions and dynamics we only imperfectly understand... We the undersigned, senior members of the world's scientific community, hereby warn all humanity of what lies ahead."[47]

—Union of Concerned Scientists
including 102 Nobel laureates

"We know that there are concerns about chloro-organic materials, and we are addressing those concerns. We will depend on credible science to point the way, and we will do the right things as good product stewardship requires."[48]

—Chlorine Institute

Ordinary salt (sodium chloride), ubiquitous throughout the earth's crust and the human body, is essential for life. Elemental chlorine (chlorine gas) does not exist in nature. Industry creates chlorine gas by passing electricity through salt-water, thereby transforming chloride into chlorine. Chlorine gas reacts with organic (carbon-containing) materials to form organochlorines. Organochlorines readily bind to fat tissues, breast milk and semen.

For millions of years, nature restricted the quantity of organochlorines in the global environment to only trace amounts. All that changed following World War II. Chlorine production now totals about 40 million tons per year.[49] Dioxin, DDT, Agent Orange, PVC plastic and 11,000 other organochlorines owe their existence to chlorine.[50]

Petrochemicals and chlorine grease the engines of industry, forming the basis of our economy. The U.S. runs on chlorine and oil. Organochlorines are valuable to industry because they're stable and resistant to natural breakdown processes. Examples:

- DDT (dichloro-diphenyl-trichloroethane) has a half-life of 57.5 years in temperate soil.[51]
- CFCs (chlorofluorocarbons) have atmospheric lifetimes ranging from 25–150 years.[52]

- In pure water, chloroform and trichloroethane remain stable for 1,850 years and 1 million years, respectively.[53]
- PCBs (polychlorinated biphenyls) will remain detectable in humans for the next six generations.[54]

Organochlorines accumulate in the environment over time, working their way up the food chain in magnified form. Industry's desire to live in harmony with chlorine ranks as one of humanity's most magnificent follies.

At least 177 organochlorines are detectable in the tissues and body fluids of North Americans.[55] Every woman's breast milk contains pesticides, dioxins and 65 isomers of PCBs.[56] American semen contains 35 PCBs, plus phenols and ethers. Even Eskimos and polar bears carry high levels of organochlorines.[57] Beluga whales in the St. Lawrence River contain such high PCB levels that dead whales are legally hazardous waste.

From the deepest ocean to the remotest ice cap, organochlorines blanket the earth with far-reaching consequences.

HEALTH RISKS

Dioxins are by-products formed during chlorine production. Dioxins are present in coffee filters, milk cartons, tampons, sanitary napkins, disposable diapers and other bleached fiber products. The level of dioxins found in preindustrial humans was less than 2% of that detected in current human tissues.[58] According to the EPA, dioxins in American fat tissues (40–60 parts per trillion or 5–10 nanograms per kilogram) are at or near levels causing reproductive damage, cancer and immune suppression.[59]

Female chemists exposed to organochlorines have higher breast cancer rates.[60] All organochlorines biodegrade into other compounds, most of which are more toxic than the original chemical.[61] Despite the risks to public health, industry deliberately releases thousands of organochlorines into the environment.

Each year, the paper industry discharges 30,000 tons of chloroforms into the air and 2 million tons of organochlorines into the world's waterways.[62] Dry cleaners release 15 million pounds of carbon tetrachloride annually. The bleaching of wood pulp products creates up to 1,000 organochlorines.

Organochlorines comprise a global biological threat on a scale without precedent. In order to preserve the life-sustaining capacity of this planet, organochlorine production must be phased-out. Since all uses of chlorine gas produce organochlorines, the production of chlorine itself must also be phased-out.[63]

SUPPORT FOR BANNING CHLORINE

The International Joint Commission recently urged the U.S. and Canadian governments to phase-out chlorine production.[64] Several other international organizations called for zero chlorine discharge into waterways:

- the Paris Commission on the North Atlantic (15 nations)
- the Barcelona Convention on the Mediterranean (21 nations)
- the International Whaling Commission (30 nations)

In 1993, the American Public Health Association called for American industry to phase-out chlorine.[65] In 1994, the White House proposed a "national strategy for substituting, reducing or prohibiting the use of chlorine and chlorinated compounds" as part of the Clean Water Act.[66] Congressman Richardson introduced the Chlorine Zero Discharge Act of 1994, which requires the paper industry to phase-out chlorine bleaches within 5 years.

INDUSTRY REACTION

In 1990, the chairman of Occidental Chemical recommended that industry become "more adept at communicating chlorine health, safety and environmental information."[67] The Chlorine Institute urged industry to "overcome negative images and concerns."[68]

The chlorine industry recently launched a PR campaign to soothe the public's fear of organochlorines, especially dioxins. Several government agencies joined in this effort.

> *"Everybody in this country has [dioxin] in their body...It is no cause for alarm."*[69]
>
> —Dr. Vernon Houk, director
> Centers for Disease Control

According to an industry spokesperson, "Dioxin is a natural product" and "absolutely no public health threat."[70] In 1991, the chlorine industry falsely reported that dioxins were less dangerous than once believed, but recent studies indicate dioxins are more toxic than previously estimated.[71]

Chlorine supporters argue that volcanoes and seawater add far more chlorine to the stratosphere than CFCs (chlorofluorocarbons), and that forest fires generate large amounts of dioxins. These positions are not supported by current evidence.[72] Chlorine from volcanoes is soluble and not found in the upper atmosphere; CFCs are insoluble and deplete the ozone layer. Forest fires generate dioxins only from dioxin pollution deposited on the trees.

The Chlorine Institute released a report which claims that banning chlorine would cost the U.S. and Canadian economies $102 billion per year.[73] Yet by industry's own estimates, over 95% of chlorine could be phased-out for $17 billion per year—far less than the $90 billion industry spends each year in waste management,[74] and the $100 billion our country spends each year in health-care costs related to toxic substances.[75]

Industry reported that banning chlorine would cost 370,000 jobs[76] when, in fact, a phase-out would create 92,500 new jobs.[77] These changes would reduce costs and improve productivity, according to the Office of Technology Assessment.[78]

American chlorine makers assert that EPA's chlorine regulations are too restrictive.[79] Meanwhile, Europe is far ahead of the U.S. in developing chlorine-free technologies.[80] Swedish paper mills no longer use chlorine gas.[81] Sweden will eliminate all chlorine in papermaking by the year 2000. British Columbia and Ontario will eliminate it by 2002. Most European countries no longer use chlorine in treating drinking water.

America must move forward to phase-out chlorine or else risk losing its competitive edge in the global marketplace. An intransigent industry must no longer be allowed to block transition to a less toxic economy.

WAKE UP CALL

Between 1986–1992, thousands of marine animals including whales, seals, dolphins and fish washed up on beaches worldwide.[82] Some were apparent victims of red tides caused by toxic algae blooms. Others were apparent victims of infections caused by weakened immune systems. During this time, half the world's green sea turtle population developed large tumors.[83]

Current evidence suggests the red tides, marine epidemics and tumors were caused by organochlorine pollution.[84] All the animals involved were heavily contaminated or lived in polluted waters. The world's fisheries are now in absolute decline while chlorine pollution worsens with each passing year.

> *"No more than one or a few decades remain before the chance to avert the threats we now confront will be lost and the prospects for humanity immeasurably diminished."*[85]
> —Union of Concerned Scientists

Organochlorines disrupt biological support systems to a degree unparalleled in recorded history. With vision and leadership, they need not defeat us. An international chlorine phase-out will eradicate humanity's most insidious environmental scourge and usher in a new era of global stewardship.

It is particularly difficult for corporations to do business with dead planets. Biological sustainability is tantamount to economic sustainability. Long-term sustainable policies will fundamentally alter the way this country does business, but such policies are imperative for survival. Since chlorine production is incompatible with sustained life on this planet, the question is not whether to phase-out chlorine, but how.

CHLORINE PHASE-OUT

Economical alternatives already exist for about 75% of U.S. industrial chlorine applications.[86] These applications include:

- Chlorine-based pesticides, solvents and paper bleaching.
- Polyvinyl chloride plastic (PVC).
- Chlorinated refrigerants (CFCs and HCFCs).
- Chlorinated drinking water (increases the risk of bladder and colon cancers).[87]
- Perchloroethylene (perc) used in dry cleaning.
- Chlorine (chlorohydrins and phosgene) used in producing epoxy resins, synthetic fibers, titanium dioxide, olefins, polycarbonates, isocyanates, propylene and ethylene oxides.

Proposed Chlorine Reform

- Establish a national program to phase-out chlorine production and prohibit dioxin discharges within 5–10 years.
- Eliminate taxpayer subsidized electrical power to chlorine production plants.
- Establish a tax on chlorine production and chlorine-containing products. Raise the tax over time to fund chlorine alternatives and worker retraining.
- Prohibit the use of persistent toxic chemicals as chlorine substitutes (fluorine, bromine, organohalogens).
- Exempt chlorine-based pharmaceuticals (accounting for less than 1% of chlorine use) until substitutes are found.

What You Can Do

- Boycott household products containing chlorine.
- Pressure national magazines to use chlorine-free paper.
- Support chlorine phase-out legislation and federal procurement mandates for purchasing chlorine-free paper.

Fluoride

"The simple truth is that there's no 'scientific controversy' over the safety of fluoridation."[88]

—*Consumer Reports*

"[The fluoridation] market potential has fluoride chemical makers goggle-eyed...it adds up to a nice piece of business on all sides."[89]

—*Chemical Week*

For over 50 years, the U.S. government and media have trumpeted fluoride as a safe and effective means of reducing cavities, especially in children. But fluoride is not the benevolent and innocuous substance the public has been led to believe.

From its inception, the issue of water fluoridation has been heavily laden with political subterfuge and chicanery. Government agencies have turned a blind eye to the adverse effects of fluoride while championing its virtues. The fluoride controversy vividly illustrates one of the greatest challenges of our time: the obfuscation of scientific integrity for political and financial gain.

Fluoride is a non-essential trace mineral,[90] and the 13th most common element found in the earth's crust.[91] Elemental fluoride is fluorine, a pale yellow gas and deadly poison used in rocket fuel and uranium production.[92] Since fluoride is non-biodegradable and more toxic than lead,[93] and since it accumulates in bone like lead,[94] logic would dictate that it be regulated like lead. Not so with fluoride. Not when corporate economic interests override public interests.

Fluoride is an industrial waste product generated during the production of aluminum, phosphate, pesticides, coal-burning power, gasoline, fertilizer, steel, copper and glass.[95] U.S. industries profit handsomely by discharging fluoride into the environment.

The weakening of environmental regulations and the resulting billion-dollar profits, are the real motives behind water fluoridation. The history of this ongoing saga provides an instructive tale of Machiavellian deception.

FLUORIDATION HISTORY

The idea to add fluoride (hydrofluosilicic acid, sodium fluoride) to drinking water came from ALCOA (Aluminum Company of America), North America's largest fluoride polluter.[96] During the early 1930s, bogus surveys appeared to reveal fewer cavities among children in naturally-fluoridated communities. These surveys were funded by the Public Health Service under the direction of Treasury Secretary Andrew Mellon (founder of ALCOA).[97] Studies were deliberately falsified to purport the benefits of fluoride.[98]

During World War II, industrial fluoride emissions increased dramatically, spurring damage claims against polluters. Something had to be done. In 1945, fluoridation began in Grand Rapids, MI. An ALCOA lawyer, appointed to head the Public Health Service, launched a disinformation campaign to change fluoride's image from rat poison and insecticide to the guardian of children.[99] This stunning transformation ranks among the classic public-relations coups of all time.

Reputable scientists who expressed concern were grouped with convicted felons and the Ku Klux Klan. Smear tactics and dogma did little to encourage open scientific debate. By 1950, with government health agencies heralding the flawed studies,[100] with cities clamoring for fluoridation while the public bowed in servile reverence, fluoride's transformation was complete.[101]

Water fluoridation has since evolved into a means of industrial waste disposal at taxpayer's expense. Each year the city of Calgary pays $230,000 for chemicals, of which 99.9% are flushed straight down the city sewers. This results in 150 tons of fluoride deposited into the Bow River and environment each year.[102] Fluoridation is the second largest source of fluoride pollution in Canada.[103]

Industries use fluoridation to circumvent pollution control laws—which in turn generates profits, jobs, taxes and political campaign contributions.

ENVIRONMENTAL RISKS

Of all major industrial pollutants, fluoride is the most toxic to plants, animals and humans.[104] According to the USDA, "Airborne fluorides have caused more worldwide damage to domestic animals than any other air pollutant."[105] In 1972, fluoride emissions were high enough to damage livestock, forests, crops, statues and glass.[106]

During 1960–75, fluoride pollution from aluminum plants destroyed the skeletons of cattle in New York, forcing these animals to crawl on their stomachs like giant snails.[107] Animals and humans accumulate high fluoride levels through plants, meat, water and air.[108]

Each year, U.S. industries discharge an estimated 155,000 tons of fluoride into the air,[109] and 500,000 tons into waterways.[110] Fluoride released into rivers can persist for 1–2 million years.[111] Contrary to popular belief, the capacity of the environment to absorb fluoride pollution is finite. The growing magnitude of fluoride effluents has led to saturation in many areas.

The same level of fluoride added to drinking water can be lethal to freshwater fish.[112] Levels above 0.2 ppm (parts per million) are fatal to salmon.[113] The legal limit for fluoride in drinking water is 4 ppm; for toothpaste, 1,100 ppm.[114]

In 1982, fluoride from an aluminum plant killed 45% of salmon on the Columbia River.[115] The fluoride concentration was 0.5 ppm. In 1985, when the fluoride level was reduced to 0.2 ppm, salmon loss dropped to 5%.

HEALTH RISKS

When fluoride enters the body, it seeks out and rapidly binds to calcium. Since every cell in the body contains calcium, fluoride binds with all tissues including the brain, heart, liver and kidneys.[116]

Fluoride is a cumulative enzyme poison which inhibits calcium metabolism and cell permeability.[117] Fluoride breaks down protein and inhibits collagen production.[118] In plants, it interferes with photosynthesis. Fluoride combines with stomach acid to form hydrofluoric acid, which dissolves protein, steel and glass.

No other substance deliberately added to food and water carries this degree of risk. Fluoride is the most toxic agent ever enjoined by government to assault the human condition. Because fluoride is so persistent, even minuscule traces can build up over time, eventually reaching levels where "age-related" afflictions occur.

Fruit juices can contain significant concentrations of fluoride from tap water, pesticide and fertilizer residues. Cow's milk and infant milk formulas contain between 0.02–0.8 ppm fluoride.[119] Soy milk contains up to 0.49 ppm. Fluoride in beverages is not labeled. Public policies which encourage fluoride contamination show little regard for biological consequences.

Exposure to multiple fluoride sources is a fact of life in America today. A large portion of the U.S. population is probably above the 4–5 mg/day level where adverse health effects likely manifest.[120] The human body removes fluoride from teeth and bones more slowly than it's deposited. If fluoride intake remains constant, fluoride deposits increase with age.[121]

FLUOROSIS

Dental fluorosis (brown mottled teeth) and skeletal fluorosis (deformity, bone/joint pain) both arise from excess fluoride. Dental fluorosis is increasing among American children.[122] The prevalence ranges from 8–81% in fluoridated communities, compared to 3–26% in nonfluoridated areas.[123] This bodes poorly for public health since dental fluorosis is an early visible sign of systemic fluoride toxicity. Dental fluorosis may foreshadow skeletal fluorosis later in life.

Most Americans lose 33–50% of their kidney function by age 80. As kidney function declines, fluoride levels in bone and blood increase.[124] Fluoride intake as low as 2–5 mg daily can cause early stage skeletal fluorosis, which can mimic arthritis.[125] Skeletal fluorosis is endemic in several nations and it behooves policymakers to prevent its occurrence here.

HIP FRACTURES

Most developed nations do not fluoridate their water supplies. Less than 1% of Western European countries are fluoridated.[126] The U.S. is the most heavily fluoridated country,[127] and has the world's highest hip fracture rate.[128] Water fluoridation is strongly linked to hip fractures.[129]

In current clinical studies, patients receive massive doses of fluoride as treatment for osteoporosis. This produces denser but weaker bones which are more prone to fractures.[130] Patients given 40–60 mg daily for 5 years had their bone strength reduced by 45%.[131] This dose is near the level most Americans receive from their diet over 50 years.[132]

CANCER

Several government studies reveal an increase in bone cancers among young males in fluoridated communities.[133] Fluoride is a potent carcinogen and causes genetic damage at 1 ppm.[134] Fluoride may react with pollutants now found in public water supplies.[135] The EPA fired their chief toxicologist after he disclosed a link between cancer, hip fractures and fluoridated drinking water.[136]

Studies implicate fluoride in the cause of brain impairment,[137] decreased fertility,[138] sperm and testosterone inhibition,[139] immune suppression,[140] blood cell alterations,[141] kidney stones,[142] thyroid depression,[143] cataracts,[144] artereosclerosis,[145] oral and pharyngeal cancers.[146] In addition, fluoride corrodes water pipes and elevates lead levels.[147]

The Maximum Contaminant Level of fluoride in drinking water is 0.8 ppm in Japan, and 4 ppm in America. Waterworks engineers, during the 1940s, warned that water containing 1 ppm fluoride was contaminated.[148] Policymakers would do well to heed this warning, now vindicated by the preponderance of current evidence.

BIASED RESEARCH

Most studies in medical journals find fluoridation to be safe and effective. This is not surprising since most funding for fluoride research originates with the Public Health Service, an organization officially mandated to promote fluoride.[149] This apparent conflict-of-interest is somehow overlooked by fluoridation proponents.

In 1990, the *Journal of the National Cancer Institute* published a curious study (funded by Procter & Gamble) which concluded that fluoridation doesn't cause cancer.[150] That same journal rejected a second study which found an increase in cancers with fluoride.[151]

In 1993, the National Research Council expert panel released its long-awaited report: *The Health Effects of Ingested Fluoride*.[152] This panel proclaimed fluoridation to be safe despite the well-documented risks of cancer, fluorosis and hip fractures. Several panel members received grant money from pro-fluoride government and industry sources.[153] A 1983 expert panel expressed concerns over fluoride's safety—concerns later deleted by the Public Health Service.[154]

An international feud has erupted between pro- and anti-fluoride forces. In 1994, nearly 300 scientists from 15 countries convened in Beijing, China, for the XXth Conference of the International Society for Fluoride Research. Studies funded by the U.S. National Institute for Dental Research promoted fluoride's safety, even at high levels. These studies conflicted sharply with those presented by experts from other countries.[155] Politically-acceptable research, sponsored by the U.S. government, is an embarrassment to the international scientific community.

TOOTH DECAY

Tooth decay in the U.S., Canada, Australia, New Zealand and Western European countries has declined sharply since 1948. This decline was virtually equal in both fluoridated and unfluoridated communities.[156] Decay rates in the fluoridated areas began to fall before fluoridation was introduced; decay rates in the unfluoridated areas began to fall before fluoridated toothpaste was introduced.[157]

Studies in the U.S. and abroad show decay rates not significantly changed by water fluoride variations.[158] The U.S. city with the lowest decay rate did not fluoridate its water.[159] Fluoride's impact on tooth decay pales compared to that of improved dental hygiene.

To reach consensus on the issue of water fluoridation, this nation must decide if the benefit of reducing tooth decay by 0.1%[160] is worth the risks. Blind acceptance of dubious ideologies must not deter us from the critical task at hand: a national fluoride policy.

Proposed Fluoride Reform

- Regulate fluoride like lead. Curtail fluoride discharges into air and waterways.
- Cease fluoridation of drinking water.
- Establish a national drinking water goal of 0.2 ppm by the year 2000. Finance the construction of defluoridation plants through a tax on industrial fluoride discharges.
- Label the fluoride content of beverages and bottled water. Limit fluoride contamination in foods, fertilizers and animal feed.
- Prohibit fluoride in dental products, medications and osteoporosis treatments.
- Eliminate the Public Health Service mandate to promote fluoride. Launch an educational campaign to counter the 50 years of pro-fluoride indoctrination.

Natural Toxins and Risk

"A few of us in Midland [Dow Chemical] have deliberately ingested small quantities of 2,4,5-T [Agent Orange] to satisfy ourselves of its safety. . . ."[161]

—V. A. Stenger
analytical scientist

"Natural carcinogens...are a far greater danger than pesticides and additives, accounting for more than 98% of the cancer risk in the diet."[162]

—Dr. Robert Scheuplein
FDA Office of Toxicological Sciences

"Organic food may be more dangerous than Safeway food. When plants get stressed, they make more of the natural pesticides."[163]

—Dr. Bruce Ames
University of California, Berkeley

According to Dr. Ames, natural plant toxins pose a far greater hazard than industrial pollutants, and are second only to cigarettes as important causes of cancer.[164] Scientists estimate we consume 10,000 times more toxins from foods than from synthetic pesticides.[165]

"When one understands that toxins, carcinogens and mutagens are everywhere in Mother Nature's own food supply, one can see the absurdity of panicking over minute levels of man-made chemicals."[166]

—American Council on Science and Health

Monsanto promoted this theme in its 1977 Chemical Facts of Life campaign under the heading "Rhubarb Can Kill."[167]

Lettuce and carrots form nitrosamines and stomach cancer. A peanut butter sandwich is 100 times more deadly than pesticides. Barbecued anything? Forget it! You name it, it causes cancer… or so they say.

FACT: Potatoes would be banned if they were judged by the same standard as pesticides.

- **Government Response:** We therefore shouldn't worry about synthetic pesticides.
- **Public Response:** Everything causes cancer.
- **Chemical Industry Response:** We need stronger laboratory rats.
- ***Long Life Now* Response:** We need more accurate cancer tests.

For ease of understanding, all pesticides and natural toxins can be divided into five groups based on how quickly they biodegrade, starting with the slowest.

Group 1 Synthetic Pesticides

- Organochlorines (DDT, Agent Orange, chlordane, heptachlor)
- Organophosphate insecticides (malathion, parathion)
- Carbamate insecticides (carbaryl, carbofuran)

Organochlorines last for decades. Synthetic pesticides form few breakdown products, thus making their residues easy to test for. The FDA's Total Diet Study detected malathion and DDE in 20–40% of food samples tested.[168] Benzene hexachloride, a pesticide 19 times more potent than DDT, is commonly found in butter, hot dogs and milk chocolate.

Group 2 Naturally-Derived Pesticides (botanicals)

- Rotenone (from a South American root)
- Pyrethrum (from chrysanthemums)
- Camphor (from camphor trees)
- D-limonene (from orange peels)

Pyrethrum is toxic to insects but relatively safe for mammals because of poor gut uptake and rapid breakdown.[169] There are no established methods for detecting the residues of botanicals because they leave no residues.[170] However, botanicals should not be considered part of organic farming because of their toxicity to beneficial insects and soil organisms.

Group 3 Pyrotoxins (by-products of cooking or fermentation)

- Benzopyrenes: charcoal broiling a 1-pound steak produces as many benzopyrenes as the smoke of 600 cigarettes.[171]

- Heterocyclic aromatic amines: form on the charred portions of burnt meat.

- Polynuclear aromatic hydrocarbons: form in the smoke after dripping fat onto hot coals.

- Urethane (ethyl carbamate): forms during the fermentation of alcohol, soy sauce and yogurt. Easily broken down and excreted.

Group 4 Mycotoxins (by-products of mold growth)

- Ergot: a fungus with a long and glorious history, possibly contributing to the French Revolution and the 17th century Salem witch trials.[172] Ergot grows on grains and produces a natural form of LSD—a good way to stir up a crowd.

- Aflatoxin: produced by two common molds (aspergillus flavus and aspergillus parasiticus) that thrive on nuts, seeds and grains. Aflatoxin causes liver cancer in rodents but its impact on humans remains unclear.[173]

Group 5 Phytotoxins (plant toxins)

When scientists estimate we consume 10,000 times more natural plant toxins than synthetic pesticides, this is the group they're referring to. Natural toxins comprise up to 10% of a plant's weight.[174] Plants generate toxins in response to invading organisms, fungus, blight, insects, grazing animals and physical damage.[175]

> *"Since plants do not have teeth or jaws to protect themselves, they employ chemical warfare."*[176]
>
> —Dr. Bruce Ames

Thousands of natural plant toxins have been isolated and identified. Examples:

- Canavanine: causes lupus in monkeys fed 40% of their calories from alfalfa sprouts.

- Quercetin: causes bladder cancer in cattle and rats fed bracken ferns.

- Cycapsin: causes liver cancer in rats fed cycad tree ferns.
- Hydrazines: cause stomach cancer in mice fed raw mushrooms. (Most hydrazines are destroyed by cooking; stomach cancer is rare in the U.S.)
- Solanine: a liver toxic alkaloid from green potato skins.
- Alkenylbenzene: causes liver cancer in rats and mice fed safrole (from sassafras oil), estragole (from tarragon, sweet basil, and fennel), and methyl eugenol (from cloves, sweet bay, and lemon grass).

Orange oil contains at least 42 chemicals including 14 hydrocarbons, 12 alcohols, 9 aldehydes, 4 ketones, and 2 esters.[177] Potatoes contain at least 150 different compounds. Other whole foods are equally complex. Natural plant components pose no significant risk to most people since they're biodegradable, utilized as nutrition, quickly excreted, or combined with other substances. Pesticides are a different matter.

> *"Many of the chemical agents introduced into the food supply, including pesticides, fertilizers, plant-growth regulators and antibiotics can be harmful to humans at high doses or after prolonged exposure at lower doses."*[178]
>
> —National Academy of Sciences

PESTICIDES VS. NATURAL TOXINS

Authorities claim that synthetic pesticides must be viewed in context of the enormous background of natural toxins.[179] This viewpoint overlooks several critical differences.

> *"Pesticides are biological poisons, and I share everyone's concern about the potential health effects of residues that may **remain** on foods. . . ."*[180]
>
> —Dr. Frank Young
> former FDA Commissioner

The key difference is the word "remain." Pesticides remain; natural toxins do not. Examples:

- Natural toxins do not persist in the environment for decades, nor do they drift through the air for thousands of miles.
- Natural toxins are not found in Arctic ice, polar bears, Great Lakes fish, cancer tumors, human breast milk, rain, snow, fog, and the poisoned groundwaters of 35 states.[181]
- Natural toxins do not damage eggshells, sperm, and fetuses.

If pesticides and natural toxins are equally dangerous, then why have cancers increased sharply following the introduction of pesticides after World War II?

BIODEGRADABILITY

Over millennia, the human body has evolved to protect itself from the chemical warfare employed by plants. The immune system neutralizes toxins by placing oxygen atoms (free radicals) inside the toxic molecules. This literally burns up toxins by the process of oxidation. Plant toxins are quickly broken down because they're normally not exposed to oxygen. But this process doesn't work with pesticides, which are formulated to resist breakdown. A pesticide's lack of biodegradability makes it valuable to farmers and toxic to humans.

Plant chemicals (phytochemicals), steroid hormones (estrogens), and dioxins (TCDD) all bind to receptors within the human body. Plant chemicals and hormones degrade after a few hours, but dioxin requires 7 years to reduce its concentration by half.[182] Because of dioxin's long half-life, the body cannot regulate this process. Thus, one dioxin molecule can continuously disrupt normal cell physiology. This distinction appears lost on certain scientists.

> *"Everyone worries about minute amounts of dioxin, but there is a lot more of a dioxin-like compound naturally in broccoli than you will ever be exposed to through dioxin contamination in the environment."*[183]
>
> —Dr. Bruce Ames

The disregard of biodegradability by otherwise knowledgeable authorities seems disingenuous at best.

CHEMICAL FORMS

The FDA recommends that kelp tablets be avoided since they contain arsenic.[184] Industrial workers exposed to arsenic have higher cancer rates. However, arsenic comes in two forms: industrial arsenic is a poison; organic arsenic may be required by humans in trace amounts.[185] Kelp tablets contain organic arsenic.

Chromium also comes in two forms: industrial chromium is a poison used in auto plating; dietary chromium is essential for blood sugar control.[186] This raises several important questions:

- Are industrial PCBs the same PCBs that naturally occur in ferns and seaweed?
- Are nitrates in cured meats the same nitrates that naturally occur in carrots and saliva?
- Are industrial formaldehydes the same formaldehydes that naturally occur in orange juice and human blood?
- Has any scientist removed the formaldehyde from his or her blood and replaced it with embalming fluid?

CANCER TESTS

Most chemicals classified as carcinogens appear not to be damaging DNA.[187] Current risk assessment methods rely on animal studies using high-level doses of single chemicals. Low-level multi-chemical exposures are largely ignored. In estimating cancer risk, animal tests may not be transferable to humans because sensitivity to chemicals varies widely by species. Examples:

- The drug Thalidomide caused birth defects in humans but not in animals.[188]
- Guinea pigs are 1,900 times more sensitive to dioxins than hamsters. Rodents are more sensitive to dioxins than humans.[189]
- B-naphthylamine causes cancer in humans but not in rats or hamsters.[190]
- UDMH (a breakdown product of Alar) causes cancer in mice but not in rats.[191]
- Saccharin causes cancer in rats but not in mice or humans.[192]

- A chemical found in orange peels (d–limonene) causes kidney cancer in male rats but not in female rats, mice or humans.[193]
- Rats and mice disarm circulating estrogens by attaching a specific protein molecule; humans attach a sulfate molecule.[194]
- Fluoride causes gene mutations in rodent and human cell cultures but doesn't induce bacteria to mutate (Ames Test).[195]

Animal and bacteria studies are of little value in determining human cancer risk. If an isolated chemical causes bacteria mutation or rodent cancer, we cannot conclude that human cancer will also develop. Current risk assessment procedures are **not accurate** in predicting human cancer risk. We simply need better tests.

AFLATOXIN RISK

The aflatoxins found on nuts and grains may, in fact, not be carcinogenic at all. Aflatoxin apparently does not cause liver cancer in humans unless the liver is damaged by other agents.[196] Consider the following:

- Mozambique, West Africa has the world's highest rates of liver cancer and aflatoxin contamination. But this region also has high rates of hepatitis B, a known cause of liver cancer.[197]
- The southeastern U.S. has the nation's highest aflatoxin contamination but lower liver cancer rates than other parts of the country.[198] (Southerners also have a low incidence of hepatitis B.)
- The China Health Project found no association between aflatoxin and liver cancer.[199]
- Aflatoxin causes liver cancer in rats but not in mice or primates.[200]

Our current understanding of aflatoxin underscores the need to develop test protocols for examining chemical breakdown products and their impact on human cells.

CHILDHOOD CANCER

Today's children face risks that did not exist in generations past. Recent studies link the household use of pesticides to childhood brain cancer and leukemia.[201] Cancer is now the leading cause of death in American children ages 1–14.[202] But unlike adult cancers, the increase cannot be explained by better diagnostic procedures.

> *"We don't understand why childhood cancer is increasing. Frankly, it's likely to be some as yet unknown factor in the environment. We could be talking about things we don't even know how to measure."*[203]
>
> —Dr. Devra Davis
> Mount Sinai Medical Center

Current federal regulatory policies are not adequate in protecting human health due to the weak scientific foundation on which those policies are based.

DETERMINING CANCER RISK

The core tenet of toxicology is "the dose makes the poison." In other words, one aspirin will relieve a headache and 1,000 will kill. This premise works fine for aspirin which is water soluble, biodegradable, rapidly excreted and does not mimic estrogen. Shortcomings quickly develop when this reasoning is applied to pesticides. Certain chemicals create toxic effects in amounts as small as 1 billionth of a gram.

The average American consumes 150 micrograms of pesticide residues and PCBs each day (547,500 micrograms per decade).[204] A chemical's ability to bioaccumulate and its endocrine-disrupting effects are ignored by our current methods of evaluating risk.[205]

One common method of determining cancer risk involves exposing a mouse to 400,000 times the level of chemical a human would receive. If no tumors appear, then 1/100th of this amount is deemed safe for daily human consumption.

Extrapolations from animal studies trouble many consumers, epidemiologists and toxicologists. The public has good reason to mistrust the current scientific methods.

"The standard carcinogen tests that use rodents are an obsolescent relic of the ignorance of past decades."[206]

—Philip Abelson
deputy editor of *Science*

Chemical companies have taken steps to enhance the biodegradability of their pesticides. However, several newer pesticides are just as harmful because their breakdown products are more toxic than the parent compounds.[207] Current risk assessment procedures ignore breakdown products.

Animal tests cannot cope with the infinitesimally small quantities that analytical chemists are able to measure: parts per milliattogram (10^{-21}) using high-performance capillary electrophoresis, and parts per attomole (10^{-18}) using accelerated mass spectrometry with radioimmunoassay.[208] Sensitivity of this magnitude allows investigators to exclude uncertain dose extrapolations for chemicals like dioxins, PCBs and pesticides. Government risk assessment tests are due for a major upgrade.

We all want to know which chemicals are safe; we all want to know the truth. Pro-pesticide scare tactics and media manipulations have no place in this search. The time has come for the government and scientific community to move forward so that self-serving exaggeration from both sides will no longer be needed to save the day.

Proposed Cancer Risk Guidelines

- Any ingested chemical not broken down or excreted by the body, will be retained by the body.
- Short-term animal cancer risk is determined by dose.
- Long-term human cancer risk is determined by cumulative dose.
- Cumulative dose is influenced by biodegradability.
- Anything that doesn't biodegrade can build up.
- Anything that builds up can damage the immune system.
- Anything that damages immune function increases cancer risk.

FOUR STEPS TO SUSTAINABLE AGRICULTURE

- Halt biotech research that develops pesticide-tolerant crops.[209]
- Shift agricultural research from pesticides (synthetic and botanical) to alternative pest controls (beneficial insects, neuropeptides, pheromones and lasers).[210]
- Supplement our current cancer tests with low-dose risk assessment at the molecular and cellular levels . . . the new toxicology.
- Sharp phaseout and ultimate ban of any chemical found to be carcinogenic using the new toxicology.

THE NEW TOXICOLOGY

- The long-term safety of a substance is directly proportional to Group A and inversely proportional to Group B.
- The cancer potential of a substance is directly proportional to Group B and inversely proportional to Group A.

Group A	Group B
1) Water solubility	1) Fat solubility
2) Low molecular weight	2) High molecular weight
3) Ease of excretion	3) Gut uptake
4) Speed of breakdown	4) Ability to bioaccumulate
5) Breakdown products	5) Hormonal and DNA activity
6) Nutritional value	6) Receptor binding capacity

The old toxicology measures what a chemical does to an animal or organism (a pig's nervous system, a rat's sperm, or a bacteria's genetic material) and then extrapolates that information to humans. The new toxicology measures the chemical itself: how the ultimate breakdown products impact human cells, genes, metabolic pathways and receptors.

Such protocols would be highly cost-effective by guarding against both overregulation and underregulation. Instead of replacing the Delaney Clause with "negligible cancer risk" based on animal tests, it makes more sense to keep Delaney and improve risk assessment. Heretical paradigms shift slowly.

THE POLITICS OF RISK ASSESSMENT

Belief: *"Pesticides are among the most rigorously tested products tested today.*[211]

—Jay J. Vroom, president
National Agricultural Chemical Association

Reality: No amount of testing can compensate for flawed methodology, mindless extrapolation, dubious applicability to humans, and bias due to a financial stake in the outcome.

Belief: *"'Natural' and 'chemical' are mythical distinctions since there is no basic difference between the substances provided by nature and those produced by industry."*[212]

—American Medical Association

Reality: Only by improving risk assessment accuracy can we know for certain.

Belief: *"The FDA, USDA and EPA make sure that any pesticide or animal drug residues that might remain in foods are at safe levels."*[213]

—Food and Drug Administration

Reality: Current risk assessment protocols do not ensure food safety. The reliance on cancer tests alone is an inappropriate basis for regulatory or public health policy.

"If you poison your boss a little bit each day its called murder; if your boss poisons you a little each day its called Threshold Limit Value."[214]

—James Keogh, M.D.

RANKING ENVIRONMENTAL HAZARDS

Most Dangerous

1) Occupational pesticide exposure
2) Smoking
3) Excess fats and proteins
4) Obesity
5) Radon gas
6) Asbestos
7) Dietary pesticide exposure (food, tap water)
8) Air pollution (indoor, outdoor)
9) Solar radiation (UVA, UVB)
10) X-ray radiation (medical, dental)
11) Non-ionizing radiation (computer screens, powerlines)
12) Natural plant toxins

Least Dangerous

Be wary of cigarette smoke, fats, radon and pesticides: the four horsemen of cancer's apocalypse. Watch out for the cars, not the lights. Lights don't kill.

> *"I do not know of a flowering plant that tastes good and is poisonous. Nature is not out to get you."*[215]
>
> —Euell Gibbons, author
> *Stalking the Wild Asparagus*

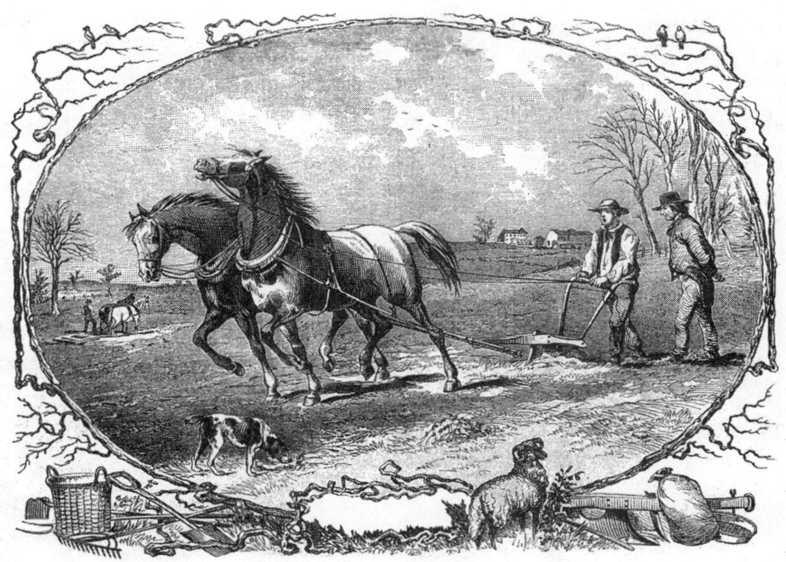

Organic vs. Conventional

"If you eliminate synthetic pesticides, you make fruits and vegetables more expensive. People will then eat less of them and more will die of cancer. . . .Organic foods are selling because Americans have been sold unreasonable fears of modern technology."[216]

—Dr. Bruce Ames
University of California, Berkeley

"The biggest threat to human food supply today, to human cancer, and to wildlife maintenance would be organic farming."[217]

—Dennis Avery
Hudson Institute

In the 1840s, a German chemist named Justus von Liebig developed the first synthetic fertilizer. Chemical farming was born, spreading quickly throughout Western nations. The reaction to von Liebig was the beginning of organic farming.[218]

No issue within the province of nutrition provokes greater controversy than questions surrounding how foods are grown in America. The U.S. has only 6% of the world's agricultural land, yet uses 50%

of the world's pesticides (2.2 billion pounds in 1993).[219] About half are used in agriculture.[220]

Every spring, farmers throughout the Midwest apply 150 million pounds of herbicides to soybean and corn fields. Rains wash large portions of these chemicals into the drinking water of 11.7 million residents.[221] During the spring run-off of 1993, the U.S. Geological Survey noted that up to 16,000 pounds of herbicides were moving down the Mississippi River each day.[222] Agricultural pesticides cause about half of all water pollution.[223]

Chemically dependent farming did not exist before World War II. Since 1945, the share of crops lost to insects increased by 20% despite a 3,300% jump in pesticide use.[224] In 1942, only seven insect species were resistant to pesticides; today there are 504.[225]

Historically, topsoil depletion has been a prime cause in the fall of civilizations. About 33% of U.S. cropland is now exhibiting declining productivity.[226] Herbicides are applied to U.S. crops on a fixed schedule regardless of need. This practice increases pesticide residues, birth defects, water pollution, soil depletion and chemical industry profits. The USDA recently warned, "Conventional agriculture places man on a collision course with nature."[227]

According to the National Academy of Sciences study *Alternative Agriculture,* "Alternative farming methods are practical and economical ways to maintain yields, conserve soil, maintain water quality and lower operating costs."[228] This report recommends restructuring federal farm subsidy programs to encourage sustainable agriculture.

Farm subsidy programs determine U.S. agricultural practices by accounting for 20–40% of all farm income since 1955. Farm programs reward farmers who apply chemicals and waste topsoil, but penalize farmers who rotate crops or convert to sustainable agriculture.[229] Certain banks and insurance companies require farmers to use pesticides.[230] The pesticide industry maintains farm subsidy programs through campaign contributions to Congress.

Organic produce appears more expensive than conventional produce…until you count the hidden costs: farm subsidy programs, taxes, cancer and environmental cleanup costs. David Pimental of Cornell estimates that a 50% reduction in pesticide use would increase food prices by 0.6%, but would save $4–10 billion in environmental and health-care costs.[231]

Fruits, vegetables and whole grains cost less than meats, dairy products and processed foods—not to mention the time and money you save on laxatives, antacids, fiber products, stool softeners, medicines, doctor bills, lost work and nursing homes.

Farming methods affect a crop's nutritional value. A recent study compared 38 minerals in organic and conventional apples, pears, corn, potatoes and wheat. The organic foods averaged about twice the nutrient content and contained 25% less mercury, 29% less lead and 40% less aluminum.[232] A British study reported similar results.[233] Synthetic fertilizers and pesticides increase the nitrate content of vegetables up to 20-fold.[234]

PRODUCE TERMS

- **Organic:** grown and processed without pesticides, synthetic fertilizers, irradiation, or genetic engineering.
- **No Detected Pesticide Residues:** no pesticides "at levels greater than those allowed by law." This is **not** the same as pesticide-free. It is legal to use this term even when there **are** detected residues. This term appears only on conventional produce.
- **Integrated Pest Management (IPM):** crops raised using selective pesticides and non-chemical pest controls (beneficial insects and crop rotation).

The Clinton Administration has mandated the use of IPM on 75% of American farmland by the year 2000. However, IPM has no clear definition. This allows farmers to ignore non-chemical methods and actually use more pesticides, not less.[235] With no clear definition, the IPM program is a sham. IPM is neither alternative nor sustainable agriculture.

Milwaukee sewage sludge is sold in all 50 states as "organic fertilizer" under the name Milorganite.[236] Sewage sludge fertilizer may contain over 60,000 toxic substances including heavy metals (lead, cadmium, mercury, arsenic), dioxins, PCBs and pesticides without disclosure. Toxic chemicals can remain in soil indefinitely and be taken up by plant roots.

Procter & Gamble offers a produce rinse (FIT) for removing pesticide residues from fruits and vegetables. Just a few squirts from a plastic bottle, "For a clean you can feel good about."[237] There's just one problem: systemic pesticides cannot be washed off. The USDA recently found systemic pesticides in 61% of washed and peeled produce samples.[238] (Procter & Gamble also makes pesticides and chemotherapy drugs.)

Conventional produce may be treated with post-harvest pesticides without disclosure. In Leavenworth, Washington, a Safeway customer saw the produce manager spray Black Flag House and Garden Insect Killer on the apricots, plums and nectarines. One Safeway employee was reportedly instructed "only to spray produce when the isle was clear of customers."[239]

Ultimately the consumer decides which business practices will die off and which will flourish. (Consumers spent $524 billion on food and beverages in 1993.) Each grocery dollar is an economic vote in determining the direction of our country.

Proposed Agriculture Reform

- Reform the farm subsidy programs. Tax the sale and use of pesticides. Encourage farmers to rotate crops.
- Provide credit assistance only to organic growers. Eliminate produce requirements for cosmetic perfection, minimum size and uniformity.
- Shift USDA research from chemical to non-chemical pest controls. Clearly define Integrated Pest Management.
- Fully disclose the level of heavy metals, pesticides and chemical contaminants in fertilizers.
- Label all fruits and vegetables grown with municipal wastes.
- Phaseout central sewage processing plants. Develop separate waste disposal and treatment systems for human and industrial wastes.

> *"The nation that destroys its soil destroys itself."*
> —Franklin D. Roosevelt, 1937

Seed Wars

"Where might a chemical company interested in agricultural chemicals go? Obviously, into seeds. Some members of the chemical industry are getting into seed development."[240]

—Chemical Manufacturers Association official

"The single most serious threat to the global food system is the threat of genetic erosion."[241]

—Al Gore

In 1846, a fungus attacked Ireland's uniform potato crop reducing it to black slime. More than a million people starved to death in the Irish potato famine and another 3 million fled the country. A crop's ability to resist disease depends upon biological diversity.

This valuable history lesson appears lost on modern agriculture as we drift toward a global cataclysm on a scale without precedent. Biodiversity is disappearing. No environmental onslaught holds greater potential for irreversible harm. The EPA ranks pollution as a lessor threat to world survival than the extinction of plant species.[242]

In 1970, half the U.S. corn crop from Florida to Texas was devastated by blight because the entire crop was spliced with a single gene.[243] In 1946, blight destroyed 86% of U.S. oats including 30 oat varieties—all bred from a single genetic parent.[244] Uniformity breeds vulnerability. The world's food system and the botanical gene pool on which it depends, are endangered by corporate vested interests and short-term greed. The problem is patents.

In recent years, multinational pesticide and pharmaceutical industries have purchased over 1,000 independent seed houses.[245] Multinational corporations operate by introducing new hybrid seeds which are patented and, at the same time, dropping non-patented heirloom seeds from their seed catalogs. Only one company sells certified organic heirloom seeds nationwide.[246] Both conventional and organic growers use hybrid seeds because nothing else is available.

Heralded as bioengineering miracles, hybrid seeds are vulnerable to diseases and dependent on pesticides which the industries produce.[247] Monsanto, manufacturer of Roundup, developed a Roundup-tolerant gene which they splice into hybrid soybeans.[248] Monsanto holds patents to the gene, the hybrid and the pesticide.

Hybrid seeds are expensive and often coated with pesticides prior to sale.[249] Hybrid seeds require large amounts of water and synthetic fertilizers, which the corporations produce. This adds to soil depletion and further increases dependence on chemicals. International lending agencies often require growers to use hybrid seeds as a condition for receiving farm credit.[250]

Hybrid seeds may be genetically tagged to prevent growers from sharing second generation seeds with each other.[251] Large seed companies have filed lawsuits against growers over this issue.[252] Lawsuits protect patents but further reduce biodiversity and self-reliance. Growers have shared seeds with each other for thousands of years.

> *"Van Gogh loved sunflowers. He painted them again and again. It's amazing that some of the sunflowers that are in Van Gogh paintings have been patented by modern seed companies."*[253]
>
> —Alan Kapuler
> plant breeder

The USDA and the American Seed Trade Association promoted passage of the seed patent laws.[254] The USDA and Forest Service are encouraging the use of herbicide-tolerant plants, thus increasing the sale of pesticides and the extinction of countless plant species.[255] Federal and state agencies have spent millions of tax dollars funding this research. Breeding pesticide-dependent plants is not in the interests of public health or planetary survival.

Bromoxynil is a herbicide that kills cotton and causes birth defects. The maker of bromoxynil, Rhone Poulenc, funded the biotech company Calgene to develop cotton resistant to this herbicide.[256] The International Rice Research Institute and eight other international agencies receive funding from chemical companies and the U.S. government to develop pesticide-tolerant hybrid seeds.

NUTRITION

Plants grown from hybrid seeds generally provide less nutrition than plants grown from heirlooms.[257] Food producers don't believe that Americans care about nutrition.[258] Consequently most U.S. food is bred for industrial traits: yield, shelf-life, bruise resistance and cosmetic appearance.[259] Iceberg lettuce is a prime example. Livestock feed, in contrast, is bred for nutrition. This agricultural agenda will change only when consumers demand that it change.

Multinational corporations have been poor guardians of the world's botanical gene pool, our living legacy. The preservation of biological diversity and the global food chain for future generations is an issue that cannot wait.

Proposed Biodiversity Reform

- Support legislation abolishing seed patents.
- Tax the sale of patented hybrid seeds. Give tax incentives to companies offering non-patented heirloom seeds.
- Halt taxpayer funding of pesticide-tolerant plants.
- Encourage growers to use heirloom seeds by restructuring the farm subsidy programs to include both nutrition-per-acre and yield-per-acre.

> *"The meaning of life, and the unique nature of life, is in its diversity. The philosophy of survival is based on the philosophy of diversity."*[260]
>
> —Mikhail Gorbachev

Industrial-Grade Hemp

"Make the most of the Indian Hemp seed and sow it everywhere."[261]

—George Washington, 1794

"Since 1937, about half the forests in the world have been cut down to make paper. If hemp had not been outlawed, most would still be standing, oxygenating the planet."[262]

—Alan Bock

Historical tradition, if not current federal law, favors hemp. The Declaration of Independence, the Gutenberg *Bible*, the sails of the U.S.S. Constitution, and Old Glory (our nation's first flag) were all made from hemp—as was the favorite fuel of Henry Ford, the reading lamp oil of Abraham Lincoln, and the parachute webbing that saved the life of George Bush.[263]

Hemp canvas covered the Westward-bound wagons, the biplanes and zeppelins of World War I, and provided the original Levi pants worn by California goldminers in 1849.[264] Hemp was so crucial to colonial America that its cultivation was mandated by law.[265]

INDUSTRIAL USES

As an agricultural commodity, hemp is arguably the world's top renewable resource for fuel, paper, cloth, paint, plastic, protein, soap, oil and over 25,000 other products.[266] Anything made from oil or wood can be made from hemp.[267]

Hemp biomass can be converted into fuels (methane, methanol, gasoline) more efficiently than fossil fuels (coal, oil) and without the sulfur or acid rain.[268] Hemp fiberboard is stronger than wood; hemp houses are as strong as cement houses and better insulated.[269] Plastic, rayon and cellophane made from hemp are biodegradable; plastic and nylon made from petrochemicals are non-biodegradable.

Grocery shoppers given the choice between paper or plastic bags must decide between spewing toxic chemicals or cutting down trees. In landfills, both biodegrade slowly if at all. Imagine an alternative: biodegradable cellophane or paper bags made from hemp.

The paper industry uses nearly half the world's timber harvest. According to the USDA, hemp produces four times the paper/acre as trees, and grows in all climate zones.[270] Hemp paper will last up to 1,500 years; hemp cloth is stronger than cotton. Cotton requires more pesticides than any other agricultural product (39 million pounds in 1993).[271] Hemp grows without pesticides, improves soil quality and reduces erosion.

ERADICATION CONSPIRACY

During the 1930s, machinery was developed for separating hemp fibers from the stalk, thus making widespread industrial applications feasible. *Popular Mechanics* called hemp a "billion-dollar crop."[272] Hemp's future looked promising, but this was not to be.

DuPont had just obtained patents for making nylon from coal, plastic from oil, and paper from trees.[273] Treasury Secretary Andrew Mellon (an oil baron) was DuPont's chief financial backer. The Hearst newspaper empire owned enormous timber tracts. The oil, timber, synthetic fiber and cotton industries stood to lose billions if hemp was not outlawed.[274]

Secret meetings were held. Andrew Mellon appointed his nephew-in-law to head the Federal Bureau of Narcotics. Hearst newspapers introduced the word "marijuana" into English and inflamed the public with outrageous stories of drug-related violence.[275] Anti-marijuana films (Reefer Madness, Assassin of Youth) fanned the flames of hysteria. The strategy worked. In 1937, Congress outlawed hemp by imposing a prohibitive tax—just as DuPont's annual report predicted:

> *"...the revenue-raising power of government may be converted into an instrument for forcing acceptance of sudden new ideas of industrial and social reorganization."*[276]
>
> —DuPont Corporation, 1937

As a model of deception and orchestrated media manipulation, the anti-hemp crusade constitutes one of the greatest hoaxes ever perpetuated on the American people. Few public-relations campaigns in history can match its success in eradicating competition while transforming citizens into unknowing pawns of big business. The legacy of Reefer Madness lives on today.

Industrial-grade hemp is worthless as marijuana since its THC (tetrahydrocannabinol) content is so low, as little as 0.06%.[277] Industrial-grade hemp varieties posses no psychoactive qualities.

High-grade marijuana strains can have THC contents exceeding 10% but are worthless for industrial purposes.[278] This vital distinction appears lost on those caught up in the anti-drug frenzy currently fashionable in this country, a frenzy perpetuated by vested interests.

The *New York Times*, for example, owns a pulp mill in Canada and benefits from wood pulp paper production.[279] DuPont, Monsanto, Dow Chemical and Standard Oil are protected from competition by the marijuana laws…as are the cotton, coal, timber, chlorine, vinyl plastic, latex paint and polyester industries. The major obstacles blocking hemp's utilization are not agricultural or botanical, but political.

PATENTED HEMP

At least 18 European and Asian countries now grow industrial-grade hemp. France, the world's largest producer of hemp, recently patented a hybrid strain containing only 0.4% THC.[280] The French hybrid is unstable causing successive generations to deteriorate.[281] This ensures ongoing seed purchases from France. French hybrid hemp requires fertilizers, growth stimulators and pesticides.[282] Patents promote the cultivation of inferior seeds which adversely affect hemp's overall commercial value.

ENERGY CONVERSION

Global climate change is the most threatening and intractable of all environmental problems we face. Carbon dioxide (CO_2) is the crucial greenhouse gas contributing to global warming. Since pre-industrial times, CO_2 levels have risen by almost 30% due to deforestation and fossil fuel combustion.[283] The U.S. burns fossil fuels for 93% of its energy needs and consumes 25% of the world's supply.[284] One tank of gasoline generates up to 400 pounds of CO_2.

During the 1930s, Henry Ford grew hemp on his estate to demonstrate the efficiency of methanol production. Both Henry Ford and Rudolph Diesel (inventor of the diesel engine) intended to power their vehicles with plant-based fuels.[285]

Hemp biomass grown for fuel would reverse global warming by converting CO_2 into oxygen during the growing cycle. Hemp is one of the richest biomass sources. Each acre of hemp yields 10 tons of biomass (1,000 gallons of methanol) in 4 months.[286]

The gas turbine generates cost-competitive electrical power using biomass fuels. Researchers at Princeton University estimate that biomass fuels combined with advanced gasifier-gas turbine technology could compete in cost with coal, nuclear and hydroelectric power in both industrialized and developing countries.[287] If vehicle fuel efficiency were doubled, biomass energy could replace all fossil fuels now used in cars and all coal burned for electricity in the U.S. To maximize efficiency, plant-based methanol, plastic, rayon and electrical production could occur at the same facility.

In 1982, U.S. nuclear power plants consumed 540 tons of nuclear fuel, and coal-fired power plants released 2,772 tons of radioactive uranium and thorium into the environment.[288] Hemp biomass farms would abate foreign oil dependency, soil erosion, acid rain, global warming and air pollution, while laying the groundwork for revitalized rural communities.

Rural pasture land (7% of U.S. acreage) could produce enough biomass to end U.S. dependence on gas and oil.[289] By converting cotton, tobacco, sugar and cattle feed production into biomass, energy independence would be within reach. The least valuable hemp product is biomass fuel. Each acre of hemp grown for fiber and pulp is worth $750—considerably more than either corn or wheat.[290]

In 1994, President Clinton issued an executive order naming hemp in the National Defense Industrial Resources Preparedness Policy.[291] In 1995, Colorado introduced the Hemp Production Act, and Kentucky appointed a hemp feasibility task force.[292]

Several American companies are using imported hemp to produce clothing, paper, oil and other products. Hemp ice cream, cheese, cookie and pancake mixes are now available. In each case, demand outstrips supply. Domestically-grown hemp would generate new job and business opportunities that benefit the environment.

Innovative economic and environmental programs can benefit communities. When Oregon restricted logging in 1991, a state retraining program turned timber workers into cabinet makers, auto mechanics, health-care workers, or accountants.[293] State programs can retrain workers now employed in the chlorine, pesticide, cotton, bleached paper, tobacco and coal industries. In the long run, every American job depends on our natural resources.

Let us uphold our forefather's traditions by restoring hemp to its rightful place as this nation's top renewable resource. Let us use its bountiful harvest to heal the mistakes of generations past and to ensure the quality of life for succeeding generations. The transition of our economy from petrochemical-based to plant-based will ease the conversion to a chlorine-free economy. Both conversions should be planned and coordinated simultaneously.

During World War II, America's prohibitionist hemp laws were suspended to meet pending material shortages.[294] Our government asked Kentucky 4-H Club youths to help in the war effort by growing hemp.[295] Farmers were encouraged to grow hemp through the USDA film "Hemp for Victory." Critical environmental pressures call for these laws to again be set aside.

Proposed Economic Reform

- Establish a program to cultivate industrial-grade hemp (1.4% THC or less).
- Tax fossil fuel production. Subsidize biomass fuels and worker retraining.
- Tax coal-based electrical production. Subsidize biomass electricity and worker retraining.
- Tax wood pulp paper production. Subsidize tree-free paper and worker retraining.
- Prohibit the patenting of hemp seeds by U.S. companies.

> *"If federal regulations can be drawn to protect the public without preventing the legitimate culture of hemp, this crop can add immeasurably to American agriculture and industry."*[296]
>
> —*Popular Mechanics,* 1938

National Media

"Those who manipulate this unseen mechanism of society constitute an invisible government which is the true ruling power of our country."

—Edward Bernays
Propaganda

"We know in the not too distant future a half dozen corporations are going to control the media. We took this step [merger] to ensure we were one of them."[297]

—Time Warner spokesperson

Corporate control of the media is nothing new. During the early 1900s, drug companies spent about $40 million each year on newspaper advertising. The Proprietary Association (representing pharmaceutical interests) inserted the following clause into each newspaper advertising contract:

"It is hereby agreed that should your State or the United States Government pass any law that would interfere with or prevent the sale of proprietary medicines, this contract shall become void."[298]

Journalistic independence of the time was quickly swayed by the persuasion of circumstance and self-interest. The same principles apply today. All major media outlets are now controlled by giant corporations, many of which produce pharmaceuticals or pesticides.

General Electric operates toxic waste dumps and owns NBC. Olin Chemicals sponsors PBS-TV's Firing Line.[299] Richard Gelb is a director of the *New York Times,* the Memorial Sloan-Kettering Cancer Center and Bristol-Myers Squibb, the world's largest maker of chemotherapy drugs.[300]

MEDIA BIAS

In 1992, the *Journal of the National Cancer Institute* and the *New England Journal of Medicine* published studies on the effectiveness of nontoxic cancer treatments.[301] The *New York Times* excluded both studies. Jane Brody, the *Times* nutrition writer, later published an article promoting chemotherapy and warning patients against alternative therapies. According to Brody, chemotherapy offers "the only chance for a lasting cure."[302]

In 1990, the U.S. Office of Technology Assessment issued its controversial report entitled "Unconventional Cancer Treatments."[303] This 3-year report contained information favorable to nontoxic alternative therapies and called for fair tests to be carried out. The *New York Times* interviewed leaders of the alternative movement but excluded those interviews and the report from publication.[304]

In 1991, the Hoechst drug company was fined $202,000 after pleading guilty to withholding information on adverse drug reactions resulting in several deaths. The guilty pleas and sentences of this case went unreported by the *New York Times*.[305]

During the debates over the North American Free Trade Agreement (NAFTA), the *New York Times* ran a series of advertisements and editorials in favor of the agreement. Simultaneously it refused to sell advertising space to those in opposition, even though the country was deeply divided. The *Times* owns a paper mill in Canada and profited greatly from NAFTA's passage.[306]

In 1993, the *Times* reported that EPA's anti-pollution rules would cost the wood-preservative industry $5.7 trillion per life saved.[307] This made the regulations seem absurdly costly. However, the EPA had previously estimated the cost at $800,000 per life saved, and the *Times* article excluded the EPA's estimate.[308] This article included unsupported claims that low level chemicals cause no harm, claims later reprinted in dozens of other newspapers.[309]

The *Times* has a personal interest in exonerating dioxins and other toxic chemicals. In 1991, the *Times* was sued for $1.3 billion over the dioxin pollution caused by their Canadian paper mill.[310]

"All the News That's Fit to Print."
—New York Times

DISCLOSURE FAILURES

In 1994, Monsanto launched TV ads promoting its bovine growth hormone in milk. The ads featured the American Medical Association and the American Dietetic Association but failed to mention that Monsanto paid for the ads.[311]

In 1994, Calgene launched a video news release promoting its genetically-engineered tomato. Over 100 million TV viewers saw the news release with no disclosure that Calgene paid for it.[312]

NBC Nightly News devoted 14 minutes of its newscast to a new machine for detecting breast cancer—with no disclosure that their parent company (General Electric) produces it.[313]

Corporate owners and sponsors directly control all national TV shows, including public television. Tough investigative reporting against corporations can be as perilous for networks as voting against drug companies is for Congress. For this reason, corporate exposé programs are rarely shown. American television fails to provide a forum for controversy, debate and the free flow of information on which true democracy thrives.

SLANTED MAGAZINES

Consumers often consult health magazines for the latest nutritional and medical information. Unfortunately not all information favors the reader's health. When dairy, meat and drug advertisements dominate a magazine's pages, corporate interests will not be lost.

According to *In Health*:

- Those who eliminate red meat and dairy products gamble with nutrient deficiencies.[314]

According to *Total Health*:

- Vegetable oils and organ meats (liver, kidney) help cancerproof your diet.[315]
- Mammography is one of the best preventative measures women can take against breast cancer.[316]
- Osteoporosis is caused by calcium deficiency. The best calcium sources are dairy products and calcium carbonate.[317]

According to *American Health*:

- Buying milk from hormone treated cows is an investment in good health.[318]
- Irradiation can make foods more wholesome rather than less.[319]
- Pesticides are not a risk factor for breast cancer.[320]
- The fear over pesticides appears exaggerated. Natural toxins pose a greater risk.[321]
- Organic foods are no better than conventional foods.[322]

American Health is owned by Reader's Digest Corporation, which has financial ties to Memorial Sloan-Kettering Cancer Center, which is interlocked with chemical companies.[323]

Trusting in health magazines can be deadly. In 1989, new workers at General Electric's PCB training school in Cincinnati were given an article from *Hippocrates* magazine suggesting that PCBs are safer than peanut butter, beer and raw mushrooms.[324] Several GE workers have been permanently disabled by PCB exposure.[325]

BOOK SABOTAGE

When the anti-pesticide book *Diet for a Poisoned Planet* was first published, the chemical lobby complained to the White House that the author:

> *". . . may pose a future threat to national security."*[326]

The chemical lobby and USDA persuaded TV and radio stations to cancel interviews with the author.[327] Former Surgeon General C. Everett Koop was persuaded to trash the book.[328] Vested interests, including the National Dairy Board, blocked media coverage of two other books: *Beyond Beef* and *Diet for a New America*.[329]

Agribusiness groups pressured the Troll Book Club to drop distribution of *Teenage Mutant Ninja Turtles: ABCs for a Better Planet* because it criticized pesticides and hormones.[330] The popular book *DuPont: Behind the Nylon Curtain* was pulled from publication because of pressure from DuPont.[331] The collusion of government, media and corporations to suppress information represents the real threat to national security.

LAWSUITS

Slander lawsuits against anti-pesticide writers are as old as *Silent Spring*, Rachel Carson's environmental classic. Veliscol Chemical Corporation (maker of DDT) sued Carson's publisher.[332] The editor of *Rachel's Environment and Health Weekly* was sued by a Monsanto scientist for quoting an EPA report critical of the scientist's methods.[333] The Clorox Corporation hired a PR firm which recommended filing slander lawsuits against anti-chlorine writers.[334]

Under the agricultural disparagement laws, journalists can be sued for educating the public on the risks of pesticides, hormones and food irradiation.[335] The agrichemical lobby promoted passage of these laws.[336] Such tactics do little to encourage open debate.

The suppression of information gives those in power license to operate with impunity. Our founding fathers well understood this corrupting influence and sought to insure freedom of the press through the Bill of Rights. Transnational conglomerates have been imperfect custodians of those ideals. When the day dawns that people can no longer speak out on matters of national concern, American blood will have been shed in vain.

Inherent conflict-of-interest is the reliable handmaiden of tainted reporting, hidden agendas and self-censorship. As long as vested interests monopolize media outlets, balanced coverage cannot exist, citizens cannot be informed and democracy cannot flourish. The time has come for direct action to safeguard the sovereign principles upon which this nation was founded.

Proposed Media Reform

- Transfer 20% of radio station licenses from corporate to non-profit ownership. Dedicate one hour of prime time on each TV network to independent public-interest programming.

- Fund non-commercial broadcasting by charging corporate TV and radio stations a commensurate license fee.

- Allow consumer groups, unions and advocacy organizations to advertise on TV and radio shows without network censorship.

- Require full financial disclosure of all TV spots, print ads, studies, surveys and video news releases.

- Require full financial disclosure of all TV, radio, newspaper and magazine ownership.

- Block government censorship of the Internet.

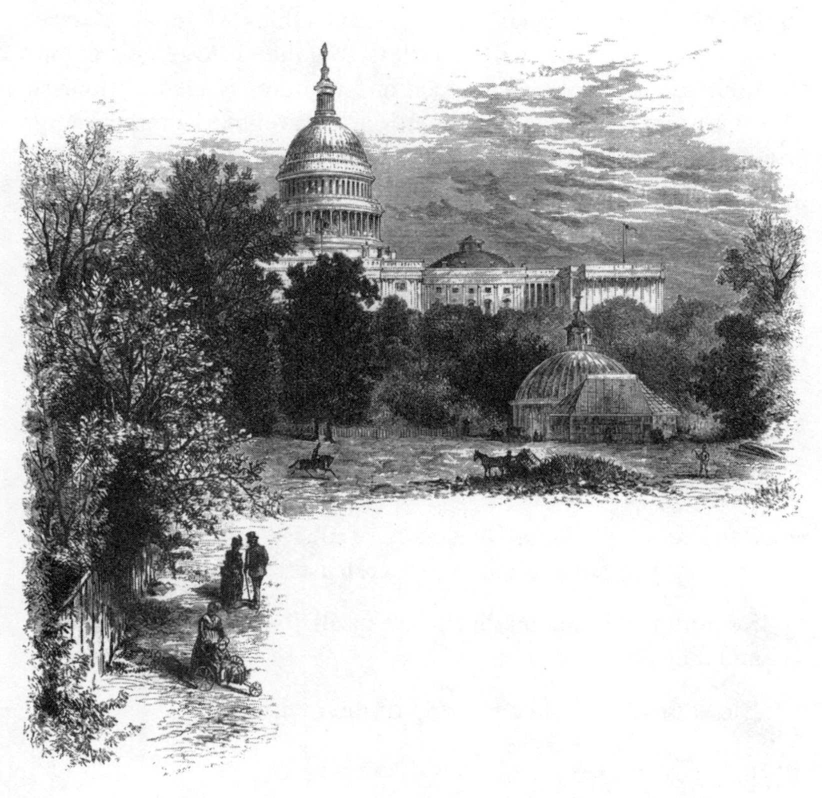

CHAPTER 8
Government

"Cherish, therefore, the spirit of the people and keep alive their attention...If once they become inattentive to public affairs, you and I, Congress and Assemblies, Judges and Governors, shall all become wolves."

—Thomas Jefferson

"It could probably be shown by facts and figures that there is no distinctly American criminal class except Congress."

—Mark Twain
Following the Equator, 1897

In 1846, construction began on Fort Jefferson, Florida, a garrison outpost designed to protect the nation's shores from marauding pirates and enemy ships. It was to be the "Gibraltar of America" and the largest unreinforced masonry structure in the country. The 50-foot-high walls surround an area the size of 20 football fields. With 400 cannons mounted in place and a building cost of $1.00 per brick, Fort Jefferson was an expensive proposition.

Unfortunately for the taxpayers, it was never used for military purposes. The fort was located so far inland that shallow waters prevented any ship from coming within cannon range.[1] Records are unclear on which contractors benefited from this fiasco. Valuable lesson: some things never change.

During the Vietnam War, our government reassured the Vietnamese people that America would be there if trouble ever came. They could always depend on us. When Saigon fell to the communists in 1972, thousands of Vietnamese all over the city climbed onto rooftops and looked skyward—waiting for the rescue helicopters that never came. More valuable lessons: not everything governments say is true, naiveté can be lethal, and rescue comes from no one but ourselves.

Much responsibility for the U.S. cancer rate lies at the doorstep of national institutions. During the 1970s, the Federal Housing Authority (FHA) required a home's foundation to be treated with the pesticide chlordane before a home loan would be approved. This mandate resulted in dying pets and convulsing babies attributed to chlordane's toxic residues.[2]

During the 1970s, insurance companies required their utility customers to use PCB transformers, thanks to aggressive marketing by the PCB manufacturers (General Electric and Westinghouse).[3] Certain banks and the Federal Crop Insurance Corporation require farmers to use pesticides. Current trade agreements (GATT) allow imported produce to contain 40 banned pesticides, including DDT levels up to 5,000% higher than allowed under U.S. laws.[4]

According to the *Wall Street Journal*, House Speaker Newt Gingrich helped launch the Progress and Freedom Foundation, a drug company supported group with the goal of giving private companies a larger role in self-regulation.[5]

By the year 2000, cancer will become America's top killer, while health-care costs are expected to rise from 15–19% of the GNP.[6] The current proclivity of Congress to roll back pesticide regulations will likely worsen cancer mortality, health-care spending and the national debt, thus damaging our competitive position in the global marketplace. Such policies seem inconsistent with national interest.

Lawmakers who advocate deregulating industrial polluters—under the guise of less government—may wish to consider public health implications in the corporate scheme of things. The self-regulation of pesticide, oil, drug and tobacco companies works to the detriment of most Americans.

Since the 13th century Magna Carta, common-law has held that property owners may not harm others through the use of property. The current political climate requires vigilance, lest Congress set aside this cornerstone of Western civilization. For the first time in human history, what we decide will simultaneously affect everyone everywhere.

LOBBIES

Environmental lobbies spend millions; corporate lobbies spend billions. A Sierra Club lobbyist can give each congressional candidate only $10,000. In contrast, a chemical industry lobbyist is backed by hundreds of companies, each of which can give that candidate $10,000.[7] Not exactly a level playing field considering that government policies favor the highest bidder.

When enormous sums of money are involved, corporate efforts to control public opinion recognize no boundaries. Public-relations representatives, skilled in the arts of deception and manipulation, apply their craft on the unwary. Powerful lobbies amass influence by holding sway over key powerbrokers and opinionmakers.

- John Dingell, Chairman of the House Energy Committee, has consistently fought against the Clean Air Act, electric car production, auto emission and fuel efficiency standards. Rep. Dingell's wife is a lobbyist for the auto industry.[8]

- Victor Neufeld, executive producer of ABC-TV's 20/20, aired shows promoting food irradiation and pesticides (while ridiculing environmental concerns). Mr. Neufeld's wife is a lobbyist for the nuclear and chemical industries.[9]

- Carol Foreman, founder of the Safe Food Coalition, helped defeat legislation which would have labeled dairy products containing bovine growth hormone (BGH). Foreman is a lobbyist for Monsanto, the maker of BGH.[10]

Corporate lobbies exclude the public voice from national debates, manipulate airwaves, undermine grassroot efforts, shield industries from accountability, secure favorable legislation and generally create mischief within the affairs of state.

Corporations exert greater control over the media in our country than in other countries because they have greater control over the politicians. A revolving door exists between former government officials and Washington lobbies. The government, corporations and media often march in ideological lockstep, inextricably intertwined by unseen forces. Information counters this troubling alliance by bridging the chasm between perception and reality.

In this age of unprecedented chemical assault, protection lies in knowing how the system works. By understanding the machinery's inner workings, citizens gain access to the controls.

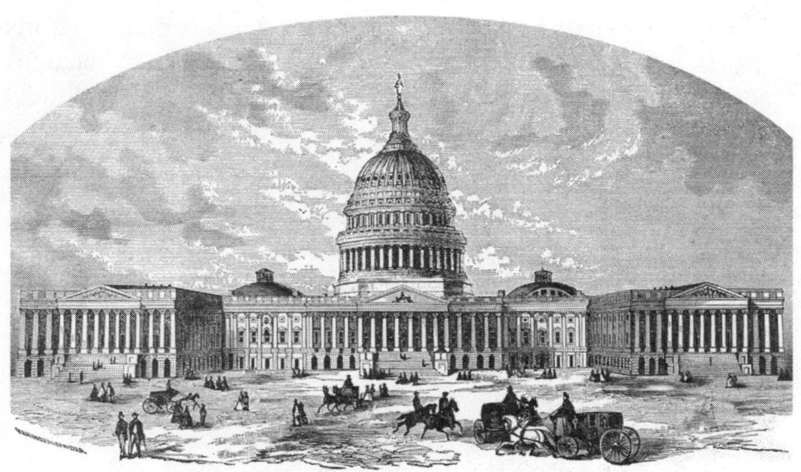

Campaign Finance Reform

"The government of the United States at present is a foster child of the special interests."
—Woodrow Wilson
campaign speech, 1912

"American politics is being held hostage by big money interests. . . . We believe it's long past time to clean up Washington."
—Bill Clinton and Al Gore
Putting People First

In 1833, a young French count named Alexis de Tocqueville visited America to witness first-hand this noble experiment in self-rule. In 1835, he published the first two volumes of his ponderous tome *Democracy in America* which described a fatal flaw, a self-destruct mechanism that would eventually lead to the downfall of this nation. Tocqueville predicted that someday Americans would realize they could have anything they wanted simply by voting for politicians who promised them anything they wanted. And from that day forward, good people would cease to exist in government.

Margaret Chase Smith served as U.S. Senator from 1949–1973. During her 24-year tenure, she observed that the caliber of people in office had declined substantially. We can safely assume a further decline since 1973. What de Tocqueville predicted and Senator Smith experienced has come to pass: a government of entrenched special interests romancing entrenched politicians...and a deepening disenchantment with the current political system.

> *"The definition of honesty in politics is staying bought once you're bought, and on Capital Hill we are, after all, honorable men."*
>
> —John L. Jackley
> *Hill Rat*

Holding elected office is no longer "the crowning achievement of one's career" as in the day of Rose Kennedy. Politicians are regarded today with the same loathing usually reserved for child molesters.

Recalcitrant politicians can be turned out by term limits and redistricting. But addressing the more fundamental problem of special interests is a far greater challenge. Vested industries have a long and nefarious history of altering events.

> *"Tobacco financed the American Revolution."*[11]
>
> —C. Everett Koop, M.D.

Railroad and livestock industries financed the slaughter of buffalo and the eradication of indigenous cultures.[12]

During the 1930s, America had one of the finest electric train systems in the world. A powerful consortium (General Motors, Standard Oil, Phillips Petroleum, Firestone Tire) financed the conversion of electric trains to GM diesel buses in 16 states.[13] GM was found guilty of criminal conspiracy in 1949, but continued replacing electric trains with diesels until 1955.[14]

The U.S. now lags behind all other industrialized nations in train electrification. The restructuring of society for corporate gain seldom furthers the greater common good. What's good for General Motors is not always good for the country.

THE POLITICS OF SAFE FOOD

Most Americans believe that federal agencies watch over the food supplies to insure their safety. But in fact, safe food is not always in the government's interest. The U.S. government is not a benevolent institution and consistently acts in its self-interest, even when that interest goes against the majority.

For example, it's clearly in the government's interest to safeguard healthy business profits, thereby ensuring expansion, greater employment and tax revenue. The best way to encourage business profits is by taking the side of business in every case. That's why the government was so quick to bailout Lockheed and so slow to stop acid rain. Pressure was applied both from union leaders fearful of losing jobs, and from business leaders fearful of losing profits.

American milk contains growth hormones; milk from Europe, Australia and New Zealand is hormone-free. U.S. beef contains antibiotics and hormones; European beef is drug-free. American cheeses contain dyes; Scandinavian cheeses are dye-free. Drugs, hormones, pesticides and dyes maintain healthy profits for the livestock, pharmaceutical and processed food industries—and healthy profits generate more taxes.

In fact, **all** decisions made by the FDA, EPA and USDA balance business profits against public health. How much will it cost business if a chemical is banned? How many people will die if it's not banned? What's the minimal acceptable risk? Consumers are on the receiving end of those decisions.

The meat, egg and dairy industries spend millions on campaign contributions—with strings attached. Their strategy paid off with the delayed release of weak dietary guidelines: avoid too much fat, saturated fat and cholesterol. The following communication was sent to Ronald Reagan's Secretary of Agriculture:

> *"Midwest Egg Producers endorsed Ronald Reagan's campaign for the presidency primarily in response to the Carter Administration's promotion of [these] dietary guidelines."*[15]
>
> —Midwest Egg Producers Association

The pharmaceutical industry uses campaign contributions to avoid regulation by the FDA:

> *"Every time we proposed action [against the farm use of antibiotics], it was Congress that directed us to do other things, or to withhold further action . . ."*[16]
>
> —Richard Teske, director
> FDA Center for Veterinary Medicine

Through campaign contributions, corporations subvert both foreign and domestic policy. In 1981, the World Health Organization adopted the "International Code of Marketing of Breast Milk Substitutes," which prevented infant formula companies from handing out promotional samples to new mothers. Of the 118 nations voting on the code, only the U.S. voted against it because of lobbying pressure from industry.[17]

DOMESTIC POLICY INFLUENCE

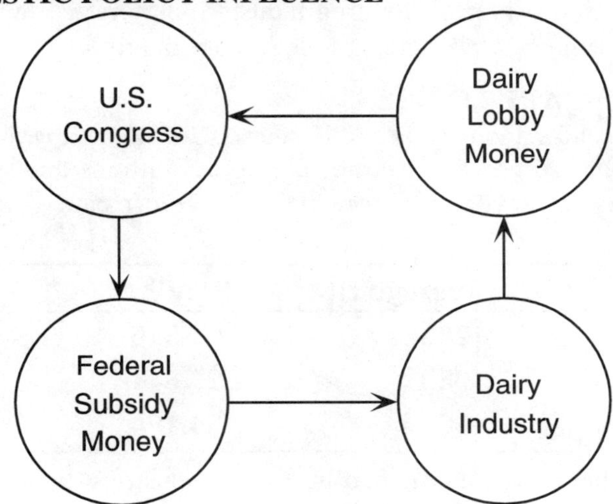

FOREIGN POLICY INFLUENCE

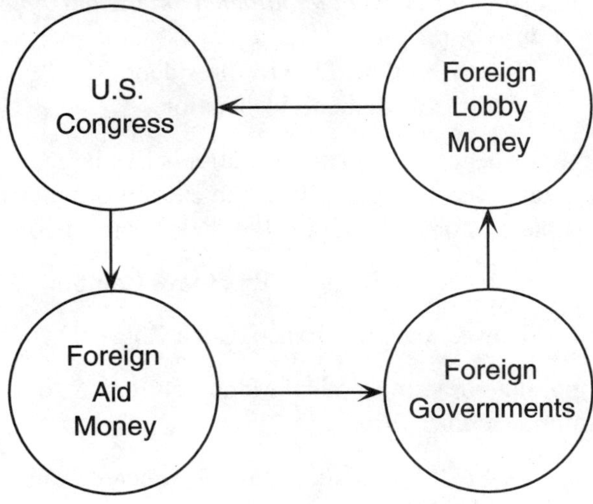

Washington's 20,000 registered lobbyists wield their enormous power by taking advantage of the system. But the system carries a heavy price: a government out of touch with its people and the lowest voter turnout of any democratic nation. Corruption creates voter apathy; voter apathy leaves corruption to reign.

While in office, Vice President George Bush lobbied the IRS for tax breaks on behalf of the drug industry, his former employer.[18] Certain members of Congress are legendary in this area.

HEALTH-CARE LOBBIES

The cancer industry is big business. Chemotherapy, radiation therapy and surgery cost billions, employ millions and generate enormous tax revenues. More people live off cancer than die from it.

Average Hospital Stay[19]	
1965	$316
1980	$1,844
1988	$4,194

In 1994, the medical, drug and insurance industries dominated the President's Task Force on National Health-Care Reform.

> *"The AMA has had good access to the administration... We have also had reasonable influence on the outcome of the final draft of the plan."*[20]
>
> —James Todd, M.D., vice president
> American Medical Association

Under Clinton's health-care plan, the nation's five largest insurance companies would have reaped billions in extra profits. Influence is revealed by the corporate affiliations of their board members:

- Aetna—Philip Morris Tobacco, Proctor & Gamble
- CIGNA—Dow Chemical, Texaco, Coca Cola
- Metropolitan—Pharmaceutical Manufacturers of America, Monsanto, Mobil
- Prudential—Pfizer Pharmaceuticals, American Cyanamid
- Traveler's—Shell Oil, Chrysler

Alternative health-care plans, which would save billions, are rarely mentioned by the national media. (Several *New York Times* board members have financial ties to insurance or drug companies.)

Pharmaceuticals are the most profitable of the Fortune 500 companies for three reasons: government-funded research, tax breaks and markups. Americans pay the highest drug prices in the Western world. In 1992, nine of the top ten Senate recipients of pharmaceutical campaign contributions voted to kill a bill aimed at reducing tax breaks for profiteering drug firms.[21]

Annual health-care spending currently exceeds $940 billion ($3,160 for each American).[22] During the 1980s, health-care costs more than doubled while Congress made little effort to reform the system. During the same decade, medical groups invested more than $60 million in congressional candidates.[23]

Our beleaguered Medicare system (heading for bankruptcy by the year 2002) stems from a government more concerned with the next election than with long-term strategic planning. Blaming politicians, however, is less productive than actually changing national priorities—a seemingly impossible task given the current realities of campaign finance.

> *"Pledges to clean up the nation's campaign financing procedures notwithstanding, Mr. Clinton has expended more energy courting well-to-do donors at fancy private receptions than prodding Congress to enact serious political reform."*[24]
>
> —*New York Times*

Nearly 33% of former House members work for Washington lobbies, and 47% of former trade negotiation staffers work for foreign governments. The magnitude of this problem calls for real reform, not tinkering.

Our level of government corruption and conflict-of-interest is not permitted by other industrialized nations. U.S. politicians extract contributions from the richest 2% of corporate elite and then purport to serve the people.

The financial advantage of House and Senate incumbents over their challengers is the greatest single threat to democracy. In 1992, Congress collected over $672 million in campaign contributions from special interest PACs (political action committees).

1992 Elections[25]	Average Expenditures	PAC Contributions
House Incumbents	$582,330	$261,976
House Challengers	$154,607	$27,621
Senate Incumbents	$4,177,459	$1,366,423
Senate Challengers	$1,753,398	$235,982

AID TO DEPENDENT CORPORATIONS[26]

- From 1985–1992, nuclear industry PACs (Westinghouse, G.E.) spent $14 million in return for $84 billion in subsidies.
- From 1985–1991, coal and oil PACs spent $26 million in return for $145 billion in subsidies.
- From 1987–1992, timber PACs spent $7 million in return for $1.5 billion in subsidies.
- From 1987–1993, cattle PACs (Chevron, Texaco) spent $1 million in return for $364 million in grazing subsidies.
- From 1987–1994, mining industry PACs spent $17 million in return for $26 billion worth of precious minerals extracted from public lands—without paying royalties or cleanup costs.
- From 1991–1994, pesticide PACs gave Congress $3.8 million in return for blocking tougher pesticide legislation.
- From 1987–1994, dirty water PACs gave Congress $56.9 million in return for blocking tougher clean water legislation.

Wealthy corporations reap profits from 153 federal programs at an estimated annual cost of $167 billion ($1,388 per U.S. taxpayer). Citizens have reason to feel disenchanted with the current system.

While politicians talk of deficit reduction, entrenched special interests marshal their resources to block reform. History suggests our government is ill-prepared to counter these forces. Politicians respond to economic pressures first, political pressures second and ethics last. Only through campaign reform will corporations be weaned from feeding at the public trough.

Campaign contributions jeopardize our representative system of government, a concept politicians have been slow to grasp. During the 1980s, Congress pressured regulators to overlook questionable loan practices by the savings and loan industry—in return for campaign contributions. The resulting S&L crisis cost taxpayers dearly.

When President Reagan left office, he was paid $2 million by the Tujisankei Corporation for two 20-minute speeches.[27] The Japanese wanted to express their appreciation for 8 years of favorable trade relations. Under Reagan, entire national forests were sold to Japan for $1.00 per tree.

ILLUSION

Voters realize there's often little difference between Democratic and Republican candidates. Both drink from the tainted waters of legalized bribery; both are wings on the same bird of prey. Political handlers also know this and consequently promote image, rather than issues. Content and substance have given way to style, illusion and candidacy by soundbite.

The 1988 election brought us images of George Bush holding an American flag ("Don't let it touch the ground"), and Michael Dukakis driving a tank. Expensive image-building advertising dominates contemporary American politics. Money, rather than issues, determines the outcome of most political races.[28]

The mass media profits from the current system by collecting millions from candidates ($230 million in 1990 for TV alone). Spending caps on congressional races would directly cut media profits. Institutions heavily supported by the current system will likely resist reforming the system.

POLITICAL PARTIES

Most Americans favor environmental protection, reduced defense spending, abortion choice, gun registration, and the separation of church and state—views not shared by the Republican Party.

Most Americans favor the balanced budget amendment, welfare limits, immigration control, and the English language—views not shared by the Democratic Party.

Most Americans feel disenfranchised by **both** political parties. Campaign contributions by extremist elements have left most Americans without adequate representation.

"There is no group in America that can withstand the force of an aroused public opinion."

—Franklin D. Roosevelt, 1933

This nation was founded on a single cherished ideal: the sovereign right of the people to govern themselves. We hold our forefather's legacy and our children's future in trust. At this moment in history, with the government no longer answerable to its people, America has reached a turning point: democracy itself is at stake.

Public opinion is clear. Americans want clean government, decisions made for the national good, and a Congress with the taxpayer's interest at heart. Ordinary citizens feel powerless under the current system because they are powerless under the current system.

Americans know what needs to be done. The time has come to take our country back.

NATIONAL CAMPAIGN FINANCE REFORM

☒ Prohibit all fundraising by political candidates and parties.

☒ Ban all campaign contributions to candidates and political parties, including gifts, honorariums and travel expenses.

☒ Ban all spending by candidates and parties, including billboards,TV ads, posters, bumper stickers, mailings and charity donations.

☒ Prohibit private spending for and against candidates.

☒ Provide public financing for national campaigns including at least 30 mandatory televised debates—issue-oriented with audience participation. (Require major TV networks to share the cost.)

☒ Prohibit former members of Congress and executive branch officials from lobbying for 10 years after leaving office.

☒ Eliminate the business tax deduction for lobbying expenses.

STRATEGY FOR REFORM

Despite years of work by dedicated grassroots organizations (Common Cause, Public Citizen) Congress has refused to consider serious campaign finance reform. To continue this approach perpetuates futility. Congress will never give up power voluntarily. Congress will never change the system. Only the American people can change it—a new strategy is called for.

True campaign finance reform must come through the initiative process at the federal level enacted by Constitutional amendment. The initiative would bypass Congress and become the fourth branch—the people's branch—of government. A national movement to recall the House and Senate speakers would convince Congress that people are serious.

INITIATIVE FRAUD

The initiative process has its pitfalls. Philip Morris Tobacco placed a pro-smoking referendum on the California ballot by setting up a front group called Californians for State Smoking Restrictions.[29] Billboards read, "Yes on 188—Tough Statewide Smoking Restrictions—The Right Choice." But in fact, a yes vote would have mandated smoking areas by outlawing local anti-smoking ordinances.[30] Nazi propagandist Joseph Goebbels would have delighted in this initiative, the legal equivalent of razor blades in Halloween candy.

The tobacco industry fights public-smoking bans by conducting fraudulent surveys through several front groups—Restaurants for a Sensible Voluntary Policy, California Business and Restaurant Alliance—with no disclosure of funding sources.[31] Valuable lessons can be learned from these examples. Without effective safeguards, similar deceptive tactics would likely occur at the federal level.

Proposed Initiative Safeguards

- Require organizations sponsoring initiatives to identify their major sponsors.
- Require groups conducting initiative advertising, telemarketing, mail solicitations, or surveys to identify their funding sources.
- Conduct spot-checks of initiative circulators to insure honest representation.
- Prohibit foreign governments and multinational corporations from sponsoring U.S. initiatives.

A second source of initiative deception is Congress itself. Any member of Congress who votes for an initiative which requires **approval of Congress** should be recalled by the voters.

The initiative process at the federal level would open the door to several areas currently off-limits to citizens. These areas include:

- Congressional salary, staff and spending cuts
- Corporate welfare and foreign aid cuts
- National referendum voting
- Proportional representation

In our democracy, no political force has more power than ordinary citizens working together with conviction for the common good. Grassroots America drives major political reform. No well-oiled campaign machine can defy an aroused electorate.

As long as power rests with entrenched special interests, there's much work to be done. The arrogance of big money has no place in a true democracy. The purging of corruption from our nation's core will be the average citizen's finest hour.

Let us now put our house in order and change the course of history on a global scale. Future generations deserve no less.

> *"The basis of our political systems is the right of the people to make and alter their constitutions of government."*
>
> —George Washington
> Farewell Address, 1796

> *"This country, with its institutions, belongs to the people who inhabit it. Whenever they shall grow weary of the existing government, they can exercise their constitutional right of amending it, or their revolutionary right to dismember or overthrow it."*
>
> —Abraham Lincoln
> Inaugural Address, 1861

> *"I just received the following wire from my generous Daddy—'Dear Jack. Don't buy a single vote more than necessary. I'll be damned if I'm going to pay for a landslide.'"*[32]
>
> —John F. Kennedy
> campaign speech, 1958

Health-Care Reform

"We must make this our most urgent priority, give every American health-care security, health-care that can never be taken away, health-care that is always there."[33]

—Bill Clinton

"Think of health-care reform as throwing a trillion-dollar pot of gold up for grabs."[34]

—Joseph Califano, former Secretary
Health, Education and Welfare

At the turn of the century, numerous health-care systems coexisted in America: homeopathy, naturopathy, chiropractic, osteopathy, herbology and others. Choices were many and the U.S. was among the healthiest of nations. Campaign contributions from medical and drug lobbies changed all that.

In 1920, Congress endorsed the Flexner Report on Medical Education (funded by Rockefeller and drug companies) which proclaimed allopathic medicine to be superior. Strict licensing laws eradicated or downgraded the other disciplines to "alternative" status.

For over 75 years, health-care reform has been one of the grand pieces of unfinished business on America's agenda. When Clinton's health-care proposal died in September 1994, it marked the sixth time this century that reformers failed to enact national health insurance.[35]

The U.S. has the finest health-care system in the world in terms of high-tech procedures—not in terms of cost, access, or life expectancy. About 40 million Americans are uninsured; others stay with undesirable jobs to maintain their coverage. The General Accounting Office estimates we waste at least $100 billion yearly to fraud and overbilling.[36] Private administrators waste another $70 billion.[37] Without reform, health-care costs could skyrocket from 15–19% of the gross national product by the year 2000.[38] Only through dramatic and sustained spending reductions will we cure the U.S. medical system.

Clinton's proposal to increase health-care spending by $100–150 billion each year[39] was less than well received. Such rarefied blank-check proclivity gives pause for concern. Politicians have a reputation for feathering their nests while looking with favor to special interests intent on dividing the spoils. Health-care reform is no exception.

Americans utilize alternative practitioners more than conventional primary care physicians.[40] The medical system loses nearly $14 billion each year to unconventional therapies. More patients are taking responsibility for their health, and fewer patients view doctors as exalted deities—a historic shift somehow overlooked by the Clinton Administration.

The Clinton plan mandated a 3.5–7% payroll tax covering allopathic medicine exclusively. This plan required patients using inexpensive, alternative remedies to subsidize high-tech procedures. Forced participation in conventional medicine is not the answer. Consumers have a fundamental right to the care that best suits their needs. Clinton's plan offered fewer choices than the current system; the single payer plan offers fewer choices still. The noble goal of universal coverage diametrically opposes choice.

Optimal health-care reform fosters more choices, lower taxes and less government. Reckless spending and vast layers of bureaucracy have brought our nation to the brink of financial ruin. A government large enough to give us everything we want is expensive enough to take everything we have—a concept politicians have been loathe to grasp.

Squandering our resources for a perverted health-care system is inconsistent with national security. A nation's ability to control costs is central to its ability to self-govern. History may judge us harshly if we fail. At first glance, it seems difficult to simultaneously reduce costs, increase access, improve quality, and lower taxes. Yet that is the goal, an end achievable only by addressing the underlying cause.

America's gargantuan medical costs arise from for-profit hospitals and fee-for-service specialists prescribing unnecessary high-risk interventions to insured patients suffering from preventable afflictions. Add overpriced drugs, predatory conglomerates, profiteering insurance companies, cavalier fiscal leadership, inherent conflict-of-interest, and stir. A recipe for disaster.

To curb abuse, each element must be dealt with decisively—banish waste, encourage competition, offer incentives for self-care and prevention. Critical milestones to keep in sight as the journey of national reform unfolds.

PROPOSED HEALTH-CARE REFORM

- Convert fee-for-service hospitals and for-profit HMOs into non-profit HMOs modeled after Kaiser Permanente. Pay HMO doctors a salary and offer stock options as an incentive to control costs. (The lower the costs, the more doctors earn.)
- Offer an enrollment option for catastrophic care only. Set premiums according to known risk factors (tobacco use, cholesterol, blood pressure, body fat) and offer cash back to patients who don't use their deductible.
- Offer an enrollment option for accident coverage only. Under this plan, medical treatments involving illness would be paid by the patient on a per-use basis.
- Encourage community hospitals by eliminating the Joint Commission on Accreditation of Health-Care Organizations.[41]
- Amend the Nurses Practices Act. License advanced specialty nurses to provide outpatient primary care, nurse-run community clinics, hospital admitting and prescriptive authority.[42]
- License midwives in all states. Require insurance companies to cover nursing and midwifery services.
- Eliminate insurance compensation for cancer and heart disease treatments which fail to improve survival.
- Reduce administrative costs by prohibiting health-care providers in private practice from accepting third-party payments. (Patients would pay their providers; insurance companies would reimburse the patients.)
- Repeal insurance company exemptions from anti-trust laws.
- Permit unconventional (non-medical) cancer clinics to operate in the U.S. without government interference or "peer" discrimination.
- Require informed consent laws to disclose the limitations of conventional and non-medical treatments.
- Expand the Patient Protection Act to include comparison information on all health insurance plans.

- Expand the National Practitioner Data Bank to include comparison information on all conventional and non-medical providers, treatments, outcomes and prices.[43]
- Require full financial disclosure of physician-owned laboratories in which the referring physician has an equity interest.
- Prohibit the patenting of medical procedures.
- Encourage self-care using doctor-staffed toll-free hotlines, consumer-initiated literature searches, fax-on-demand and on-line self-help groups.
- Allow consumers access to their medical records. Permit laboratory diagnostic tests without prescriptions.
- Lower drug prices by allowing the importation, promotion and sale of foreign-made drugs without prescription (except Schedule I and II narcotics).
- Halt taxpayer funding of drug research (NIH grants and tax credits) leading to additional drug company profits. Amend the Orphan Drug Act.
- Restrict "pain and suffering" malpractice settlements.
- Issue vouchers to Medicare and Medicaid recipients to buy private insurance. Raise the Medicare eligibility age to 70.
- Eliminate motorcycle helmet laws. (Spinal cord injuries cost more than funerals.)
- Allow individual tax-free medical savings accounts (medical IRAs) to be used without penalty for health-care expenses.
- Provide a 100% tax credit for day-care expenses to all working parents.
- Offer tax breaks to health-care professionals who provide medical care for low-income patients.
- Eliminate the tax-exempt status of churches; offer tax breaks to churches which provide food, clothing and shelter for low-income citizens.

- Block licensing moves by the American Dietetic Association to give registered dietitians a monopoly to provide nutritional advice.
- Ban tobacco advertising, cigarette vending machines and smoking in public places. Fund adequate prenatal care by raising the cigarette tax. (Each prenatal $1 invested saves $3.50 in special education and Medicaid costs.)[44]
- Allow the sale of nicotine gum and patches to smokers without prescription.
- Lift the ban on clean needle exchanges. Fund drug education and rehabilitation programs by raising the alcohol tax.
- Limit hospital services to American citizens, legal visitors and legal immigrants.
- Amend the 14th Amendment to limit U.S. citizenship to children born of U.S. citizens.
- Require each birth certificate to include the father's name, and hold the father responsible.

Until we restructure the fundamental meaning and basis of health-care, until we eliminate the fee-for-service system, prevention will continue to receive only lipservice—a divisive folly this nation can ill afford.

> *"The health of the people is really the foundation upon which all their happiness and all their powers as a state depend."*
> —Benjamin Disraeli

The EPA

"The public perceives its interests are not being looked at because of the process we have to follow, and my sympathies are with the public."[45]

—Jack Moore
former EPA deputy administrator

After Cleveland's Cayahoga River caught fire in 1969, Congress passed the Clean Water Act, the Clean Air Act, and the Toxic Substances Control Act. But after spending billions of tax dollars since EPA's inception, the dream of a clean environment remains elusive.

In 1970, Congress gave the Environmental Protection Agency authority to set maximum tolerance levels for pesticide residues in food. The EPA also establishes maximum chemical levels for water and air. These are critical responsibilities upon which public health depends. Unfortunately the EPA's record of balancing corporate interests with public interests seems a less-than-stellar model of evenhandedness.

WATER QUALITY

In 1990, about one-third of America's rivers, half its estuaries and half its lakes were unsafe for swimming and fishing.[46] Lake Ontario is so full of chemicals it develops photographs.[47] In 1992, 20% of Americans consumed water contaminated with unlawfully high levels of toxic chemicals.[48] More than 700 pollutants are detected in U.S. drinking water, including pesticides, solvents and radioactive substances.[49] At least 35 pesticides leached into the groundwaters of 35 states.[50] Herbicides are found in Midwestern rain, snow and fog.

In 1986, the EPA approved the use of weed killer (Sonar) in drinking-water reservoirs even though one of its breakdown products (monomethyl formamide) persists in water and causes severe birth defects.[51]

In 1988, Monsanto dumped its never-registered herbicide (Machete) into the Mississippi River.[52] The Procter & Gamble pulp mill in Perry, Florida, discharges 50 million gallons of chlorinated effluent into the Fenholloway River each day.[53]

INDOOR AIR QUALITY

In 1987, the EPA began installing 27,000 square yards of new carpeting in its Washington headquarters. At least 1,141 EPA employees have since become ill while EPA officials refused to even acknowledge the problem. EPA scientists have taken their employer to court over this issue.

> *"We now have a health emergency at EPA headquarters with adverse health effects likely in the long-term among EPA employees."*[54]
>
> —Mark Bradley, M.D.

EPA air quality studies established a link between carpet emissions and health problems among its employees[55] Yet the EPA denies the association between toxic carpet emissions and ill health.[56] At least 1,000 chemicals are used in carpeting.[57]

Thousands of people including infants have developed severe neurological reactions to toxic carpet emissions. But despite the well-documented hazard, carpet chemicals remain unregulated. In fact, the EPA, the Consumer Product Safety Commission and carpet industry launched a public relations campaign promoting the safety of carpeting.[58]

Indoor air pollution is a public health issue that touches everyone. Over 100 employees at Harvey's Casino at Lake Tahoe were sickened by pesticide applications at their workplace.[59] Neurotoxic chemicals can permanently damage brain and nerve function.[60] A good thing to keep in mind the next time your home or workplace is sprayed.

There are many reasons why the EPA has failed in its mission to clean up America. Foremost among them is conflict-of-interest: the revolving door between EPA officials and the industries they regulate. EPA chief William Ruckelshaus joined Union Carbide after leaving his EPA position.[61] Environmental protection tends to suffer when careers are at stake.

> *"[I am] mad that some scientists are saying that dioxin is the most deadly chemical known to man. That's not true. It depends on the concentration. In the right concentration, table salt is just as deadly."*[62]
>
> —Rita Lavelle
> former Superfund administrator

In 1991, the EPA reassessed dioxin toxicity based on flawed research suggesting that dioxin was less dangerous than previously thought. This research was funded by the chlorine and paper industries, which produce dioxins as byproducts.[63] Increased pollution during the 12-year Reagan-Bush administration may have caused an estimated 600,000 additional U.S. cancers.[64]

The EPA recently published *The Environmental Consumer's Handbook*, which describes non-toxic alternatives to conventional cleaning products. Despite the handbook's popularity, the EPA halted distribution because of pressure from industry.[65]

THE POLITICS OF OZONE

Each chlorine atom will destroy 100,000 ozone molecules. EPA head William Reilly led the push to replace ozone-destroying CFCs (chlorofluorocarbons) with ozone-damaging HCFCs.[66] DuPont manufactures both and profited handsomely from this conversion. After leaving the EPA, Reilly joined the board of directors of DuPont.[67]

The U.S. now lags behind Europe in developing ozone-safe technology. Westinghouse offers ozone-safe refrigeration in Europe, but not America. The incestuous relationship between government officials and corporations is not in our nation's best interest.

At least 70,000 chemicals are used commercially with another 700 added each year.[68] Most industrial chemicals have never been tested for adverse health effects.[69] Many are known carcinogens or neurotoxins allowed by the EPA. Examples:

- Nail polish remover contains toluene.
- Room deodorizers and mothballs contain para-dichlorobenzene.
- Dry-cleaned clothes contain perchloroethylene.

Humans are designed to easily handle small amounts of toxins for short time periods. However, the cumulative exposure to low-level chemicals—a whiff of formaldehyde here, a splash of benzene there—can eventually damage even the strongest immune system.

Studies estimate that 15% of Americans are hypersensitive to common household chemicals,[70] and 7–17% of health-care workers are allergic to latex.[71] Autoimmune and environmental illnesses are commonplace. For many of these disorders, there's no real cure—only prevention, avoidance and remission.

In this era of acceptable risk, how deep a person swims in the chemical soup ultimately determines long-term health. Individuals can either sleep in the backseat while the government drives or take responsibility for the food, water and air entering their body. Placing that trust with politicians may carry a heavy price.

All things are connected. The act of taking responsibility carries the power to change who you are and the world around you. And once you see the clarity of the game, once you raise your awareness and make your stand, there's no turning back. You will not stand alone.

> *"Dear Mr. President. Please will you do something to stop pollution? I want to keep on living till I am 100 years old."*[72]
> —Melissa Poe, age 9

Proposed EPA Reform

- Prohibit former EPA officials from joining the industries they regulated for 10 years after leaving government service.
- Give citizens the right to sue polluters for damages. Impose prison terms on business executives who violate pollution control laws.
- Prohibit the use of pesticides in or near drinking-water.
- Phase-out ozone-depleting chemicals by 1998 (CFCs, HCFCs, halons, methyl bromide, methyl chloroform and carbon tetrachloride).
- Phase-out greenhouse gases (HFCs) and enact a carbon tax on fossil fuels. Phase-out diesel-powered cars and trains.
- Support ozone-safe refrigeration technology (Greenfreeze).

What You Can Do

- Buy non-toxic cleaning products, garden supplies, furniture and building materials.
- Advocate train electrification, electric vehicles and more bicycle paths.

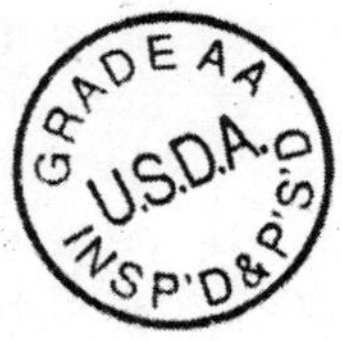

The USDA

"The best sources of calcium in the United States are milk, yogurt and cheese. Everyone should include two servings of milk, yogurt and cheese daily."
—U.S. Department of Agriculture

When Abraham Lincoln created the U.S. Department of Agriculture in 1862 to develop the best seeds, it had 9 employees. Today the USDA has grown to the most far-reaching agency in government with the fourth largest budget and over 120,000 employees.[73]

The USDA's 1992 budget of $78 billion roughly equaled the value of all U.S. crops.[74] No one knows how many employees or offices the USDA has, not even the Secretary of Agriculture.[75] Past efforts by Congress to downsize the USDA have seen little success.

PROMOTION BOARDS

The USDA is mandated to increase the consumption of agricultural products through the national promotion boards. These boards are created by Congress and regulated by the USDA. Each board collects an assessment from its members backed by the full power of the USDA.

- Cattlemen's Beef Promotion and Research Board ($1.00/head of cattle sold)
- National Dairy Promotion and Research Board (15 cents/100 pounds of milk sold)
- National Pork Board (35 cents/$100.00 sold)
- American Egg Board (5 cents/30 dozen eggs sold)

The boards use this money to fund their advertising campaigns. Examples:

- Beef. Real food for real people.
- Everybody needs milk.
- Pork. The other white meat.
- The incredible edible egg.

YOUR TAX DOLLARS AT WORK

The USDA and promotion boards spend an estimated $500 million each year influencing consumers, nutritionists and doctors. Board-sponsored studies appear in several medical journals. The Egg Board sponsored research claiming that cholesterol restriction has little effect on most diets.[76] The Dairy Board funds studies claiming that calcium prevents cancer,[77] osteoporosis,[78] and hypertension.[79] The Dairy Board conducted campaigns promoting growth hormones in milk.

McDonald's, General Mills, Miller beer and other corporations receive millions from the USDA to promote their products overseas.[80] The beef and dairy industries receive about $23 billion annually in government price support and subsidy programs.[81] The USDA sells water to cattlemen at below-market rates. Over half of U.S. water is used for livestock. USDA farm subsidy programs encourage fraud and waste.

The USDA spends $3–4 billion each year buying surplus foods for the school lunch program. In 1991, 90% of these foods were butter, cheese, whole milk, eggs, beef and pork—all high in fat.[82] This guarantees profits for the meat and dairy industries. Schools are required to offer whole milk. The USDA distributed these same high-fat foods to the Pima Indians of Arizona, thus contributing to their incidence of diabetes, the highest in the world. Taxpayers are then asked to pay for the health problems created by these foods.

The USDA's Rural Electrification Administration provides below-market rate loans to electric utilities. This program subsidizes waste and pollution with no incentive for energy efficiency. The USDA artificially doubles domestic sugar prices using import quotas and price support programs.

CAMPAIGN CONTRIBUTIONS AT WORK

The House Agriculture Committee, which oversees USDA programs, received nearly $3.8 million in campaign contributions from agricultural interests between 1991–1993. The following were the top 20 contributors:[83]

1) Associated Milk Producers
2) ConAgra
3) Nabisco
4) American Veterinary Medicine Association
5) Chicago Mercantile Exchange
6) American Crystal Sugar Corporation
7) Mid-America Dairymen
8) American Sugarbeet Growers Association
9) Philip Morris Tobacco
10) National Rural Electric Co-op Association
11) Farm Credit Council
12) National Cotton Council
13) Food Marketing Institute
14) American Association of Crop Insurers
15) National Cattlemen's Association
16) National Broiler Council
17) Chicago Board of Trade
18) National Pork Producers Council
19) Southern Minnesota Beet Sugar Co-op
20) American Meat Institute

PESTICIDES

During the 1960s, the USDA stepped up its efforts to promote pesticides. Farmers responded by tripling their pesticide use to 500 million pounds each year.[84] Pesticide residues concentrate in high-fat foods, especially meat and milk.

When milk is recalled by state regulators due to pesticide contamination, the USDA compensates dairy farmers. This creates an incentive for dairy farmers to purchase the cheapest feed available, feed that may be contaminated. Heptachlor-laced milk was sold to the public at least twice as a direct result of pesticide-contaminated feed.[85]

CLOSE INDUSTRY TIES

Nowhere is conflict-of-interest more apparent than in the USDA's regulation of meat. The USDA Food Safety and Inspection Service, which administers federal meat inspections, was recently headed by a trustee from the Live Stock Industry Institute.[86] The USDA Marketing and Inspection Services was formerly headed by Jo Ann Smith, past president of the National Cattlemen's Association, the National Live Stock and Meat Board, and the Beef Board.[87]

In recent years, USDA meat inspections have been "streamlined" with fewer inspectors, higher production line speeds and lower health standards. Much media attention has focused on the recent deaths caused by salmonella and E. coli in tainted beef. Salmonella poisonings claim 2,000 lives annually.[88] Faced with a lawsuit, the USDA established a telephone hotline and placed warning labels on packaged meats.[89]

> *"I have seen abscesses full of green pus and pathological lesions that were perhaps tumors or cysts."*[90]
>
> —Bill Lehman
> USDA meat inspector

Congress has given the USDA inherently contradictory mandates: to both promote and regulate agricultural products. In light of rising health-care costs, the time has come for some needed changes at the USDA.

Proposed USDA Reform

- Appoint an independent USDA office closure commission to downsize the USDA bypassing Congress.
- Cut USDA ties to all promotion boards.
- Eliminate livestock, poultry, egg, feed grain, sugar, dairy and tobacco subsidies.
- Prohibit compensation to dairy farmers for contaminated milk.
- Prohibit fast-food restaurants from accepting food stamps.
- Restructure the farm subsidy programs to encourage sustainable agriculture.

Food Safety

"What disturbs me is that people think the Food and Drug Administration is protecting them. It isn't. What the FDA is doing and what people think they are doing are as different as night and day."[91]

—Dr. Herbert Ley, Jr.
former FDA Commissioner

"The federal government's decision-making process for pesticides does not pay sufficient attention to the protection of public health. . . ."[92]

—Philip Landrigan, M.D.
National Research Council

Each year, the USDA spends about $558 million on federal meat and poultry inspectors, yet its consumer safety record falls somewhat short of perfection. Each year, foodborne illnesses kill about 9,000 Americans and sicken another 6.5–80 million, mostly from contaminated meat and poultry.[93] Several USDA-approved chickens were found to be putrid. The USDA now wants chicken feces defined as an acceptable part of the diet—to prevent imposing a hardship on the poultry industry.[94] The General Accounting Office criticized the USDA's inspection methods.[95] Taxpayers, it seems, are not getting their money's worth.

Most American consume 150 micrograms of pesticide residues and PCBs each day.[96] Evidence suggests these chemicals mimic the body's estrogens, disrupt reproductive function and contribute to cancer. The EPA does not test for hormone disrupting chemicals.

If the U.S. is ever to be competitive in the global marketplace, it must weigh the costs of foodborne illnesses, cancers, reproductive disorders and environmental afflictions against the costs of prevention. Dollar costs represent tragedies without the tears. The loss of trust by the American people in their government is one cost that cannot be calculated. Prevention is indeed less expensive.

THE CURRENT SYSTEM

- The EPA sets maximum limits for pesticide residues in whole and processed foods.
- The FDA enforces those limits. The FDA also regulates additives, food irradiation, dietary supplements and antibiotic residues in milk.
- The USDA regulates agricultural production and administers national organic standards.

In Belgium, the legal limit for dioxins in milk is 8 parts per million. Based on this, nearly all milk sold in the U.S. would be unfit for sale there.[97] The U.S. legal limit for heptachlor in milk is twice the level allowed by the World Health Organization.[98]

In setting maximum pesticide limits, the EPA assumes each adult eats no more than 7½ ounces **per year** of either avocados, artichokes, eggplants, melons, mushrooms, nectarines, squash, cantaloupe, or Brussels sprouts.[99] These levels were set decades ago.

The FDA inspects only 1% of the nation's produce shipments and has no authority to delay shipments pending analysis results. The FDA tests for only half of the 600 commonly used pesticides and usually recommends against fines when violations are discovered.[100]

The National Academy of Sciences found the current system lacking in protecting children against pesticides.[101] The General Accounting Office (GAO) reported the current system inadequate in protecting against drug residues in milk and unsafe chemicals in food.[102]

In 1984, the House Committee on Government Operations concluded that the EPA violated its own regulations by not removing toxic pesticides from use.[103] In 1994, the House Subcommittee on Human Resources and Intergovernmental Relations criticized the FDA's food safety efforts.[104]

The Senate Committee on Government Affairs cited glaring deficiencies in U.S. food safety.[105] It stated there was no rationale to justify maintaining separate, inconsistent and fragmented food regulatory agencies. The Vice President's Food Safety Working Group and the GAO both recommended a unified food safety system.

Proposed Food Safety Reform

- Establish an independent food safety agency (FSA).
- Transfer the EPA's pesticide tolerance functions to the FSA.
- Transfer the FDA's dietary supplement and food regulatory functions to the FSA.
- Transfer the USDA's food regulatory functions to the FSA including:
  —Food Safety and Inspection Service
  —Federal Grain Inspection Service
  —Animal and Plant Health Inspection Service
  —National organic standards (Agricultural Marketing Service)

These proposals would enable the EPA to focus its resources on water pollution, air pollution and toxic waste dumps. The FDA would concentrate on medical devices, blood banks and drug safety. The USDA would focus on agricultural research and assistance.

All three agencies could be downsized and streamlined accordingly. FDA officials should not own stock in the companies they regulate and should not join those companies for 10 years after leaving government service.

National media reports of food contaminated with fecal matter, pesticides, hormones and drugs have done little to build public trust in government. An truly independent food safety agency dedicated to consumer protection—rather than corporate profits—would go far in rebuilding that trust.

> *"Do you know what was the most thrilling moment for me in the eradication of smallpox? It wasn't when we completed it. It was the moment I realized it was possible."*[106]
>
> —Bill Foege
> Global 2000

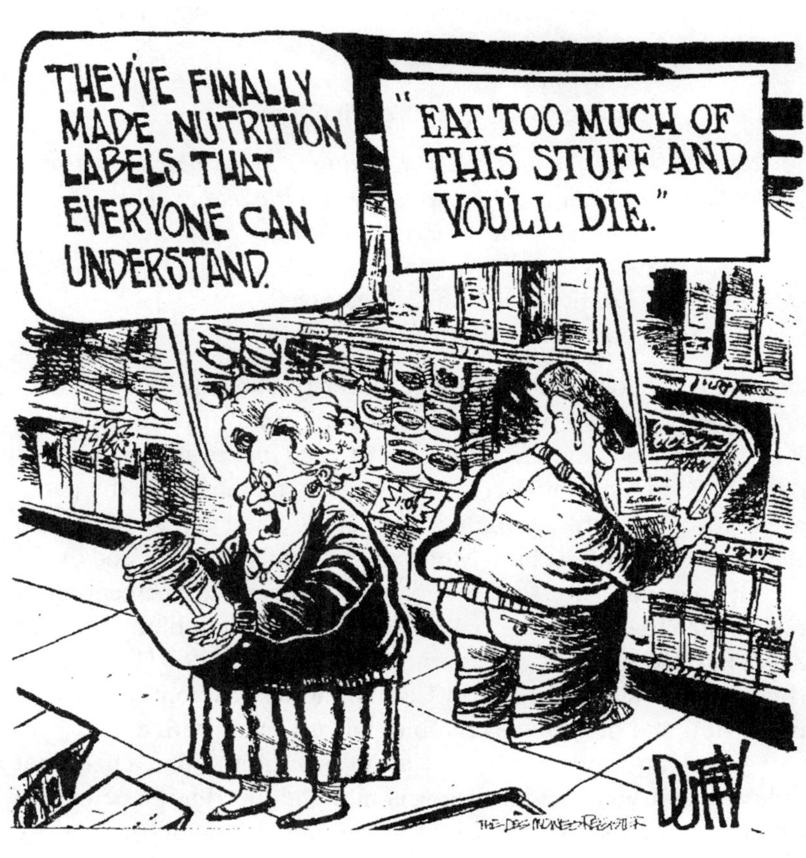
THEY'VE FINALLY MADE NUTRITION LABELS THAT EVERYONE CAN UNDERSTAND.
"EAT TOO MUCH OF THIS STUFF AND YOU'LL DIE."
DUFFY

Food Labels

"The meat industry wants to keep the public in the dark about fat content."[107]

—Sen. Howard Metzenbaum

"[Food labeling is another example of] the heavy hand of government on the activities of America."[108]

—Clayton Yeutter
former Secretary of Agriculture

"To me, extensive nutritional labeling is pretty much a waste of time and money... Why go to the trouble and expense of labeling them except to satisfy the whims of a few noisy consumer activists."[109]

—Dr. Fredrick Stare, former chair
Harvard Department of Nutrition

Each year, the food industry markets over 16,000 new food and beverage items, and spends over $36 billion in advertising. In 1992, Kellogg spent $47 million promoting Frosted Flakes and Fruit Loops cereals. Food labels reflect the ethical considerations of the packaged food industry, which is largely owned by alcohol and tobacco companies. (Philip Morris owns Kraft General Foods.)

It's far easier for food companies to change the perception of reality than to change reality itself. By adding a thimbleful of oil to a glass of water, the glass could be labeled **99.9% fat-free** (by weight)—even though 100% of its calories are from fat. Like so much fluff and filler, hype crumbles when viewed with a wary eye.

American food retailing is a multi-billion-dollar, cut-throat industry, and your grocery store is now the meeting place of two opposing forces: one force is consumer demand for healthy products at a low price; the other force is profits.

The resulting food label deception is elevated to high art...a veiled masterpiece of slickly-worded enticement, the consumer's much-heralded Tower of Babel. Welcome to the nebulous shifting world of "All Natural" food labels.

☞ P.T. BARNUM FOOD CHART ☜

Product	**Label**	**Translation**
Louis Rich Turkey Bologna	82% Fat-Free	75% calories from fat[110]
Dunkin' Donuts	No Cholesterol	50% calories from fat[111]
Mrs. Paul's Fish Fillets	Light	Fattier than the regular[112]
Nabisco Crackers	Whole Wheat	Mostly white flour[113]
Pillsbury Pumpkin Bread	Made With Real Pumpkin	1 teaspoon per serving[114]
High fiber bread	Microcrystalline Cellulose	Sawdust
Pasta	Golden Amber Durum Wheat	White flour
Refried beans	All Natural	May contain lard, BHT, BHA
Barbecue sauce	No Sugar Added	May contain sugar alcohols
Cocktail Sauce	No Salt Added	May contain added sodium

FOOD LABEL TRANSLATIONS

Fat

- **Fat Free** – less than ½ gram of total fat per serving.
- **Saturated Fat Free** – less than ½ gram of saturated fat per serving.
- **Low Fat** – maximum 3 grams of total fat per serving and per 50 grams of food (2% milk is exempt).
- **Low in Saturated Fat** – maximum 1 gram of saturated fat per serving; maximum 15% of calories from saturated fat.
- **X% Fat Free** – meets criteria for "low fat."
- **Light or Lite** – at least 50% reduction in total fat.
- **Reduced Fat** – at least 25% reduction in total fat.

Calorie

- **Calorie Free** – less than 5 calories per serving.
- **Low Calorie** – maximum 40 calories per serving and per 50 grams of food.
- **Light or Lite** – at least 33% reduction in calories.
- **Reduced Calorie** – at least 25% reduction in calories.

Cholesterol

- **Cholesterol Free** – less than 2 mg of cholesterol per serving.
- **Low Cholesterol** – maximum 20 mg per serving and per 50 grams of food.
- **Reduced Cholesterol** – at least 25% reduction in cholesterol.

Sugar

- **Sugar Free** – less than ½ gram of sugar per serving.
- **No Added Sugar** – may contain added sugar other than sucrose.
- **Naturally Sweetened** – may be sweetened with fruit juice, fructose, sucrose, or any other naturally-occurring sugar.
- **Reduced Sugar** – at least 25% reduction in sugar.

Salt

- **Salt Free or Sodium Free** – less than 5 mg of sodium per serving.
- **Unsalted or No Added Salt** – may contain added salt other than sodium chloride.
- **Very Low Sodium** – maximum 35 mg per serving and per 50 grams of food.
- **Low Sodium** – maximum 140 mg per serving and per 50 grams of food.
- **Light or Lite** – at least 50% reduction in sodium.
- **Reduced Sodium** – at least 25% reduction in sodium.

Other Terms

- **Fresh** – may be irradiated but not heated. "Fresh" chicken may be frozen down to 1 degree.
- **More** – at least 10% more of a nutrient than the comparison.
- **Good Source Of** – 10% to 19% of a nutrient's Daily Value.
- **High In** – at least 20% of a nutrient's Daily Value.
- **Cold Pressed Oil** – no legal definition except in Switzerland.
- **Natural** – no legal definition except for meats and poultry.
- **Natural Flavoring** – may be derived from any plant or animal product.
- **Pure or Real** – no legal definition.
- **Enriched** – contains added thiamin, niacin, riboflavin and iron.
- **Fortified** – contains nutrients not originally in the food.
- **Lean** – less than 10 grams of fat, 4 grams of saturated fat, and 95 mg of cholesterol per serving.
- **Extra Lean** – less than 5 grams of fat, 2 grams of saturated fat, and 95 mg of cholesterol per serving.

FOOD LABEL CAVEATS

- Manufacturers may list hydrogenated fats as polyunsaturated or monounsaturated oils.
- Manufacturers often use multiple sugars, multiple salts, or multiple fats to prevent them being listed as the first ingredient.
- Genetically altered foods and irradiated ingredients may be sold without disclosure.
- Non-dairy creamers labeled "Fat–Free" may contain more fat per cup than whole milk if each serving contains under ½ gram of fat. Be wary of serving sizes.
- Foods labeled "No MSG Added" may contain MSG from hydrolyzed vegetable protein, yeast extract, or natural flavorings.
- Food labels do not disclose the percentage of calories from fat. (To calculate, divide the calories from fat by the calories per serving.)

> *"Polished brass will pass upon more people than rough gold."*
> —Lord Chesterfield (1694–1773)

The RDA

"...if you don't eat Milk Group foods, you could have a difficult time getting all the calcium your body needs."[115]
—National Dairy Council

"And I would further suggest that nutritionists in poor countries would be well advised not to blindly accept nutrient recommendations formulated by rich countries because these values...reflect a serious lack of concern for nutrient-linked diseases of affluence, perhaps because of an intense interest within rich countries to maintain the status quo."[116]
—Dr. T. Colin Campbell
China Health Project

The RDAs (Recommended Dietary Allowances) are the American nutritional standard against which all diets are measured. A recent USDA study of 21,500 people found that none received the full RDA for 20 nutrients.[117] National surveys report Americans falling short in meeting the RDAs.[118] Such findings help push vitamin sales to record levels. But no one considers the RDA itself. So deeply ingrained is the RDA's cultural authority that to question it seems tantamount to blasphemy.

Contrary to popular belief, a varied diet that's low in the RDAs will not collapse the skeleton like a wet cardboard box, will not transform the body into a Bangladesh poster child, nor shatter it like a broken TV tube. The minimum nutritional intake needed to prevent deficiencies (the Minimum Daily Requirement) is 2–6 times lower than the RDA.[119] The RDAs are established by a curious hierarchy:

- the Committee on Dietary Allowances of
- the Food and Nutrition Board of
- the Commission of Life Sciences of
- the National Research Council of
- the National Academy of Sciences.

The American RDA for calcium was set about 50% higher than allowances established by Canada, England and the United Nations even though all allowances were based on the same data.[120] The U.S. calcium standard was set artificially high to compensate for

America's meat and dairy-based diet. Most Americans absorb only 20–40% of their calcium intake while losing 320 mg of calcium each day.[121]

> *"A country with a restricted food supply can't be as liberal as others. It needs stronger evidence of a genuine need for high levels. Calcium is one example. America has a very large milk supply."*[122]
>
> —D. Mark Hegsted, administrator
> USDA Human Nutrition Service

The RDAs are designed primarily for animal product consumers. Different standards are needed for Americans who cut back on meat and dairy products. Fortunately different standards already exist:

- The RDIs (Recommended Dietary Intakes) set by the World Health Organization.
- The PRIs (Population Reference Intakes) set by the European Community.

The following table compares all three standards. The values are set for 174-pound males and 138-pound females, ages 25–50. Values in parentheses are for women only; values without parentheses are the same for both sexes.

Nutritional Standards

	RDA[123]	RDI[124]	PRI[125]
Protein (g)	63 (50)	45 (33)	59 (47)
Vitamin A (mcg)	1,000 (800)	750	700 (600)
Vitamin D (mcg)	5	2.5	0–10
Vitamin B_{12} (mcg)	2	2	1.4
Calcium (mg)	800	500	700
Phosphorus (mg)	800	—	550
Iron (mg)	10 (15)	5–9 (14–28)	9 (16)

For Americans who reduce their intake of animal products, the optimal recommendations could include all three standards:

- •• RDIs (Recommended Dietary Intakes) – protein, vitamin D, calcium and iron.
- • PRIs (Population Reference Intakes) – vitamin A, vitamin B12 and phosphorus.

RDAs (Recommended Dietary Allowances) – all other nutrients.

Split Nutritional Standards

	Male	Female
Protein (g) ••	45	33
Vitamin A (mcg) •	700	600
Vitamin D (mcg) ••	2.5	2.5
Vitamin E (mg)	10	8
Vitamin K (mcg)	80	65
Vitamin C (mg)	60	60
Vitamin B1 (mg)	1.5	1.1
Vitamin B2 (mg)	1.7	1.3
Niacin (mg)	19	15
Vitamin B6 (mg)	2	1.6
Folate (mcg)	200	180
Vitamin B12 (mcg) •	1.4	1.4
Calcium (mg) ••	500	500
Phosphorus (mg) •	550	550
Magnesium (mg)	350	280
Iron (mg) ••	5	14
Zinc (mg)	15	12
Iodine (mcg)	150	150
Selenium (mcg)	70	55

RDA vs. U.S. RDA

- The RDAs (Recommended Dietary Allowances) are set by the National Academy of Sciences for six categories: infants, children, men, women, pregnant and nursing women.
- The U.S. RDAs (U.S. Recommended Daily Allowances) are found on food/vitamin labels and use the highest RDA for each nutrient. The U.S. RDAs are set by the Food and Drug Administration.
- There's an "RDA" for selenium, but not for pantothenic acid, copper or biotin.
- There's a "U.S. RDA" for copper, biotin and pantothenic acid, but not for selenium.

RDI VS. RDI

- The RDIs (Reference Daily Intakes) are set by the FDA to average the difference between the U.S. RDAs and the RDAs for each nutrient.
- The RDIs (Recommended Dietary Intakes) are set by the World Health Organization and are designed mostly for vegetarians.

Calcium Standards			
U.S. RDA	**RDI (FDA)**	**RDA**	**RDI (WHO)**
1,200 mg	1,000 mg	800 mg	500 mg

In dealing with this alphabet soup, it's important to keep in mind two things:

- All nutritional standards established by the U.S. government are designed for the average American diet (which is 44% animal products).
- Diseases of affluence arise primarily from dietary excess and toxicity, not deficiency.

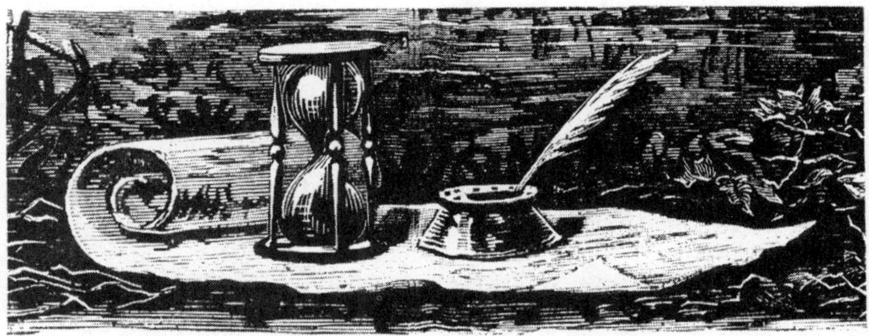

Final Thoughts

"Come, my friends, 'Tis not too late to seek a newer world."
—Alfred Tennyson
Ulysses

Mind and body are one. The day will come when we harness the full potential of the human mind and look back on this era as we now look back on the Dark Ages. Action quickens the pace of transition.

By applying the unifying principles within this book, by taking consumer action at the personal level, you reclaim your birthright: freedom from disease. By taking citizen action at the national level, you touch the lives of generations yet to come.

If your heart calls out to leave this world a better place, whether by planting gardens, raising healthy children, teaching by example, or bringing to a graceful close this troubled chapter of history—honor the voices within. Do what's right for you and keep peace within your soul.

CITIZEN ACTION

In this increasingly hostile environment, humanity has reached a critical juncture in time. Sinister elements have been released upon the earth by an indentured government and perverted science. Elements that, if left unchecked, will doom all we hold dear. Impending ecological cataclysms bode poorly for sustained life on this planet.

Citizens banding together at the community level, united in purpose and vision, will galvanize a movement that cuts across lines of generation, class and race. Only then may we part ways with old paradigms as our collective voices turn the tide. Here's how:

- Pick an issue and make your stand. Join a supportive national organization. Order educational materials and make copies.
- Talk to friends and co-workers about this issue. Hold monthly discussion groups. Start a mailing list of those who attend and send it to the national organization. Print and distribute flyers of future meetings. Formulate plans.
- As attendance grows, hold meetings in your community center, school, library, or church. Bring in other groups, hold dual meetings and share information.
- Launch a petition drive on your issue. Set up tables at shopping malls, health food stores and community events. Hand out flyers and gather signatures. Stage publicity stunts.
- Armed with signed petitions and materials, visit your city, county, state, or national representatives. Push for their commitment on favorable legislation and hold them accountable. Such action entails responsibility. Use it wisely.

> *"And as a truth eternal I say unto you, that there are three things which bring the end of civilization, even the mightiest that have ever been and shall ever be. . . impure air, impure water and impure food."*
>
> —Zend Avesta, 3000 B.C

Appendix

PERSONAL LEVEL

Center for Science in the Public Interest
1875 Connecticut Ave., NW
Washington, DC 20009

University of California Berkeley Wellness Letter
P.O. Box 420148
Palm Coast, FL 32142

Tufts University Diet and Nutrition Letter
P.O. Box 57857
Boulder, CO 80322

Consumer Reports On Health
P.O. Box 52148
Boulder, CO 80321

Mayo Clinic Health Letter
P.O. Box 53889
Boulder, CO 80322

Harvard Health Letter
P.O. Box 420300
Palm Coast, FL 32142

NATIONAL LEVEL

Pesticide Reform

Food & Water
Depot Hill Road
R.R. 1, Box 114
Marshfield, VT 05658

National Coalition Against the Misuse of Pesticides
701 E Street, SE, Suite 200
Washington, DC 20003

Pure Food Campaign
1130 17th Street, NW
Washington, DC 20036

Greenpeace
1436 U Street, NW
Washington, DC 20009

Citizens Clearinghouse for Hazardous Waste
P.O. Box 6806
Falls Church, VA 22040

Pesticide Action Network
116 New Montgomery, Suite 810
San Francisco, CA 94105

Political Reform

Common Cause
2030 M Street, NW
Washington, DC 20036

Public Citizen
2000 P Street, NW, Suite 610
Washington, DC 20036

Project Vote Smart
129 NW Fourth Street, #204
Corvallis, OR 97330

Concord Coalition
1019 19th Street, NW, Suite 810
Washington, DC 20036

National Taxpayers Union
404 8th Street, NE
Washington, DC 20002

Citizens Against Government Waste
1301 Connecticut Ave., NW
Washington, DC 20036

Health-Care Reform

Citizens For Health
P.O. Box 1195
Tacoma, WA 98401

The Cancer Chronicles
144 St. John's Place
Brooklyn, NY 11217

Cancer Prevention Coalition
520 North Michigan Ave.
Chicago, IL 60611

People Against Cancer
P.O. Box 10
Otho, IA 50569

Y–ME
18220 Harwood Ave.
Homewood, IL 60430

Women's Health Network
514 10th Street, NW, Suite 400
Washington, DC 20004

Environmental Reform

Natural Resources Defense Council
1350 New York Ave., NW
Washington, DC 20005

EarthSave
706 Frederick Street
Santa Cruz, CA 95062

Friends of the Earth
1025 Vermont Ave., NW
Washington, DC 20005

Earth Island Institute
300 Broadway, Suite 28
San Francisco, CA 94133

References

Introduction

1 —Hawkes, E., "Gentle heart, tough guy," *San Francisco Chronicle*, Parade, July 12, 1992, pg 5
Curreri, J., "Once a maverick…," *Senior Magazine*, Feb. 1993, pg 7
2 —Wolinsky, H., *The Serpent on the Staff*, Tarcher, 1994, pg 152
3 —Kell, G., "Cancer schmancer!," *Health Freedom News*, Nov. 1993, pg 32
4 —McNamara, J., "Coronary artery disease in combat casualties in Vietnam," *JAMA,* 216:1185, 1971
5 —Enos, W., "Pathogenesis of coronary disease in American soldiers killed in Korea," *JAMA,* 158:912, 1955
6 —National Cancer Institute, *Surveillance, Epidemiology and End Results: Incidence and Mortality Data, 1973–1977,* Monograph 57, June 1981, pg 4
7 —Collins, G., "Frugal gourmet: food is his mission," *New York Times,* Feb. 10, 1989, pg C–4
8 —Benderly, B., Gland illusion," *American Health*, Dec. 1990, pg 71

Chapter 1—New Thinking

1 —Crawford, M., "The role of essential fatty acids in neural developement: implications for perinatal nutrition," *Am J Clin Nutr,* 57: 703, 1993
"Present-day feeding practice report," US Department of Public Health, Nov. 9, 1974
2 —Paulsen, M., "The cancer business," *Mother Jones*, May/June 1994, pg 41
3 —Quoted in Golab, J., "Ted Nugent's wilderness workout," *Men's Fitness,* Dec. 1990, pg 113
4 —US Department of Agriculture, *USDA Today,* PA–1503, Dec. 1992, pg 5
5 —Quoted in Krakauer, J., "Brown fellas," *Outside,* Dec. 1991, pg 70
6 —Lyford, J., "Names that lie: laundering anti-environmentalism," *Propaganda Review*, Number 11, 1994, pg 70
Deal C., *The Greenpeace Guide to Anti-Environmental Organizations*, Odonian Press, 1993
Bloyd-Peshkin, S., "The health-fraud cops," *Veg Times,* Aug. 1991, pg 55
7 —Ibid
8 —Clorfene-Casten, L., "Unhappy meals," *Mother Jones*, July/Aug. 1992, pg 33
9 —Shuchman, L., *San Francisco Chronicle,* Sunday Punch, Sept. 15, 1991, pg 2
10 —Deal C., as per note 6
11 —As per note 6
12 —"Public-interest pretenders," *Consumer Reports,* May 1994, pg 316
13 —Deal C., as per note 6
14 —*Earth Island Journal,* Summer 1994, pg 4
As per note 12
15 —Deal C., as per note 6

16 —Ibid
17 —Stauber, J., *Corporate Crime Reporter*, Sept. 27, 1993, pg 4
18 —"Public-interest pretenders," *Consumer Reports*, May 1994, pg 320
19 —As per note 6
20 —Ibid
21 —Ornish, D., *Dr. Dean Ornish's Program for Reversing Heart Disease,* Ballantine Books, 1990, pg 53
22 —Levine, S., "Coronary angioplasty: clinical and angiographic follow-up," *Am J Cardiol*, 55:673, 1985
Ibid
23 —Graboys, T., "Results of a second-opion trial among patients recommended for coronary angiogram," *JAMA*, 268:2537, 1992
Alderman, E., "Ten-year follow-up of survival and myocardial infarction in the randomized coronary artery surgery study," *Circulation*, 82:1629, 1990
24 —Drummond, H., *Mother Jones*, Jan. 1978
Kirkpatrick, S., *Human Scale*, Coward & Geoghegan, 1980, pg 268
25 —Zimmermann, M., "Isn't it time to teach nutrition to medical students?," *Am J Clin Nutr*, 58:828, 1993
26 —Winick, M., "Nutrition education in medical schools," *Am J Clin Nutr*, 58:825, 1993
27 —Ibid
28 —McDougall, J., *The McDougall Plan,* New Century, 1983, pg 7
29 —Cornell University Medical College survey reported in "Most doctors ignore nutrition," *San Francisco Chronicle*, Jan. 29, 1993
30 —Quoted in Liebman, B., "Taking supplements seriously," *CSPI Nutr Action Healthletter,* Oct. 1991, pg 5
31 —McNamee, K., *The Chiropractic College Admissions & Curriculum Directory,* 2nd ed., 1990, pgs 65–157
Author review of the 16 U.S. chiropractic college curriculums
32 —"Fast food survey," American Dietetic Association, Chicago, Oct. 16, 1990
"Vital statistics," *In Health,* July/Aug. 1991, pg 14
33 —Quoted in Clark, A., "Healthy by choice," *Veg Times*, June 1993, pg 96
34 —Henry, H., "Increasing calcium intake lowers blood pressure: the literature reviewed," *JADA*, 85:182, 1985
35 —"Food & nutrition briefs," *Spectrum*, May/June 1993, pg 7
Good Medicine, Winter 1993
36 —Quoted in Moll, L., *Veg Times,* Dec. 1991, pg 23
37 —Keys, A., "The diet and 15–year death rate in the seven countries study," *Am J Epidem*, 124:903, 1986
Armstrong, B., "Environmental factors and cancer incidence and mortality in different countries," *Int J Cancer,* 15:617, 1975
38 —Quoted in *Veg Times*, Nov. 1991, pg 26
39 —Fletcher, J., "The occasional vegetarian," *San Francisco Chronicle*, Food section, Sept. 27, 1995, pg 1
Robertson, L., *The New Laurel's Kitchen*, Ten Speed Press, 1986, pg 353
40 —Stauber, J., "PR spy operation costs Kaufman million dollar-a-year account," *PR Watch*, Oct./Dec. 1993, pg 7

41 —Kaplan, S., "Lobby-PR giant Porter/Novelli plays all sides," *PR Watch*, Jan./Mar. 1994, pg 4

42 —Young, J., "California Cancer Registry, January 1993, Death Records," presented at Controversies in Breast Cancer Conference, San Francisco, Sept. 10, 1993

43 —Davis, D., "Agricultural exposures and cancer trends in developed countries," *Environ Health Persp*, 100:39, 1992

Morrison, H., "Herbicides and cancer," *JNCI*, 84:1866, 1992

Blair, A., "Cancer among farmers," *Occupat Med*, 6:335, 1991

44 —Schwartz, D., "Parental occupation and birth outcome in an agricultural community," *Scand J Work Environ*, 12:51, 1986

Schwartz, D., *Physician's Handbook on Pesticides*, UCSD Medical Center, 1980

45 —Cotts, C., "Hard sell in the drug war," *Nation*, Mar. 9, 1992, pg 300

Blow, R., "Partnership for a truth-free America," *Propaganda Review*, Number 9, 1992, pg 38

46 —Stauber, J., "From Earth Day to earth pay," *PR Watch*, April/June 1994, pg 4

47 —Food & Water, "Monsanto: one of the 'good guys?,'" *Safe Food News*, Winter 1995, pg 7

48 —Bleifuss, J., "Science in the public interest," *PR Watch*, Jan./Mar. 1995, pg 11

Kurtz, H., *Columbia Journalism Review*, Mar. 1990

"The ACSH: forefront of science, or just a front?," *Consumer Reports*, May 1994, pg 319

49 —Ibid

50 —Epstein, S., *The Politics of Cancer*, Sierra Club Books, 1978, pg 261

Moss, R., *The Cancer Industry,* Paragon House, 1989, pg 348

Junk Science

51 —Whelan, E. and Stare, F., *The Nutrition Hoax*, Atheneum, 1983, pg 282

52 —Kanis, J., "Calcium supplementation in the diet: not justified by present evidence," *Br Med J*, 298:137 and 205, 1989

Nordin, B., "Calcium supplementation in the diet: justified by present evidence," *Br Med J*, 300:1056, 1990

53 —Willett, W., "Dietary fat and fiber in relation to risk of breast cancer: an 8-year follow-up," *JAMA*, 268:2037, 1992

Willett, W., "Dietary fat and the risk of breast cancer," *N Engl J Med*, 316:22, 1987

54 —Kradjian, R., *Save Yourself from Breast Cancer,* Berkley Books, 1994, pg 206

55 —Hunninghake, D., "The efficacy of intensive dietary therapy alone or combined with lovastatin in outpatients with hypercholesterolemia," *N Engl J Med*, 328:1213, 1993

56 —Sox, H., "Screening for lipid disorders under health system reform," *N Engl J Med*, 328:1269, 1993

Ibid

57 —Ornish, D., "Can lifestyle changes reverse coronary heart disease? The Lifestyle Heart Trial," *Lancet*, 336:129, 1990

58 —Quoted in *Tufts U Diet Nutr Letter*, Dec. 1991, pg 4

59 —Sacks, F., "Effect on coronary atherosclerosis of decrease in plasma cholesterol concentrations in normocholesterolaemic patients," *Lancet*, 344:1182, 1994
60 —Ibid
61 —Schneider, E., "Life extension," *N Engl J Med*, 312:1159, 1985
Walford, R., *The 120 Year Diet*, Pocket Books, 1986, pgs 56–67
62 —Kahn, C., "His theory is simple: eat less, live longer," *Longevity*, Oct. 1990, pg 61
63 —Tierney, J., "The three secrets of Shangri-La," *In Health*, July/Aug. 1990, pg 45
64 —Hu, J., "Dietary calcium and bone density among middle-aged and elderly women in China," *Am J Clin Nutr*, 58:219, 1993
65 —"Mom was right," *CSPI Nutr Action Healthletter,* Oct. 1993, pg 4
66 —Edelstein, S., "Relation between body size and bone mineral density in elderly men and women, *Am J Epidemiol*, 138:160, 1993
67 —Personal communication with T. Colin Campbell, Nov. 16, 1993
Campbell, T., interview on Dr. John McDougall Show, Los Angeles, Nov. 7, 1993
68 —Harris, M., "The dairy debate," *Veg Times*, April 1994, pg 83
69 —Calvo, M., "Elevated secretion and action of serum parathyroid hormone in young adults consuming high phosphorus, low calcium diets assembled from common foods," *J Clin Endocrinol Metab*, 66:823, 1988
70 —Tarasoff, L., "Monosodium L-glutamate: a double-blind study and review," *Fd Chem Toxicol*, 31:1019, 1993
71 —Samuels, J. and A., "MSG: truth and consequences," *Search For Health*, Sept./Oct. 1993, pg 28
72 —Ibid, pg 38
73 —"Prostate cancer," *Harvard Health Letter,* Sept. 1988, pg 4
74 —Ibid
75 —Pak, C., "Slow-release sodium fluoride in the management of postmenopausal osteoporosis," *Ann Intern Med*, 120:625, 1994
76 —Ibid
77 —Riggs, B., "Effect of fluoride treatment on the fracture rate in postmenopausal women with osteoporosis," *N Engl J Med,* 322:802, 1990
78 —Hileman, B., "Fluoridation of water," *Chem Engineer News,* Aug. 1, 1988, pg 37
79 —As per note 75, pg 631
80 —Simon, G., "Immunologic, psychological and neuropsychological factors in multiple chemical sensitivity," *Ann Intern Med*, 119:97, 1993
81 —Baker, G., "Medical update: a rebuttal to the Simon study published previously in Our Toxic Times," *Townsend Letter for Doctors,* June 1994, pg 616
82 —Ibid
83 —As per note 80
84 —As per note 81
85 —"Why pharmaceutical drugs injure & kill because they are fraudulently tested," *Townsend Letter for Doctors*, Jan. 1994, pg 30

Braithwaite, J., *Corporate Crime in the Pharmaceutical Industry*, Routledge & Kegan Paul, 1984, pg 105

86 —*Health*, May/June 1994, pg 16

American Association of Poison Control Centers, *Annual Report*, 1992

87 —Coppolino, E., "Pandora's box," *Sierra*, Sept./Oct. 1994, pg 41

Thornton, J., "The dioxin deception," *Propaganda Review*, No. 9, 1992, pg 23

88 —Thornton, J., Ibid

89 —*Food Chemical News*, Jan. 30, 1995

Safe Food News, Spring 1995, pg 4

90 —Kassirer, J., "Financial conflicts of interest in biomedical research," *N Engl J Med,* 329:570, 1993

91 —Renaud, S., "Alcohol and platelet aggregation: The Caerphilly Prospective Heart Disease Study," *Am J Clin Nutr*, 55:1012, 1992

Hurley, J., "A drink a day?," *CSPI Nutr Action Healthletter,* Nov. 1992, pg 5

92 —Bonaa, K., "Habitual fish consumption, plasma phospholipid fatty acids and serum lipids: the Tromso Study," *Am J Clin Nutr,* 55:1126, 1992

Houwelingen, R., "Effect of a moderate fish intake on blood pressure, bleeding time, hematology, and clinical chemistry in healthy males, *Am J Clin Nutr*, 46:424, 1987

93 —Lyle, R., "Iron status in exercising women: the effect of oral iron therapy vs increased consumption of muscle foods," *Am J Clin Nutr,* 56:1049, 1992

Worthington-Roberts, B., "Iron status of premenopausal women in a university community and its relationship to habitual dietary sources of protein," *Am J Clin Nutr*, 47:275, 1988

94 —Turnlund, J., "Milk's effect on the bioavailability of iron from cereal-based diets in young women by use of in vitro and in vivo methods," *Am J Clin Nutr*, 52:373, 1990

95 —Potter, S., "Depression of plasma cholesterol in men by consumption of baked products containing soy protein," *Am J Clin Nutr*, 58:501, 1993

Laine, D., "Lightly hydrogenated soy oil versus other vegetable oils as a lipid-lowering dietary constituent," *Am J Clin Nutr*, 35:683, 1982

96 —Sabate, J., "Effects of walnuts on serum lipid levels and blood pressure in normal men," *N Engl J Med,* 328:603, 1993

97 —As per note 55

98 —Trichopoulou, A., "Consumption of olive oil and specific food groups in relation to breast cancer risk in Greece," *JNCI*, 87:110, 1995

99 —Barger-Lux, M., "Effects of moderate caffeine intake on the calcium economy of premenopausal women," *Am J Clin Nutr*, 52:722, 1990

100 —"Scientific analysis indicates that the available data do not support a causal relationship between chlorinated organic compounds and human breast cancer," prepared by CanTox for the Chlorine Institute, Dec. 4, 1992

Austin, H., "A prospective follow-up study on cancer mortality in relation to serum DDT," *Am J Pub Health*, 79:43, 1989

Chapter 2—Dietary Components

Proteins

1 —"Meat–packer defends beef," *Riverside Herald,* May 8, 1976, pg A–1
Robbins, J., *Diet For A New America,* Stillpoint, 1987, pg 262

2 —Obituary, *Riverside Herald,* Mar. 14, 1982, pg C–11
Robbins, J., Ibid

3 —Dowie, M., "Reagan: hold the steroids," *Mother Jones,* Oct. 1984, pg 9

4 —Woteki, C. and Thomas, P., *Eat For Life: The Food & Nutrition Board's Guide to Reducing Your Risk of Chronic Disease*, National Academy Press, 1992, pg 6

5 —Davis, A., *Let's Eat Right To Keep Fit,* Harcourt, 1954, pg 34

6 —Quoted in Liebman, B., "Lessons from China," *CSPI Nutr Action Healthletter,* Dec. 1990, pg 6

7 —World Health Organization, *Diet, Nutrition and the Prevention of Chronic Diseases*, Technical Report Series 797, WHO, Geneva, 1990, pg 108
USDA, *Nationwide Food Consumption Survey. Nutrient Intakes: Individuals in 48 States 1977–78,* Report No. I–1, Human Nutrition Information Service

8 —Hegsted, D., "Minimum protein requirements of adults," *Am J Clin Nutr,* 21:355, 1968

9 —FAO/WHO/UNU Committee, *Energy and Protein Requirements*, Technical Report Series 724, World Health Organization, Geneva, 1985

10 —National Research Council, Food and Nutrition Board, *Recommended Dietary Allowances,* 10th ed., National Academy Press, 1989, pg 66

11 —Coats, C., "Negative effects of a high-protein diet," *Family Practice Recertification*, 12:80, 1990
Jones, M., "The effect of dietary protein on glomerular filtration rate in normal subjects," *Clin Nephrology,* 27:71, 1987
Brenner, B., "Dietary protein intake and the progressive nature of kidney disease," *N Engl J Med,* 307:652, 1982

12 —Zemel, M., "Calcium utilization: effect of varying level and source of dietary protein," *Am J Clin Nutr,* 48:880, 1988

13 —Committee on Diet, Nutrition and Cancer of the National Research Council, *Diet, Nutrition and Cancer,* 1982

14 —Hall, A., "Epidemiology of gout and hyperuricemia: a long-term population study," *Am J Med*, 42:27, 1967

15 —Vahlensieck, W., "Review: the importance of diet in urinary stones," *Urological Res,* 14:283, 1986
Robertson, P., "The effect of high animal protein intake on the risk of calcium stone-formation in the urinary tract," *Clin Sci*, 57:285, 1979

16 —Kjeldsen-Kragh, J., "Controlled trial of fasting and one-year vegetarian diet in rheumatoid arthritis," *Lancet*, 338:899, 1991

17 —Whitney, E., *Understanding Normal and Clinical Nutrition,* 2nd ed., West Publishing, 1987, pgs 129–130
Carroll, K., "Dietary protein and heart disease," *Nutrition and the MD,* June 1985
Muscari, A., *Ann Ital Med Int,* 7:7, 1992

18 —As per note 8
As per note 10, pgs 58, 68
19 —ADA, "Position of the American Dietetic Association: vegetarian diets," *JADA*, 88:353, 1988
McDougall, J., *The McDougall Plan,* New Century, 1983, pg 96
20 —Lappe, F., *Diet for a Small Planet,* 10th ed., Ballantine Books, 1982, pg 17
21 —Adapted from Rose, W., "The amino acid requirements of adult man," *Nutr Abstr Rev*, 27:631, 1957
McDougall, J., as per note 19, pg 99
22 —Campbell, W., "Increased protein requirements in elderly people: new data and retrospective reassessments," *Am J Clin Nutr,* 60:501, 1994
23 —Ibid
24 —McDougall, J., as per note 19
25 —*Tufts U Diet Nutr Letter*, Dec. 1993, pg 2
26 —National Live Stock and Meat Board, Beef Promotion and Research Board, and National Pork Board, *Nutrition Strategies,* 1990

Fats

27 —Quoted in Liebman, B., "Putting the squeeze on saturates," *CSPI Nutr Action Healthletter*, May 1993, pg 5
28 —National Center for Health Statistics, Advance Report of Final Mortality Statistics, 1992, *Monthly Vital Statistics Report,* Vol. 41, No. 13, Sept. 28, 1993
US Department of Health and Human Services, *The Surgeon General's Report on Nutrition and Health,* US Government Printing Office, 1988
29 —Phinney, S., "Potential risk of prolonged gamma-linolenic acid use," *Ann Int Med*, 120:692, 1994
Kelley, D., "Dietary alpha-linoleic acid and immunocompetence in humans," *Am J Clin Nutr,* 53:40, 1991
30 —American Heart Association, "Position statement: dietary guidelines for healthy American adults," *Circulation*, 77:721A, 1988
World Health Organization, *Diet, Nutrition and the Prevention of Chronic Diseases*, Technical Report Series 797, WHO, Geneva, 1990, pg 108
31 —Winitz, M., "Studies in metabolic nutrition employing chemically defined diets," *Am J Clin Nutr,* 23:525, 1970
32 —World Health Organization, *Dietary Fats and Oils in Human Nutrition,* WHO/FAO, 1989
33 —Pritikin, N., *The Pritikin Program for Diet and Exercise,* Bantam Books, 1979, pg 9
34 —McDougall. J., *The McDougall Program,* NAL Books, 1990, pg 40
35 —Walford, R., *The 120 Year Diet,* Pocket Books, 1986, pg 116
36 —Ornish, D., *Dr. Dean Ornish's Program for Reversing Heart Disease,* Random House, 1990, pgs 255, 257
37 —Carroll, K., "Fat and cancer," *Cancer,* 58:1818, 1986
Rose, D., "International comparison of mortality rates for cancers of the breast, ovary, prostate, and colon, and per capita food consumption," *Cancer,* 58:2363, 1986

38 —Adapted from Carroll, K., "Nutrition and cancer: fat," in Rowland, I., *Nutrition, Toxicity, and Cancer,* CRC Press, 1991, pg 445

39 —Ibid

40 —Adapted from Reddy, B., "Nutrition and its relationship to cancer," *Adv Cancer Res,* 32:237, 1980

41 —Ziegler, R., "Migration pattern and breast cancer risk in Asian-American women," *JNCI,* 85:1819, 1993

Shimizu, H., "Cancer of the prostate and breast among Japanese and white immigrants in Los Angeles County," *Br J Cancer,* 63:963, 1991

42 —Carroll, K., "Dietary fats and cancer," *Am J Clin Nutr,* 53:1064, 1991

43 —Hursting, S., "Types of dietary fat and the incidence of cancer at five sites," *Prev Med,* 19:242, 1990

Scholar, E., "The effect of dietary fat on metastasis of the Lewis lung carcinoma," *Nutr Cancer,* 12:109, 1989

Ibid

44 —Erikson, K., "Dietary fat and tumor metastasis," *Nutr Rev,* 48:6, 1990

Pearce, M., "Incidence of cancer in men on a diet high in polyunsaturated fat," *Lancet,* 1:464, 1971

45 —Nestel, P., "Lowering of plasma cholesterol and enhanced sterol excretion with the consumption of polyunsaturated ruminant fats," *N Engl J Med,* 228:379, 1973

46 —Robertson, T., "Epidemiologic studies of coronary heart disease and stroke in Japanese men living in Japan, Hawaii and California," *Am J Cardiol,* 39:239, 1977

47 —Blankenhorn, D., "The influence of diet on the appearance of new lesions in human coronary arteries," *JAMA,* 263:1646, 1990

Felton, C., "Dietary polyunsaturated fatty acids and composition of human aortic plaques," *Lancet,* 344:1195, 1994

48 —Berner, L., "Roundtable discussion on milkfat, dairy products, and coronary heart disease risk," *J Nutr,* 123:1175, 1993

"News in review," *JADA,* 93:1343, 1993

49 —McDougall, J., *The McDougall Plan,* New Century, 1983, pg 77

Vergroesen, A., *The Role of Fats in Human Nutrition,* Academic Press, 1975, pg 19

50 —Crawford, M., "Essential fatty acid requirements in infancy," *Am J Clin Nutr,* 31:2181, 1978

51 —Quoted in Krizmanic, J., "Why bother?," *Veg Times,* Nov. 1991, pg 20

52 —Browner, W., "What if Americans ate less fat?," *JAMA,* 265:3285, 1991

53 —Ornish, D., "Can lifestyle changes reverse coronary heart disease? The Lifestyle Heart Trial," *Lancet,* 336:129, 1990

54 —Quoted in Pati, K., "Fat free diets can be hazardous to your health," *Health World,* May/June 1989, pg 19

55 —As per note 33, 34, 36

56 —Willett, W., "Intake of trans fatty acids and risk of coronary heart disease among women," *Lancet,* 341:581, 1993

Enig, M., "Dietary fat and cancer trends—a critique," *Fed Proc,* 37:2215, 1978

57 —Simopoulos, A., "The Mediterranean food guide," *Nutr Today*, 30:54, 1995
58 —Yetiv, J., "Clinical applications of fish oils," *JAMA*, 260:665, 1988
59 —Demke, D., "Effects of fish oil concentrate in patients with hypercholesterolemia," *Atherosclerosis,* 70:73, 1988
Harris, W., "Effects of a low saturated fat, low cholesterol fish oil supplement in hypertriglyceridemic patients," *Ann Intern Med*, 109:465, 1988
60 —Meydani, M., "Effect of long-term fish oil supplementation on vitamin E status and lipid peroxidation in women," *J Nutr,* 121:484, 1991
Endres, S., "The effect of dietary supplementation with n–3 polyunsaturated fatty acids on the synthesis of interleukin–1 and tumor necrosis factor by mononuclear cells," *N Engl J Med*, 320:265, 1989
61 —"Mono and di what?," *Veg Times,* Sept. 1991, pg 12

Carbohydrates

62 —Hertwig, R., quoted in Stern, J. and M., *The Encyclopedia of Bad Taste,* HarperCollins, 1990, pg 328
63 —Quoted in Hoffman, J., *Hunza: 15 Secrets of the World's Healthiest and Oldest Living People,* Professional Press, 1968, pg 152
64 —Miller, H., "The staff of life," *Remember to Remember*, 1947
65 —World Health Organization, *Diet, Nutrition and the Prevention of Chronic Diseases*, Technical Report Series 797, WHO, Geneva, 1990, pg 108
American Heart Association, "Position statement: dietary guidelines for healthy American adults," *Circulation*, 77:721A, 1988
66 —Asimov, I., *Isaac Asimov's Book of Facts*, Wings Books, 1979, pg 477
67 —*UC Berkeley Wellness Letter,* Jan. 1991, pg 3
68 —*Tufts U Diet Nutr Letter*, Dec. 1993, pg 2
American Health, Sept. 1989, pg 119
In Health, Sept./Oct. 1991, pg 12
69 —Quoted in Cader, M., *Eat These Words*, HarperCollins, 1991, pg 139

Additives

70 —*American Institute for Cancer Research Newsletter,* Summer 1990, Issue 28, pg 8
71 —*Beyond Beef Newsletter*, Spring 1993, pg 4
Food and Water, *Safe Food News*, Summer 1995, pg 4
72 —Mason, J. and Singer, P., *Animal Factories*, Harmony Books, 1990, pg 73
Barnard, N., *The Power of Your Plate*, Book Publishing Co., 1990, pg 106
73 —Marsh, R., "Transmissible mink encephalopathy, scrapie and downer cow disease: potential links," presented at the Third International Workshop on BSE, Bethesda, MD, Dec. 1992
74 —Mindell, E., *Safe Eating,* Warner Books, 1993, pg 124
75 —Quoted in Hausman, P., *Jack Sprat's Legacy—The Science and Politics of Fat and Cholesterol*, Richard Mauk Publishers, 1981, pg 207
76 —Quoted in Sapon, S., "Milk: the perfect food—Oh yeah? Says who?," *Vegetarian Voice*, Summer 1995, pg 15
77 —Gower, J., "The oxidation of benzopyrene mediated by lipid peroxidation in irradiated synthetic diets," *Int J Radiat Biol,* 49:471, 1986

Food and Drug Administration, "Irradiation in the production, processing and handling of food; Final rule: denial of request for hearing and response to objection," *Federal Register*, 53:53176, 1988

78 —Louria, D., "Zapping the food supply," *Bull Atomic Scientists,* Sept. 1990, pg 35

"The brave new world of food irradiation," *UC Berkeley Wellness Letter,* May 1992, pg 1

79 —Maxcy, R., "Significance of residual organisms in foods after substerilizing doses of gamma radiation: a review," *J Food Safety,* 5:203, 1983

80 —Bhaskaram, C., "Effects of feeding irradiated wheat to malnourished children," *Am J Clin Nutr*, 28:130, 1975

81 —Shanghai Institute of Radiation Medicine and Shanghai Institute of Nuclear Research, "Safety evaluation of 35 kinds of irradiated human foods," *Chinese Med Journal,* 100:715, 1987

82 —Shaw, M., "Effect of irradiated sucrose on the chromosomes of human lymphocytes," *Nature*, 211:1254, 1966

Brunetti, A., "Recommendations for evaluating the safety of irradiated foods," Final report prepared for the Director, Bureau of Foods, FDA, July 1980, pg IV–1

83 —Fairness & Accuracy in Reporting, *Extra!*, Jan./Feb. 1994

Stauber, J., *PR Watch*, Jan./Mar. 1994, pg 11

84 —Food and Drug Administration, "Irradiation in the production, processing and handling of food; Final rule," *Federal Register*, 51:13399, 1986

85 —Lustgarden, S., "Infectious technology," *Veg Times*, July 1994, pg 18

86 —Vanderpan, S., "A look inside a new tomato," *Sci Food Agricul Environ*, Jan. 1994, pg 4

87 —Walker, M., "Frankenstein foods," *Townsend Letter for Doctors*, May 1993, pg 424

88 —Adler, T., "Crop-weed offspring show hardy streak," *Science News*, 145:151, 1994

Union of Concerned Scientists, *Perils Amidst the Promise*, Washington D.C., Dec. 1993

89 —Falk, B., "Will transgenic crops generate new viruses and new diseases?," *Science*, 263:1395, 1994

Greene, A., "Recombination between viral RNA and transgenic plant transcripts," *Science*, 263:1423, 1994

90 —Raphals, P., "Disease puzzle nears solution," *Science*, 249:619, 1990

91 —Lustgarden, S., "Update: the year's hottest stories," *Veg Times*, Dec. 1994, pg 65

92 —Quoted in The Foundation on Economic Trends, *The Grassroots & Public Policy*, Summer 1994, pg 3

93 —Lee, J., *Optimal Health Guidelines*, 2nd ed., BLL Publishing, 1993, pg 101

Werbach, M., "Nutritional influences on illness," *Townsend Letter for Doctors*, Feb./Mar. 1994, pg 144

94 —Neri, L., "Aluminum, Alzheimer's disease and drinking water," *Lancet*, 338:390, 1991

Martyn, C., "Geographical relation between Alzheimer's disease and aluminum in drinking water," *Lancet*, 1:59, 1989
95 —McLachlan, D., "Intramuscular desferrioxamine in patients with Alzheimer's disease," *Lancet*, 337:1304, 1991
96 —Mullarkey, B., "Sweet delusion," *Informed Consent*, Sept./Oct. 1994, pg 35
US Air Force, "Aspartame alert," *Flying Safety*, 48:20, 1992
97 —Louis R., *Sax's Dangerous Properties of Industrial Materials*, 8th ed., Van Nostrand Reinhold, 1992, pg 2251
98 —Potenza, D., "Aspartame: clinical update," *Connecticut Medicine*, 53:395, 1989
99 —Roberts, H., "Does aspartame cause human brain cancer?," *J Advance Med*, 4:236, 1991
Gross, A., *Congressional Record*, SID 835:131, Aug. 1, 1985
100 —US Department of Health and Human Services, "Report on adverse reactions in the adverse reaction monitoring system," Feb. 28, 1994
101 —US General Accounting Office, "Report to the Honorable Howard M. Metzenbaum, US Senate: FDA Food Additive Approval Process Followed for Aspartame," GAO/HRD–87–46, June 1987
Bressler, J., FDA, "The Bressler Report: Investigation of Searle Laboratories," Aug. 7, 1977
102 —"Aspartame approved despite risks," *Science*, 213:984, 1981
Federal Register, July 24, 1981, pg 38285
103 —Mullarkey, B., as per note 96, pg 37
104 —"American Dietetic Association under attack," *Spectrum*, May/June 1995, pg 7
105 —Rowe, K., "Synthetic food coloring and behavior: a dose response effect in a double-blind, placebo-controlled, repeated-measures study," *J Pediatrics*, 125:691, 1994
106 —Segal, M., "Ingredient labeling: what's in a food?," *FDA Consumer*, April 1993, pg 17
107 —Morris, S., *The Emperor Who Ate the Bible and More Strange Facts and Useless Information*, Doubleday, 1991
108 —As per note 69, pg 24

Dairy Products

109 —Quoted in *JADA*, 86:1345, 1986
110 —Quoted in *The Prevention Total Health System: Food and Nutrition*, Rodale Press, 1983, pg 158
111 —Ensminger, A., *Food For Health—A Nutrient Encyclopedia*, Pegus Press, 1986, pg 694
Kitt, D., *Nutr Quarterly*, 14:28, 1990
112 —Scrimshaw, N., "The acceptability of milk and milk products in populations with a high prevalence of lactose intolerance," *Am J Clin Nutr*, 48:1140, 1988
113 —Whitney, E., *Understanding Normal and Clinical Nutrition*, 2nd ed., West Publishing, 1987, pg 75
UC Berkeley Wellness Letter, May 1988, pg 8
114 —Ensminger, A., as per note 111, pg 695
115 —Dairy milk values from *UC Berkeley Wellness Letter*, May 1990, pg 8

Goat, soy and rice milk values from author survey
116 —Bahna, S., *Allergies to Milk*, Grune and Stratton, 1980
117 —Dosch, H., "Lack of immunity to bovine serum albumin in insulin-dependent diabetes mellitus," *N Engl J Med*, 330:1616, 1994
Verge, C., "Environmental factors in childhood IDDM," *Diabetes Care*, 17:1381, 1994
118 —Couet, C., "Lactose and cataract in humans: a review," *J Am Coll Nutr,* 10:79, 1991
Simoons, F., "A geographic approach to senile cataracts: possible links with milk consumption, lactose activity, and galactose metabolism," *Digestive Diseases and Sciences*, 27:257, 1982
119 —Oski, F., *Don't Drink Your Milk*, 9th ed., Teach Services, 1992, pg 62
120 —LaVecchia, C., "Dairy products and the risk of prostatic cancer," *Oncology*, 48:406, 1991
Cramer, D., "Galactose consumption and metabolism in relation to the risk of ovarian cancer," *Lancet*, 2:66, 1989
121 —Ziegler, E., "Cow milk feeding in infancy: further observations on blood loss from the gastrointestinal tract," *J Pediatrics,* 116:11, 1990
122 —Ursin, G., "Milk consumption and cancer incidence: a Norwegian prospective study," *Br J Cancer,* 61:456, 1990
Cunningham, A., "Lymphomas and animal protein consumption," *Lancet*, 2:1184, 1976
123 —Parke, A., "Rheumatoid arthritis and food: a case study," *Br Med J,* 282:2027, 1981
Welsh, C., *Int Arch Allergy Appl Immunol*, 80:192, 1986
Clinica Chimica Acta, 203:153, 1991
124 —Hallberg, L., "Calcium: effect of different amounts of nonheme- and heme-iron absorption in humans," *Am J Clin Nutr,* 53:112, 1991
Oski, F., *Pediatrics*, 75 (Suppl):182, 1985
125 —Boat, J., "Hyperreactivity to cow milk in young children with pulmonary hemosiderosis and cor pulmonale secondary to nasopharyngeal obstruction," *J Pediatrics*, 87:23, 1975
126 —Recker, R., "The effect of milk supplements on calcium metabolism and calcium balance," *Am J Clin Nutr,* 41:254, 1985
127 —Cramer, D., "Adult hypolactasia, milk consumption and age-specific fertility," *Am J Epidemiol*, 139:282, 1994
128 —Bienenstock, J., "Mucosal barrier functions," *Nutr Rev*, 42:105, 1984
Johnson, L., *Physiology of the Gastrointestinal Tract*, Raven Press, 1981, pgs 1271–89
Hemmings, W., *Protein Transmission through Living Membranes,* Elsevier, 1979, pg 429
129 —Clyne, P., "Human breast milk contains bovine IgG. Relationship to infant colic?" *Pediatrics*, 87:439, 1991
130 —"Effects, Uses, Control and Research of Agricultural Pesticides," A Report by the Surveys and Investigations Staff of USDA, Part 1, pg 174
131 —Smith, J., "Hawaiian milk contamination creates alarm, a sour response by state regulators," *Science*, 217:137, 1982

132 —US General Accounting Office, "FDA strategy needed to address animal drug residues in milk," 1992
US General Accounting Office, "Food safety and quality. FDA surveys not adequate to demonstrate safety of milk supply," Nov. 1990
Begley, S., "The end of antibiotics," *Newsweek*, Mar 28, 1994, pg 48
133 —Fontaine, R., "Epidemic salmonellosis from cheddar cheese: surveillance and prevention," *Am J Epidemiol*, 111:247, 1980
Katz, S., *J Food Protection*, 56:229, 1993
134 —Marie-Liesse, G., "Effect of brucellosis vaccination and dehorning on transmission of bovine leukemia virus in heifers on a California dairy," *Can J Vet Res*, 54:184, 1990
Ferrer, J., "Milk of dairy cows frequently contains a leukemogenic virus," *Science*, 213:1014, 1981
135 —Gonda, M., "Bovine immunodeficiency virus," *AIDS*, 6:759, 1992
Cockerell, G., "Seroprevalence of bovine immunodeficiency-like virus and bovine leukemia virus in a dairy cattle herd," *Vet Microbiology,* 31:109, 1992
136 —Jacobs, R., "Detection of multiple retroviral infections in cattle and cross-reactivity of bovine immunodeficiency-like virus and human immunodeficiency virus type 1 proteins using bovine and human sera in a Western blot assay," *Can J Vet Res*, 56:353, 1992
137 —Young, F., "Weighing food safety risks," *FDA Consumer*, Sept. 1989, pg 8
138 —Roberts, J., "US milk cannot be labelled hormone free, says FDA," *BMJ*, 308:495, 1994
Daughaday, W., "Bovine somatotropin supplementation of dairy cows," *JAMA*, 264:1003, 1990
Townsend Letter for Doctors, Aug./Sept. 1990, pg 536
139 —"BGH firm says promotion, not give-away, is priority," *Nutr Week*, Nov. 26, 1993, pg 7
140 —Mepham, T., "Safety of milk from cows treated with bovine somatotropin," *Lancet*, 344:197, 1994
Kronfeld, D., "Bovine somatotropin," *JAMA*, 265:1389, 1991
141 —Stauber, J., "Shut up and eat your 'Frankenfoods,'" *PR Watch*, Jan./Mar. 1994, pg 8
142 —Madigan, D., "Hormones: dead…for now," *Veg Times*, Nov. 1993, pg 19
143 —As per note 141
144 —Food & Water, "Shame on them," *Safe Food News*, Fall 1994, pg 2
145 —Katzenstein, L., "Sour milk," *American Health*, Oct. 1994, pg 7
146 —Quoted in Lustgarden, S., "Milk: it does a body good?," *Veg Times*, Jan. 1993, pg 16

Seafood

147 —Quoted in Jaroff, L., "Is your fish really foul?," *Time*, June 29, 1992, pg 71
148 —Quoted in *Time,* Feb. 18, 1985
149 —Steinman, D., *Diet For a Poisoned Planet,* Harmony Books, 1990, pg 1
Steinman, D., "How I came clean," *California,* June 1990, pg 76
CSPI Americans for Safe Food, *Guess What's Coming To Dinner,* 1987, pg 42
150 —Robbins, J., *Diet For A New America,* Stillpoint, 1987, pg 331

Regenstein, L., *How to Survive in America the Poisoned,* Acropolis Books, 1982, pg 298
151 —Swain, W., "Human health consequences of consumption of fish contaminated with organochlorine compounds," *Acquatic Toxicol,* 11:357, 1988
152 —"The Tenth Annual Report of the Council on Environmental Quality," Washington DC, Dec. 1979, pgs 11, 99, 448
Ibid
153 —Goldbeck, N. and D., *The Goldbeck's Guide to Good Food,* NAL Books, 1987, pg 268
Rochlitz, S., *Allergies and Candida with the 21st Century Solution,* Human Ecology Balancing Sciences, 1988, pg 39
154 —"A Brief Review of Selected Environmental Contamination Incidents with a Potential for Health Effects," Prepared by the Library of Congress for the Committee on Environment and Public Works, US Senate, Aug. 1980, pgs 173, 284
Congressional Quarterly, Sept. 6, 1980, pg 2643
155 —Holt, S., "The food resources of the ocean," *Scientific Amer,* 221:178, 1969
Robbins, J., as per note 150
156 —Rauber, P., "Sierra Club fights PCBs in the Great Lakes," *Sierra*, Sept./Oct. 1994, pg 45
157 —CSPI Americans for Safe Food, as per note 3
158 —As per note 156
159 —As per note 147, pg 70
160 —Martin, G., "Farming of salmon now an issue," *San Francisco Chronicle*, Jan. 25, 1993, pg E-9
Corey, B., "Life on a fish farm," *FDA Consumer*, July/Aug. 1992, pg 19
161 —Quoted in "Eat a burger, save a trout," *Outside,* Dec. 1991, pg 25

Vitamin Wars

162 —Testimony before the House Subcommittee on Intergovernmental Relations, reported in "Who blocks testing of anti-cancer agents," *Alameda Times-Star*, Aug. 3, 1970
163 —National Research Council, *Diet and Health: Implications for Reducing Chronic Disease Risk,* National Academy of Sciences, 1989
164 —Recer, P., Associated Press, "US says no to vitamin pills: they won't help, may hurt," *Sacramento Bee*, Mar. 2, 1989
165 —Slutsker, L., "Eosinophilia-myalgia syndrome associated with exposure to tryptophan from a single manufacturer," *JAMA*, 264:213, 1990
166 —Leibovitz, B., "Nutrition: at the crossroads," *J Optimal Nutr*, 1:79, 1992
167 —Windsor, R., "Are (medical) drugs worth the risks?," *Spectrum*, Jan./Feb. 1995, pg 22
168 —Department of Health and Human Services, Food and Drug Administration, *Dietary Supplements Task Force Final Report,* May 1992, pgs 10–11, 33–36
169 —Ibid, pgs 2, 71
170 —Interview on "Larry King Live," CNN–TV, 1992
Quoted in Salaman, M., "Would you hire the FDA?," *Health Freedom News*, Mar. 1994, pg 14

171 —Fackelmann, K., "Beta carotene may slow artery disease," *Science News*, 138:308, 1990

172 —Nelson, R., "Body iron stores and risk of colonic neoplasia," *JNCI*, 86:455, 1994

Christensen D., "High iron stores may increase cancer risk," *Science News*, 145:132, 1994

173 —Magnuson, T., "Oral calcium promotes pigment gallstone formation," *Am J Clin Nutr*, 53:112, 1991

Aprcella, L., "Increased risk of urinary track infections associated with the use of calcium supplements," *Urological Res*, 18:213, 1990

174 —Black, M., "Zinc supplements and serum lipids in young adult white males," *Am J Clin Nutr*, 47:970, 1988

Song, M., "Possible link between zinc intake and colon cancer," *JNCI*, 85:667, 1993

Hollingsworth, J., "Immunodeficiency and lymphocyte ecto-5-nucleotidase activity in the elderly: a comparison of the effect of a trace mineral supplement with high zinc," *Nutri Res,* 7:801, 1987

Kaiser, J., "Alzheimer's: could there be a zinc link?," *Science*, 265:1365, 1994

175 —Herbert, V., "The antioxidant supplement myth," *Am J Clin Nutr*, 60:157, 1994

176 —Xu, M., "Reduction in plasma or skin alfa-tocopherol concentrations with long-term oral administration of beta-carotene in humans and mice," *JNCI*, 84:1559, 1992

177 —Galloe, A., "Influence of oral magnesium supplementation on cardiac events among survivors of an acute myocardial infarction," *Br Med J,* 307:585, 1993

178 —Herbert, V., "Recommended dietary intakes (RDI) of vitamin B12 in humans," *Am J Clin Nutr,* 45:671, 1987

Robertson, L., *The New Laurel's Kitchen*, Ten Speed Press, 1986, pg 363

179 —Lindenbaum, J., "Prevalence of cobalamin deficiency in the Framingham elderly population," *Am J Clin Nutr*, 60:2, 1994

180 —Dagnelie, P., "Vitamin B12 from algae appears not to be available," *Am J Clin Nutr*, 53:695, 1991

Langley, G., *Vegan Nutrition: A Survey of Research*, England, Vegan Society, 1988, pg 56

"The B12 question," *AHIMSA,* American Vegan Society, July/Dec. 1981, pg 1

181 —Herbert, V., "Vitamin B12: plant sources, requirements, and assay," *Am J Clin Nutr*, 48:857, 1988

182 —McDougall, J., *The McDougall Plan*, New Century, 1983, pg 40

183 —McDougall, J., *The McDougall Program,* NAL Books, 1990, pg 46

184 —Robertson, L., as per note 178, pg 397

185 —Moran, V., "Compassion: the ultimate ethic," *AHIMSA,* American Vegan Society, July/Dec. 1981, pg 1

186 —Quoted in "Revolution in medicine and diet," *Spectrum*, May/June 1992, pg 28

187 —*Consumer Reports*, Feb. 1981, pg 68

188 —Liebman, B., "Getting your vitamins?," *CSPI Nutr Action HealthLetter*, June 1990, pg 5
189 —McGurk, M., "Gulping down vitamins may not be helping," *Senior Spectrum*, Jan. 1992, pg 14
190 —Southgate, D., *Nutrient Availability: Chemical and Biological Aspects,* Royal Society of Chemistry, Thomas Graham House, UK, 1989, pg 125
Vinson, J., "Comparison of the bio-availability of combination vitamin and mineral supplements," University of Scranton, PA, unpublished study, Aug. 6, 1981
191 —Quoted in Armstrong, D. and E., *The Great American Medicine Show,* Prentice Hall, 1991, pg 222

Chapter 3—Dietary Components

1 —Hindhede, M, "The effect of food restriction during war on mortality in Coppenhagen," *JAMA*, 74:381, 1920
2 —Ingram, D., "Trends in diet and breast cancer mortality in England and Wales, 1928–1977," *Nutr and Cancer*, 3:75, 1982
Strom, A., "Mortality from circulatory diseases in Norway 1940–1945," *Lancet,* 1:126, 1951
Malmros, H., "The relation of nutrition to health: a statistical study of the effect of the war-time on arteriosclerosis, cardiosclerosis, tuberculosis and diabetes," *Acta Med Scand Suppl*, 246:137, 1950
3 —Wynder, E., "Comparative epidemiology of cancer between the United States and Japan," *Cancer*, 67:746, 1991
Okubo, I., "Cost-effectiveness analysis of mass screening for breast cancer in Japan," *Cancer*, 67:2021, 1991
Lands, W., "Changing dietary patterns," *Am J Clin Nutr*, 51:991, 1990
4 —Quoted in Hammond, M., "The decline of the Japanese diet," *East West Journal*, Oct. 1990, pg 74
5 —Chen, J., *Diet, life-style, and mortality in China: a study of the characteristics of 65 Chinese counties*, Oxford University Press, Cornell University Press, China People's Medical Publishing House, 1991
6 —Sussman, V., "A fresh attack on red meat," *US News & World Report,* Dec. 31, 1990, pg 67
7 —Harrington, G., *Real Food–Fake Food,* Macmillan Publishing, 1987, pg 338
8 —"The graphic truth," *East West Journal,* July 1990, pg 11
Wholesome Diet, Time-Life Books, 1981, pg 13
9 —Ibid
10 —Quoted in Ebert, M. and Mitric, J., "Race is on for healthy fast food," *Maturity News Service: Senior News & Views,* April 1991, pg 17
11 —Quoted in Byrne, R., *1,911 Best Things Anyone Ever Said,* Ballantine Books, 1988, pg 324
12 —"US appetite for meat continues to grow: USDA," *Nutrition Week*, Mar. 17, 1995, pg 6
13 —USDA Nationwide Food Consumption Survey, Nutrient Intakes: Individuals in 48 States, Year 1977–78, Report No. I–2, May 1984

Williams, S., *Nutrition and Diet Therapy*, 6th ed., Times Mirror/Mosby College Publishing, 1989, pg 790

14 —National Research Council, Food and Nutrition Board, *Recommended Dietary Allowances,* 10th ed., National Academy Press, 1989, pg 40

American Heart Association, "Position Statement: Dietary Guidelines for Healthy American Adults," *Circulation*, 77:721A, 1988

USDA Human Nutrition Information Service, Food Consumption Research Survey, Food and Nutrient Intake by Individuals in the United States, 1987–1988, Table 4.1

Marston, R., "Nutrient content of the U.S. food supply," *Nat Food Rev*, 36:18, 1987

As per note 5

15 —*Health*, Jan./Feb. 1994, pg 29

16 —USDA Economic Research Service, Survey of Food Consumption, Prices and Expenditures, 1989

17 —Ibid

18 —UN Food and Agriculture Organization, *FAO Food Balance Sheets, 1984–86 average*, Rome, 1991

19 —US Bureau of the Census, *Statistical Abstract of the United States: 1992*, 112th ed., US Government Printing Office, 1992, pg 134

Gallup Survey, *US News & World Report,* Nov. 13, 1989

National Research Council, 1989

USDA Economic Research Service, 1989

FDA Consumer, Oct. 1988, pg 5 and Feb. 1989, pg 16

Am Inst Cancer Res Newsletter, Summer 1990, pg 8

Tufts U Diet Nutr Letter, Sept. 1991, pg 2

CSPI Nutr Action Healthletter, June 1995, pgs 8–9

20 —Rankin, M., "Animal fat for diesel fuel," *Sci Food Agriculture*, 5:9, 1993

21 —Raloff, J., "Cholesterol: up in smoke," *Science News,* July 27, 1991, pg 61

Cass G., *Environ Sci Technol,* June 1991

22 —U.S. National Association of Pizza Operators, 1990

23 —Boyd, L., *San Francisco Chronicle,* Sunday Punch, April 12, 1992, pg 5

24 —Moser, P., "There's always room for . . .," *Health*, May/June 1992, pg 25

25 —Clorfene-Casten, L., "Unhappy meals," *Mother Jones*, July/Aug. 1992, pg 34

26 —Quoted in American Medical Association, *Let's Talk About Food,* Publishing Services Group, 1974, pg 110

Choices

27 —"Position of the American Dietetic Association: Vegetarian Diets," *JADA*, 88:351, 1988

28 —Colbin, A., *Food and Healing*, Ballantine Books, pg xiv

29 —Quoted in Crowley, S., "Nurturing body and soul," *AARP Bulletin,* April 1990, pg 20

30 —Feldman, B., "Compass," *East West Journal,* July/Aug. 1991, pg 10

31 —"Revolution in medicine and diet," *Spectrum*, May/June 1992, pg 28

32 —*Time*, May 11, 1992, pgs 16–17

"Beef or bull," *Veg Times*, July 1991, pg 22

San Francisco Chronicle, April 28, 1992, pg A1

33 —Quoted in “USDA’s pyramid scheme,” *CSPI Nutr Action Healthletter*, June 1991, pg 3

Quoted in Burros, M., “Plain talk on eating right,” *San Francisco Chronicle*, This World, Jan. 12, 1992, pg 7

34 —Quoted in National Live Stock and Meat Board, “Why didn’t the industry respond?,” *The Veal Checkoff Report*, July 1991

35 —“Carrot and stick,” *Veg Times,* Oct. 1990, pg 73

36 —Willett, W., “Diet and health: what should we eat?,” *Science*, 264:532, 1994

37 —Schardt, D., “Going Mediterranean,” *CSPI Nutr Action Healthletter,* Dec. 1994, pg 9

38 —United Nations, *FAO Food Balance Sheets, 1984–86 average*, Rome, 1991

USDA, Nutrient Content of the USA Food Supply, HNIS Adm Rep. No. 299–21, Aug. 1988

1992 Demographic Yearbook, 44th issue, United Nations Publications, 1994, pgs 118–123

39 —Briggs, J., “Coronary heart disease in France,” *Br Med J,* 309:611, 1994

40 —Marlin, J. and Collins, S., *Book of World City Rankings*, The Free Press, 1986, pg 580

41 —Mazess, R., “Bone mineral content of North Alaskan Eskimos,” *Am J Clin Nutr,* 27:916, 1974

Ho, K., “Alaska Arctic Eskimos: responses to a customary high fat diet,” *Am J Clin Nutr,* 25:737, 1972

42 —Dewailly, E., “Inuit exposure to organochlorines through the aquatic food chain in Arctic Quebec,” *Environ Health Perspect,* 101:618, 1993

43 —Eaton, S., “Paleothic nutrition,” *N Engl J Med,* 313:283, 1985

Eaton, S., “Diet: paleolithic genes and twentieth century health,” *Leakey Foundation Anthroquest*, Winter 1985, pg 19

44 —Gould, G., *Anomalies and Curiosities of Medicne,* Julian Press, 1954, pg 405

45 —National Center for Health Statistics, “Life expectancy at birth and at 65 years of age, by sex: selected countries, 1982 and 1987,” *Health, United States, 1990*, Public Health Service, 1991, Table 22

46 —Ibid

47 —*United Nations Demographic Yearbook,* 1986

48 —Joossens, J., “Salt intake and mortality from strokes,” *N Engl J Med*, 300:1396, 1979

49 —Quoted in *Awake*, Dec. 8, 1989, pg 6

50 —As per note 28, pg 64

51 —Ibid

52 —Carter, J., “Hypothesis: dietary management may improve survival from nutritionally linked cancers based on analysis of representative cases,” *J Am Coll Nutr*, 12:209, 1993

53 —Wigmore, A., *The Hippocrates Diet,* Avery Publishing, 1984, pg 174

54 —Douglass, J., “Effects of a raw food diet on hypertension and obesity,” *South Med J,* 78:841, 1985

55 —Robertson, L., *The New Laurel’s Kitchen,* Ten Speed Press, 1986, pg 397

Longevity Centers

56 —Quoted in Kadison, E., "Forever young!," *Let's Live*, Sept. 1991, pg 20

57 —Quoted in Leaf, A., "Getting old," *Scientific American,* Sept. 1973, pg 46

58 —Leaf, A., "Unusual longevity: the common denominators," *Hospital Practice*, Oct. 1973, pg 75

59 —Leaf, A., "Every day is a gift when you are over 100," *National Geographic*, Jan. 1973, pg 96

60 —Quoted in *Los Angeles Times*, July 16, 1973

61 —As per note 58, pg 82

62 —Andrade, M., *San Francisco Chronicle*, This World, Dec. 13, 1989, pg 13

63 —Ibid

64 —Ibid

65 —Mazess, R., "Bone mineral content in Vilcabamba, Ecuador," *Am J Roentgenol*, 130:671, 1978

Pelletier, K., *Longevity: Fulfilling Our Biological Potential,* Delacorte, 1981, pg 286

66 —Wallechinsky, D. and Wallace, I., *The People's Almanac*, Doubleday, 1975, pg 1066

67 —Classic, C., *Secret To Hunza Superior Health,* Center for Human Natural Nutrition, 1989, pg 40

68 —McCarry, J., "High road to Hunza," *National Geographic*, Mar. 1994

69 —Tierney, J., "The three secrets of Shangri-La," *In Health*, July/Aug. 1990, pg 42

70 —As per note 66, pg 1065

71 —As per note 69

72 —As per note 59, pg 102

73 —As per note 59, pg 108

74 —As per note 59, pg 110

75 —Walford, R., *The 120 Year Diet,* Pocket Books, 1986, pg 120

76 —Hoffman, J., *Hunza: 15 Secrets of the World's Healthiest and Oldest Living People*, Professional Press, 1968, pg 81

77 —As per note 66, pg 1070

78 —As per note 57, pg 47

79 —As per note 66, pg 1070

80 —As per note 59, pg 102

81 —USDA Nationwide Food Consumption Survey, Nutrient Intakes: Individuals in 48 States, Year 1977–78, Report No. I–2, May 1984

82 —Leaf, A., "Observations of a peripatetic gerontologist," *Nutr Today,* Sept./Oct. 1973, pg 4

Pelletier, K., as per note 10, pg 294

83 —As per note 57

84 —Ibid

85 —As per note 66, pg 1069

86 —Banik, A. and Taylor, R., *Hunza Land*, Whitehorn Publishing, pg 121

Taylor, R., *The Hunza-Yoga Way To Health And Longer Life*, Lancer Books, 1969, pg 23

As per note 66, pg 1066

As per note 67, pg 53

Chapter 4—Personal Application

1 —Interview on the Larry King Show, daytime radio, Feb. 8, 1993
2 —Quoted in "Overheard," *Newsweek*, Aug. 26, 1991, pg 15
3 —Pennisi, E., "Food cravings tied to brain chemicals," *Sci News,* 144:310, 1993
4 —MacFie, H., "Assessment of sensory properties of food," *Nutr Reviews,* 48:87, 1990
5 —Mattes, R., "Fat preference and adherence to a reduced-fat diet," *Am J Clin Nutr,* 57:373, 1993
6 —Quoted in Thomson, B., "Marvelous Mollie Katzen: still life after Moosewood," *East West Journal*, Sept. 1988, pg 70
7 —Quoted in DeSilver, D., "Halloween with Elvira," *Veg Times*, Oct. 1991, pg 46
8 —*UC Berkeley Wellness Letter,* June 1989
9 —*UC Berkeley Wellness Letter,* April 1989
10 —*Family Circle* survey of 35,000 women, reported in *Psychology Today*, June 1989, pg 12
11 —Ibid
12 —Tribole, E., *Eating on the Run,* 2nd ed., Leisure Press, 1992, pg 1
13 —"Vital statistics," *In Health,* Jan./Feb. 1990, pg 12
14 —"Vital statistics," *Health*, April 1992, pg 12
15 —Raper, N., *Nutrient Content of the U.S. Food Supply 1908–1988*, Washington D.C., USDA, Home Economics Research Report #50, 1992

Chapter 5—The Human Body

Weight Control

1 —Quoted in *People Weekly*, Jan. 14, 1991, pg 88
2 —Taylor, E., "From fat to fabulous," *Good Housekeeping*, Mar. 1988, pg 1
3 —Interview on KGO Radio, San Francisco, CA, April 25, 1991
4 —Robbins, J., *Diet For A New America*, Stillpoint Press, 1987, pg 287
Friday, S., *The Food Sleuth Handbook*, Athenum Publishers, 1982
5 —Mark Clements Research Group, reported in *Earth Island Journal,* Spring 1994, pg 16
6 —Herbert, V., *The Mount Sinai School of Medicine Complete Book of Nutrition,* St. Martin's Press, 1990, pg 271
"Very low-calorie diets," *UC Berkeley Wellness Letter*, Jan. 1989, pg 4
7 —Kuczmarski, R., "Increasing prevalence of overweight among US adults," *JAMA*, 272:205, 1994
Robison, J., "Obesity, weight loss and health," *JADA*, 93:446, 1993
USDA Human Nutrition Information Service, *Food and Nutrient Intake by Individuals in the United States, 1987–88*, Table 4.1
8 —Quoted in Hausman, P., *Jack Sprat's Legacy—The Science and Politics of Fat and Cholesterol*, Richard Mauk Publishers, 1981, pg 207
9 —US Department of Health and Human Services, *The Surgeon General's Report on Nutrition and Health,* 1988
10 —Brody, J., "Huge study of diet indicts fat and meat," *New York Times,* May, 8, 1990, pg C–1

11 —Miller, W., "Dietary fat, sugar and fiber predict body fat content," *JADA*, 94:612, 1994

12 —Marx, J., "Catching up with the world's fastest human," *Runner's World*, Aug. 1992, pg 62

13 —Swinburn, B., "Energy balance and fat balance?," *Am J Clin Nutr*, 57:766, 1993

Oliver, O., "Oxidative and nonoxidative macronutrient disposal in lean and obese subjects after mixed meals," *Am J Clin Nutr*, 55:630, 1992

Suter, P., "The effect of ethanol on fat storage in healthy subjects," *N Engl J Med*, 326:983, 1992

Hellerstein, M., "Measurement of de novo hepatic lipogenesis in humans using stable isotopes," *J Clin Invest,* 87:1841, 1991

14 —Tjonneland, A., "Adipose tissue fatty acids as biomarkers of dietary exposure in Danish men and women," *Am J Clin Nutr,* 57:629, 1993

Schafer, L., "Subcutaneous adipose-tissue fatty acids and vitamin E in humans: relation to diet and sampling site," *Am J Clin Nutr,* 52:486, 1990

London, S., "Fatty acid composition of subcutaneous adipose tissue and diet in postmenopausal US women," *Am J Clin Nutr,* 54:340, 1991

Thomas, L., "Hydrogenated oils and fats: the presence of chemically-modified fatty acids in human adipose tissue," *Am J Clin Nutr,* 34:877, 1981

15 —Blundell, J., "Dietary fat and the control of energy intake: evaluating the effects of fat on meal size and postmeal satiety, *Am J Clin Nutr,* 57:722, 1993

16 —Campbell, T. reported in Mead, N., "The champion diet," *East West Journal,* Sept. 1990, pg 49

17 —Barnard, N., *Food for Life*, Harmony Books, 1993, pgs 87–88

Scanlon, D., *Diets That Work*, Lowell House, 1991, pgs 24–56

18 —Foster, G., "Controlled trial of the metabolic effects of a very-low-calorie diet: short- and long-term effects," *Am J Clin Nutr,* 51:167, 1990

Weigle, D., "Weight loss leads to a marked decrease in nonresting energy expenditure in ambulatory human subjects," *Metabolism Clin Exp*, 37:930, 1988

Blackburn, G., "Weight cycling: the experience of human subjects," *Am J Clin Nutr,* 49:1105, 1989

19 —Quoted in Armstrong, D. and E., *The Great American Medicine Show*, Prentice Hall, 1991, pg 255

20 —Spielman, A., "The cost of losing: an analysis of commercial weight-loss programs in a metropolitan area," *J Am Coll Nutr*, 11:36, 1992

21 —Interview on the Larry King Show, daytime radio, Los Angeles, Mar. 24, 1993

22 —Quoted in Cader, M., *Eat These Words*, HarperCollins Publishers, 1991, pg 75

23 —Orphanidou, C., "Accuracy of subcutaneous fat measurement: comparison of skinfold calipers, ultrasound, and computed tomography," *JADA*, 94:855, 1994

Stout, J., "Validity of percent body fat estimations in males," *Med Sci Sports Exercise*, 26:632, 1994
24 —*Guinness Book of World Records*, Bantam Books, 1986, pg 9
25 —Manchester, R., *Incredible Facts*, Bristol Park Books, 1985, pg 103
Guinness Book of World Records, Bantam Books, 1991, pg 12

Exercise

26 —Quoted in *Newsweek*, Aug. 6, 1956
27 —Jones, T., "Cost-benefit analysis of walking to prevent coronary heart disease," *Arch Fam Med*, 3:703, 1994
28 —Ibid
29 —Sussman, V., "Muscle bound," *San Francisco Chronicle*, This World, Oct. 13, 1991, pg 18
30 —Wuntch, P., "A filmmaker's apocalypse," *Marin Independent Journal*, Oct. 8, 1991, pg D-1
31 —Quoted in Tanny, A., "72 and going strong," *Muscle and Fitness,* May 1993, pg 191
32 —Saltin, B., "Free fatty acids and exercise," *Am J Clin Nutr,* 57(Suppl): 752, 1993
33 —Shephard, R., *Physical Activity and Aging*, 2nd ed., Aspen, 1987
34 —*Canada Health Survey*, Ottawa: Health and Welfare Canada, 1982
35 —Shephard, R., "Exercise and aging: extending independence in older adults," *Geriatrics*, 48:62, 1993
36 —Ibid
37 —Lee, I., "Exercise intensity and longevity in men," *JAMA*, 273:1179, 1995
Fries, J., "Running and the development of disability with age," *Ann Intern Med*, 121:502, 1994
38 —White, J., "Enhanced sexual behavior in exercising men," *Arch Sexual Behavior,* 19:193, 1990
39 —Duncan, J., "Women walking for health and fitness: how much is enough?," *JAMA*, 266:3295, 1991
40 —*UC Berkeley Wellness Letter,* Nov. 1994, pg 8
41 —Bernstein, L., "Physical exercise and reduced risk of breast cancer in young women," *JNCI*, 86:1403, 1994
Helmrich, S., "Physical activity and reduced occurence of non-insulin-dependent diabetes mellitus," *N Engl J Med*, 325:147, 1991
As per note 27

Biological Age

42 —*Life*, Feb. 1989, pg 61
43 —*UC Berkeley Wellness Letter,* June 1989, pg 2
Brenner, B., "Dietary protein and the progressive nature of kidney disease," *N Engl J Med*, 307:652, 1982
Leaf, A., "Getting old," *Scientific American*, Sept. 1973, pg 52
Merz, B., "Why we get old," *Harvard Health Letter*, Supplement, Oct. 1992, pg 10
44 —Liebman, B., "The HDL/triglyceride trap," *CSPI Nutr Action Healthletter,* Sept. 1990, pg 5
45 —Pritikin, N., *The Pritikin Program for Diet & Exercise*, Bantam Books, 1979, pg 21

46 —Pollock, M., *Health and Fitness Through Physical Activity*, John Wiley and Sons, 1978, pg 420
47 —Bechtel, S., "How old are you really?," *Esquire*, May 1990, pg 134
48 —American College of Sports Medicine, *The Y's Way to Fitness,* Human Kinetics, 1982
Eller, D., "Flex time," *American Health*, April 1993, pg 72
49 —Morris, J., "Prediction nomograms (BTPS), spirometric values in normal males," *Am Rev Respir Dis*, 103:57, 1971, (values for 170 cm height)
50 —Bruce Treadmill Stress Test (VO_2 Max)
As per note 46
51 —As per note 46
52 —Walford, R., *The 120 Year Diet*, Pocket Books, 1986, pg 54
53 —McDougall, J., *The McDougall Plan*, New Century, 1983, pg 65
54 —Bagshaw, J., quoted in Thomas, R., "New medicine for a nation of health nuts," *San Francisco Chronicle*, This World, Oct. 13, 1991, pg 8
55 —Ibid
56 —Fries, J., "Reducing health care costs by reducing the need and demand for medical services," *N Engl J Med*, 329:321, 1993
57 —Raskin, D., "Premium fitness," *American Health,* April 1991, pg 79
58 —"Tangible benefits for better health," *Veg Times*, April 1992, pg 22
59 —"Shape up – or else!," *Newsweek*, July 1, 1991, pgs 42–43
60 —Hulley, S., "Health policy on blood cholesterol: time to change directions," *Circulation*, 86:1026, 1992
Goldman, L., "Cost-effectiveness of HMG-CoA reductase inhibition for primary and secondary prevention of coronary heart disease," *JAMA*, 265:1145, 1991
Ravnskov, U., "Cholesterol lowering trials in coronary heart disease: frequency of citation and outcome," *Br Med J*, 305:15, 1992
Ramsay, L., "Dietary reduction of serum cholesterol concentration: time to think again," *Br Med J*, 303:953, 1991
61 —Ornish, D., "Can lifestyle changes reverse coronary heart disease? The Lifestyle Heart Trial," *Lancet*, 336:129, 1990
62 —Drummond, H., "On growing old," *A Sourcebook on Health & Survival,* Foundation for National Progress, 1981, pg 44

Slowing the Clock

63 —De Ropp, R., *Man Against Aging*, St. Martin's Press, 1960, pg 4
64 —Tierney, J., "Buying time," *Hippocrates*, Jan./Feb. 1990, pg 59
65 —*UC Berkeley Wellness Letter*, Sept. 1992, pg 8
66 —Young, R., "Biological renewal, applications to the eye: the Bowman lecture," *Trans Ophthalmol Soc UK*, 102:42–67, 1982
67 —Quoted in Kahn, C., "A day in the life of a longevity physician," *Longevity*, Aug. 1990, pg 43
68 —Quoted in Pitts, W., "Cancer and the power of positive thinking," *Total Health,* June 1993, pg 38
69 —Quoted in Kahn, C., "Are illness and aging one and the same?," *Longevity*, April 1991, pg 45

American Seniors

70 —Quoted in DeRopp, R., *Man Against Aging,* St. Martin's Press, 1960, pg 267
71 —US Bureau of the Census, Current Population Reports, Special Studies, P23–178, *Sixty-Five Plus in America*, US Government Printing Office, 1992, pg 2–1
72 —Olshansky, S., "In search of Methuselah: estimating the upper limits to human longevity," *Science,* 250:635, 1990
73 —Kemper, P., "Lifetime use of nursing home care," *N Engl J Med*, 324:595, 1991
74 —Drummond, H., *A Sourcebook On Health & Survival,* Foundation for National Progress, 1981, pg 43
"Setting loose old folks," *Spectrum*, July/Aug. 1993, pg 25
"Harper's index," *San Francisco Chronicle,* This World, June 9, 1991, pg 6
75 —*Longevity*, Sept. 1991, pg 36
CSPI Nutr Action Healthletter, June 1992, pg 6
76 —Drummond, H., as per note 74, pg 42
77 —Lubitz, J., "Trends in Medicare payments in the last year of life," *N Engl J Med*, 328:1092, 1993
78 —Shephard, R., "Exercise and aging: extending independence in older adults," *Geriatrics*, 48:63, 1993
Canada Health Survey, Ottawa: Health and Welfare Canada, 1982
79 —"The rate of disability in old age is dropping," *John Hopkins Medical Letter,* July 1993, pg 1
80 —Popcorn, F., *The Popcorn Report,* Doubleday, 1991
81 —Quoted in Kahn, C., *Longevity,* Oct. 1990, pg 66
82 —US Bureau of the Census, Current Population Reports, P25–1092, *Population Projections of the United States by Age, Sex, Race and Hispanic Origin: 1992–2050*, US Government Printing Office, Nov. 1992, Table G
83 —Reported on ABC Radio News, Paul Harvey News, Oct. 17, 1991
84 —*Time,* Aug. 19, 1991, pg 55
Newsweek, Aug. 19, 1991, pg 57

Chapter 6—Survival Skills

1 —Mann, G., "Physical fitness and immunity to heart disease in Masai," *Lancet*, Dec. 25, 1965, pg 308
2 —"Healthy hearts out of Africa," *Hippocrates*, Mar./April 1988, pg 12
3 —Mann, G., "Diet–heart: end of an era," *N Engl J Med*, 297:644, 1977
Mann, G., "Atherosclerosis in the Masai," *Am J Epidemiol*, 95:26, 1972
4 —Burros, M., "Calcium, fat and sodium: caveats for teen-agers," *New York Times,* Feb. 14, 1987, pg 52
5 —National Center for Health Statistics, Advance Report of Final Mortality Statistics, 1993, *Monthly Vital Statistics Report,* Vol. 42, No. 13, Oct. 11, 1994
6 —US Department of Health and Human Services, *The Surgeon General's Report on Nutrition and Health,* 1988

Heart Disease

7 —Quoted in Armstrong, D. and E., *The Great American Medicine Show*, Prentice Hall, 1991, pg 139

8 —Ibid, pg 230

9 —Patlak, M., "Women and heart disease," *FDA Consumer*, Nov. 1994, pg 7

10 —*Nutrition Week*, Feb. 11, 1994, pg 7

11 —"The population approach: nutritional recommendations for healthy children and adolescents," National Cholesterol Education Program Report of the Expert Panel on Blood Cholesterol Levels in Children and Adolescents, Pub. No. 91–2732:11, 1991

12 —Johnson, C., "Declining serum total cholesterol levels among US adults," *JAMA*, 269:3002, 1993

Brody, J., "Huge study of diet indicts fat and meat," *New York Times,* May 8, 1990, pg C–1

Chen, J., *Diet, Life-Style, and Mortality in China: A Study of the Characteristics of 65 Chinese Counties*, Oxford University Press, Cornell University Press, China People's Medical Publishing House, 1991

13 —Castelli, W. in Liebman, B., "The HDL/triglycerides trap," *CSPI Nutr Action Healthletter*, Sept. 1990, pg 7

14 —Walford, R., *The Anti-Aging Plan*, Four Walls Eight Windows, 1994, pg 5

15 —Roberts, W., "Atherosclerotic risk factors," *Am J Cardiol,* 64:552, 1989

16 —Pooling Project Resource Group, "Relationship of blood pressure, serum cholesterol, smoking habit, relative weight and ECG abnormalities to incidence of major coronary events: final report of the Pooling Project," *J Chronic Dis*, 31:201, 1978

17 —Blackburn, G., "The ups and down of your cholesterol," *Prevention*, Sept. 1989, pg 120

18 —Yano, K., "Serum cholesterol and hemorrhagic stroke in the Honolulu Heart Program," *Stroke*, 20:1460, 1989

19 —Neaton, J., "Serum cholesterol level and mortality findings for men screened in the Multiple Risk Factor Intervention Trial," *Arch Int Med,* 152:1490, 1992

20 —Tornberg, S., "Cancer incidence and cancer mortality in relation to serum cholesterol," *JNCI*, 81:1917, 1989

Isles, C., "Plasma cholesterol, coronary heart disease and cancer in the Renfrew and Paisley Survey," *Br Med J,* 298:920, 1989

21 —Davey Smith, G., "Plasma cholesterol concentration and mortality: the Whitehall Study, *JAMA*, 267:70, 1992

Winawer, S., "Declining serum cholesterol levels prior to diagnosis of colon cancer," *JAMA*, 263:2083, 1990

22 —Lindberg, G., "Low serum cholesterol concentrations and short-term mortality from injuries in men and women," *Br Med J,* 305:277, 1992

As per note 19

23 —Engelburg, H., "Low serum cholesterol and suicide," *Lancet*, 339:727, 1992

Muldoon, M., "Lowering cholesterol concentrations and mortality: a quantitative review of primary prevention trials," *Br Med J,* 301:309, 1990

24 —Davey Smith, G., "Lowering cholesterol concentrations and mortality," *Br Med J*, 301:552, 1990

MRFIT Research Group, "Mortality rates after 10.5 years for participants in the Multiple Risk Factor Intervention Trial," *JAMA*, 263:1795, 1990

Pekkanen, J., "Serum cholesterol and risk of accidental or violent death in a 25-year follow-up: the Finnish cohorts of the Seven Countries Study," *Arch Intern Med,* 149:1589, 1989

25 —Pearce, M., "Incidence of cancer in men on a diet high in polyunsaturated fat," *Lancet,* 1:464, 1971

26 —Steering Committee of the Physicians' Health Study Research Group, "Final report of the aspirin component of the ongoing Physicians' Health Study," *N Engl J Med*, 321:129, 1989

Peto, R., "Randomised trial of prophylactic daily aspirin in British male doctors," *Br Med J*, 296:13, 1988

27 —Mensink, R., "Effect of dietary cis and trans fatty acids on serum lipoprotein levels in humans," *J Lipid Res*, 33:1493, 1992

Willett, W., "Intake of trans fatty acids and risk of coronary heart disease among women," *Lancet*, 341:581, 1993

Enig, M., "Dietary fat and cancer trends," *Fed Proc*, 37:2215, 1978

28 —Truswell, A., "ABC of nutrition. Reducing the risk of coronary heart disease," *Br Med J,* 291:34, 1985

United Nations, *FAO Food Balance Sheets 1979–1981*, 1984

29 —Kummerow, F., "Additive risk factors in atherosclerosis," *Am J Clin Nutr,* 29:579, 1976

Whitney, E., *Understanding Normal and Clinical Nutrition,* 2nd ed., West Publishing, 1987, pgs 129–130

Carroll, K., "Dietary protein and heart disease," *Nutrition and the MD*, June 1985

30 —Felton, C., "Dietary polyunsaturated fatty acids and composition of human aortic plaques," *Lancet*, 344:1195, 1994

31 —Morin, R., "The role of cholesterol oxidation products in the pathogenesis of atherosclerosis," *Ann Clin Lab Sci*, 19:225, 1989

Hattersley, J., "Acquired atherosclerosis: theories of causation, novel therapies," *J Orthomol Med*, 6:83, 1991

Ibid

32 —Matsumura, F., "Mechanism of action of dioxin-type chemicals, pesticides and other xenobiotics affecting nutritional indexes," *Am J Clin Nutr*, 61:695S, 1995

33 —Ornish, D., "Can lifestyle changes reverse coronary heart disease? The Lifestyle Heart Trial," *Lancet*, 336:129, 1990

34 —Hunninghake, D., "The efficacy of intensive dietary therapy alone or combined with lovastatin in outpatients with hypercholesterolemia," *N Engl J Med*, 328:1213, 1993

35 —Vorster, H., "Egg intake does not change plasma lipoprotein and coagulation profiles," *Am J Clin Nutr*, 55:400, 1992

McNamara, D., "Heterogeneity of cholesterol homeostasis in man," *J Clin Invest,* 79:1729, 1987

Dawber, T., "Eggs, serum cholesterol and coronary heart disease," *Am J Clin Nutr*, 36:617, 1982

Flaim, E., "Plasma lipid and lipoprotein cholesterol concentrations in adult males consuming normal and high cholesterol diets under controlled conditions," *Am J Clin Nutr*, 34:1103, 1981

Flynn, M., "Effect of dietary egg on human serum cholesterol and triglycerides," *Am J Clin Nutr*, 32:1051, 1979

36 —Porter, M., "Effect of dietary egg on serum cholesterol and triglyceride of human males," *Am J Clin Nutr*, 30:490, 1977

37 —Clifton, P., "Relationship between sensitivity to dietary fat and dietary cholesterol," *Arteriosclerosis*, 10:394, 1990

38 —Kestin, M., "Effect of dietary cholesterol in normolipidemic subjects is not modified by nature and amount of dietary fat," *Am J Clin Nutr*, 50:528, 1989

39 —McNamara, D., as per note 35

40 —Vuoristo, M., "Absorption, metabolism and serum concentrations of cholesterol in vegetarians: effects of cholesterol feeding," *Am J Clin Nutr*, 59:1325, 1994

41 —Ibid

42 —Karanja, N., "Plasma lipids and hypertension: response to calcium supplementation," *Am J Clin Nutr*, 45:60, 1987

43 —Bell, L., "Cholesterol-lowering effects of calcium carbonate in patients with mild to moderate hypercholesterolemia," *Arch Intern Med*, 152:2441, 1992

44 —Denke, M., "Short-term dietary calcium fortification increases fecal saturated fat content and reduces serum lipids in men," *J Nutr,* 123:1047, 1993

45 —O'Dea, K., "Cholesterol-lowering effect of a low-fat diet containing lean beef is reversed by the addition of beef fat," *Am J Clin Nutr*, 52:491, 1990

46 —As per note 34

47 —Gravlee, G., *Cardiopulmonary Bypass: Principles and Practice*, Williams & Wilkins, 1993, pg 546

Tinker, J., *Cardiopulmonary Bypass: Current Concepts and Comtroversies,* WB Saunders Co., 1989, pg 32

48 —Waldhausen, J., *Complications in Cardiothoracic Surgery,* Mosby-Yearbook, 1991, pg 46

49 —Ornish, D., *Dr. Dean Ornish's Program for Reversing Heart Disease,* Ballantine Books, 1990, pg 53

50 —Levine, S., "Coronary angioplasty: clinical and angiographic follow-up," *Am J Cardiol*, 55:673, 1985

Ibid

51 —Graboys, T., "Results of a second-opion trial among patients recommended for coronary angiogram," *JAMA*, 268:2537, 1992

Alderman, E., "Ten-year follow-up of survival and myocardial infarction in the randomized coronary artery surgery study," *Circulation*, 82:1629, 1990

52 —Ornish, D., "Effects of stress management training and dietary changes in treating ischemic heart disease," *JAMA*, 249:54, 1983
As per note 33
53 —Quoted in National Live Stock and Meat Board, *Exploring Meat and Health*, 1991, pg 23
54 —AMA VideoClinic ad, "Practical strategies for improving dietary compliance in hypercholesterolemia," *American Medical News*, Oct. 26, 1992, pg 25

Cancer

55 —Drummond, H., "On growing old," *A Sourcebook on Health and Survival,* Foundation for National Progress, 1981, pg 42
56 —Reported on ABC Radio News, July 29, 1991
57 —Osler, W., *Principles and Practice of Medicine*, Appleton Company, 1909
58 —Kilburn, K., "Epidemics then and now: chemicals replace microbes and degenerations oust infections," *Arch Environ Health*, 49:3, 1994
59 —Harrison, T., *Principles of Internal Medicine*, 13th ed., McGraw-Hill, 1994
60 —Davis, D., "Decreasing cardiovascular disease and increasing cancer among whites in the United States from 1973 through 1987," *JAMA*, 271:431, 1994
61 —Bailar, J., "Progress against cancer?," *N Engl J Med,* 314:1231, 1986
62 —*Healthline*, Dec. 1991
63 —Cole, P., "The evolving picture of cancer in America," *JNCI*, 87:160, 1995
American Hospital Association, *Meditrends,* 1991–1992
64 —As per note 60
65 —American Cancer Society, *Cancer Facts & Figures—1993*, pg 1
Friend, T., "Storm warning!," *American Health*, Dec. 1990, pg 8
66 —Reis, L., *SEER Cancer Statistics Review: 1973–1991*, NIH Pub. No. 94–2789, National Cancer Institute, 1994
67 —American Cancer Society, as per note 65, pg 14
68 —Davis, D., "Agricultural exposures and cancer trends in developed countries," *Environ Health Persp*, 100:39, 1992
Cole, P., as per note 63
69 —"Dioxin toxicity research: studies show cancer, reproduction risks," *Chem Engineer News*, Sept. 6, 1993, pg 5
70 —Thorton, J., "The dioxin deception," *Propaganda Review*, Number 9, 1992, pg 22
71 —As per note 66
72 —Renneker, M., *Understanding Cancer,* Bull Publishing, 1988, pg 49
Moss, R., "Cancer—what you need to know," *Spectrum*, Mar./April 1993, pg 27
73 —Bruning P., "Insulin resistance and breast cancer risk," *Int J Cancer,* 52:511, 1992
74 —Freiss, G., "Anti-steroidal and anti-growth factor activities of anti-estrogens," *J Steroid Biochem*, 37:777, 1990
75 —Ingram, D., "Effects of low-fat diet on female sex hormone levels," *JNCI,* 79:1225, 1987

76 —Rose, D., "High-fiber diet reduces serum estrogen concentrations in premenopausal women," *Am J Clin Nutr,* 54:520, 1991

77 —Ames, B., "Ranking possible carcinogenic hazards," *Science*, 236:272, 1987

78 —Harris, J., "Breast cancer," *N Engl J Med*, 327:319, 1992

Hortobagyi, G., "Current status of adjuvant systemic therapy for primary breast cancer: progress and controversy," *CA Cancer J Clin,* 45:199, 1995

79 —Feuer, E., "The lifetime risk of developing breast cancer," *JNCI*, 85:892, 1993

Swanson, G., "Breast cancer risk estimation: a translational statistic for communication to the public," *JNCI*, 85:848, 1993

80 —Sacks, N., "Primary management of carcinoma of the breast," *Lancet*, 342:1402, 1993

Holland, R., "The presence of an extensive intraductal component following a limited excision correlates with prominent residual disease in the remainder of the breast," *J Clin Oncol*, 8:113, 1990

Renneker, M., as per note 72, pg 144

81 —Spratt, J., "Mammographic assessment of human breast cancer growth and duration," *Cancer*, 71:2020, 1993

Gullino, P., "Natural history of breast cancer—progression from hyperplasia to neoplasia as predicted by angiogenesis," *Cancer*, 39:2697, 1977

82 —Nystrom, L., "Breast cancer screening with mammography: overview of Swedish randomised trials," *Lancet*, 341:973, 1993

83 —Kolata, G., "New ability to find earliest cancers: a mixed blessing?," *New York Times,* Nov. 8, 1994, pg C–1

84 —Hetelekidis, S., "Management of ductal carcinoma in situ," *CA Cancer J Clin,* 45:244, 1995

Jatoi, I., "American and European recommendations for screening mammography in younger women: a cultural divide?," *Br Med J,* 307:1481, 1993

Harris, J., as per note 78, pg 391

85 —Debonis, D., "Survival of patients with metastatic breast cancer diagnosed between 1955 and 1980," *J Surg Oncol*, 48:158, 1991

Todd, M., "Survival of women with metastatic breast cancer at Yale from 1920 to 1980," *J Clin Oncol*, 6:406, 1983

86 —Skrabanek, P., "False premises and false promises of breast cancer screening," *Lancet*, 2:316, 1985

87 —"Breast cancer: have we lost our way?," *Lancet*, 341:344, 1993

Plotkin, D., "Breast cancer—biology and malpractice," *Am J Clin Nutr*, 14:254, 1991

Patel, J., "Does more intense palliative treatment improve survival in metastatic breast cancer patients?," *Cancer*, 57:567, 1986

Ibid

88 —Quoted in Hunt, D., "Mammogram alert," *East West Journal*, Sept./Oct. 1991, pg 109

89 —Page, D., "Controversies in the local management of invasive and noninvasive breast cancer," *Cancer Letters*, 90:91, 1995

Fisher, E., "Conservative management of intraductal carcinoma of the breast," *J Surg Oncol,* 47:139, 1991

Sacks, N., as per note 80

90 —Devitt, J., "Breast cancer: have we missed the forest because of the tree?," *Lancet*,344:734, 1994

91 —Boice, J., "Cancer in the contralateral breast after radiotherapy for breast cancer," *N Engl J Med*, 326:781, 1992

Mattsson, A., "Radiation-induced breast cancer: long-term follow-up of radiation therapy for benign breast disease," *JNCI*, 85:1679, 1993

Haybittle, J., "Postoperative radiotherapy and late mortality: evidence from the Cancer Research Campaign trial for early breast cancer," *Br Med J*, 298:1161, 1989

92 —Curtis, R., "Risks of leukemia after chemotherapy and radiation treatment for breast cancer," *N Engl J Med,* 326:1745, 1992

Boogerd, W., "Brain metastases in breast cancer: natural history, prognostic factors and outcome," *J Neurooncol,* 43:165, 1993

Penn, I. review of Coleman, M., "Cancer risk after medical treatment," *N Engl J Med*, 326:1298, 1992

Bodey, G., "Infections in cancer patients," *Cancer Treat Rev*, 2:89, 1975

93 —Benner, S., "A stopping rule for standard chemotherapy for metastatic breast cancer: lessons from a survey of Maryland oncologists," *Cancer Invest*, 12:451, 1994

94 —Holm, L., "Treatment failure and dietary habits in women with breast cancer," *JNCI*, 85:32, 1993

Boyar, A., "Response to a diet low in total fat in women with postmenopausal breast cancer," *Nutr Cancer*, 11:93, 1988

95 —Bailar, J., "Mammography: a contrary view," *Ann Intern Med*, 84:77, 1976

Greenberg, D., "Medicine and public affairs," *N Engl J Med*, 295:739, 1976

96 —Miller, A., "Canadian national breast screening study: public health implications," *Can J Public Health*, 84:14, 1993

Tabar, L., "Update of the Swedish Two-Country Program of mammographic screening for breast cancer," *Radiol Clin North Am*, 30:187, 1992

Anderson, I., "Mammographic screening and mortality from breast cancer: the Malmo mammographic screening trial," *Br Med J,* 297:943, 1988

Verbeek, A., "Mammographic screening and breast cancer mortality: age-specific effects in Nijmegen project 1975–82," *Lancet*, 1:865, 1985

Shapiro, S., "Ten to fourteen year effect of breast cancer screening on mortality," *JNCI,* 69:349, 1982

97 —GAO/PEMD 89-9, "The survival of breast cancer patients," US GAO Report to the Chairman, Subcommittee on Health and the Environment, Committee on Energy and Commerce, House of Representatives, Feb. 1989

Powles, T., "Failure of chemotherapy to prolong survival in a group of patients with metastatic breast cancer," *Lancet*, 15:580, 1980

98 —Epstein, S., "Evaluation of the National Cancer Program and proposed reforms," *Int J Health Services,* 23:30, 1993

99 —Netten, J., "Physical trauma and breast cancer," *Lancet*, 343:978, 1994

Watmough, D., "X-ray mammography and breast compression," *Lancet*, 340:122, 1992

100 —Cancer Prevention Coalition, "Breast cancer unawareness month," *Cancer Prevention News,* Oct. 21, 1994, pg 2

101 —Wright, C., "Screening mammography and public health policy: the need for perspective," *Lancet*, 346:29, 1995

102 —Gitts, R., "Carcinoma of the prostate," *N Engl J Med,* 324:236, 1991

103 —Krahn, M., "Screening for prostate cancer," *JAMA*, 272:773, 1994

Chodak, G., "Results of conservative management of clinically localized prostate cancer," *N Engl J Med*, 330:242, 1994

Fleming, C., "A decision analysis of alternative treatment strategies for clinically localized prostate cancer," *JAMA*, 269:2650, 1993

104 —Johansson, J., "High 10-year survival rate in patients with early, untreated prostate cancer," *JAMA*, 267:2191, 1992

Hanks, G., "Radiotherapy or surgery for prostate cancer? Ten and fifteen-year results of external beam therapy," *Acta Oncol*, 30:231, 1991

105 —Freidman, G., "Case-control study of screening for prostate cancer by digital rectal examination," *Lancet*, 337:1526, 1991

106 —Schmid, H., "Observations on the doubling time of prostate cancer," *Cancer*, 71:2031, 1993

107 —Carter, J., "Hypothesis: dietary management may improve survival from nutritionally linked cancers based on analysis of representative cases," *J Am Coll Nutr*, 12:209, 1993

108 —DeCosse, J., "Effect of wheat fiber and vitamins C and E on rectal polyps in patients with familial adenomatous polyposis," *JNCI*, 81:1290, 1989

109 —Stryker, S., "Natural history of untreated colonic polyps," *Gastroenterol*, 93:1009, 1987

110 —Ahlquist, D., "Accuracy of fecal occult blood screening for colorectal neoplasia," *JAMA*, 269:1262, 1993

111 —Haubrich, W., *Bochus Gastroenterology*, 5th ed., W.B. Saunders Co., 1995, pg 320

Atkins, S., "Prevention of colorectal cancer by once-only sigmoidoscopy," *Lancet*, 341:736, 1993

Selby, J., "A case-control study of screening sigmoidoscopy and mortality from colorectal cancer," *N Engl J Med,* 326:653, 1992

Bombi, J., "Polyps of the colon in Barcelona, Spain," *Cancer*, 61:1472, 1988

112 —Wargovich, M., "Inhibition of the promotional phase of azoxymethane-induced colon carcinogenesis in the F344 rat by calcium lactate: effect of stimulating two human nutrient density levels," *Cancer Letters*, 53:17, 1990

Lipkin, M., "Colonic epithelial cell proliferation in responders and nonresponders to supplemental dietary calcium," *Cancer Res,* 49:248, 1989
113 —Gann, P., "Low-dose aspirin and incidence of colorectal tumors in a randomized trial," *JNCI*, 85:1220, 1993
Thun, M., "Aspirin use and reduced risk of fatal colon cancer," *N Engl J Med,* 325:1593, 1991
114 —Carroll, K., "Calcium and carcinogenesis of the mammary gland," *Am J Clin Nutr*, 54:206, 1991
Jacobson, E., "Effects of dietary fat, calcium and vitamin D on growth and mammary tumorigenesis…," *Cancer Res*, 49:6300, 1989
115 —Cancer Prevention Coalition, *Cancer Prevention News,* Fall 1994, pg 4
116 —Chowka, P., "Cancer 1988," *East West Journal,* Dec. 1987, pg 47
117 —Kaplan, S., "Lobby-PR giant Porter/Novelli plays all sides," *PR Watch*, Jan./Mar. 1994, pg 4
118 —National Cancer Institute, *Cancer Rates and Risks,* 1985
Committee on Diet, Nutrition and Cancer, National Research Council, *Diet, Nutrition and Cancer*, National Academy Press, 1982
119 —"Report to Congress from the Office of Techology Assessment: assessment of technologies for determining cancer risks from the environment," June 1981
120 —Quoted in Chowka, P., "Cancer research: the $20 billion failure," *East West Journal,* Mar. 1981, pg 18
121 —Ibid, pg 13
122 —Epstein, S., "Evaluation of the National Cancer Program and proposed reforms," *Int J Health Services*, 23:15, 1993
123 —Bleifuss, J., "Science in the public interest," *PR Watch*, Jan./Mar. 1995
Epstein, S., "Losing the war against cancer," *Int J Health Services*, 20:53, 1990
124 —Moss, R., *The Cancer Industry*, Paragon Books, 1991, pg 358
The Cancer Chronicles, Equinox Press, Feb. 1995, pg 2
As per note 122, pg 21
125 —As per note 122, pg 25
126 —Austin, H., "A prospective follow-up study of cancer mortality in relation to serum DDT," *Am J Public Health*, 79:43, 1989
127 —Morris, R., "Chlorination, chlorination by-products and cancer: a meta-analysis," *Am J Public Health*, 82:955, 1992
128 —Quoted in Begley, S., "Is science censored?," *Newsweek*, Sept. 14, 1992, pg 63
129 —Barnard, N., *Food for Life*, Harmony Books, 1993, pg 67
Paulsen, M., "The politics of cancer," *Utne Reader*, Nov./Dec. 1993, pg 87
130 —Fink, D., "Executive notice for unit routing," American Cancer Society of California, Aug. 20, 1993
Wilt, T., Letter to the editor, *JAMA*, 268:3198, 1992
131 —Moss, R., as per note 124, pg 428
132 —Moss, R., as per note 124, pg 395
133 —Quoted in Motavalli, J., "Killing us softly," *E Magazine*, May/June 1995, pg 4

134 —Rutqvist, L., "Adjuvant tamoxifen therapy for early stage breast cancer and second primary malignancies," *JNCI*, 87:645, 1995

Kedar, R., "Effects of tamoxifen on uterus and ovaries of postmenopausal women in a randomised breast cancer prevention trial," *Lancet*, 343:1318, 1994

Phillips, D., "Safety of prophylactic tamoxifen," *Lancet*, 341:1485, 1993

135 —Griffith, H., *Complete Guide to Prescription & Non-Prescription Drugs*, Body Press/Perigee Books, 1993, pg 378

136 —Pike, M., "Chemoprevention of breast cancer by reducing sex-steroid exposure: perspectives from epidemiology," *J Cell Biochem,* 17G:26, 1993

137 —Lear, M., *Heartsounds*, Simon & Schuster, 1980

Osteoporosis

138 —Clinton, H., "The fight for women's health," *Ladies' Home Journal,* Nov. 1993

139 —Blackburn, G., "Shake down your cholesterol and blood pressure," *Prevention*, Aug. 1992, pg 101

140 —Dixon, A., "The National Osteoporosis Society," *Lancet*, 2:55, 1986

141 —Heaney, R., "Thinking straight about calcium," *N Engl J Med,* 328:503, 1993

Heaney, R., "Nutritional factors in osteoporosis," *Ann Rev Nutr*, 13:287, 1993

142 —Nelson, M., "A 1-y walking program and increased dietary calcium in postmenopausal women: effects on bone loss," *Am J Clin Nutr,* 53:1304, 1991

Matkovic, V., "Factors that influence peak bone mass formation: a study of calcium balance and the inheritance of bone mass in adolescent females," *Am J Clin Nutr*, 52:878, 1990

Recker, R., "The effect of milk supplements on calcium metabolism and calcium balance," *Am J Clin Nutr*, 41:254, 1985

Calvo, M., "Elevated secretion and action of serum parathyroid hormone in young adults consuming high phosphorus, low calcium diets assembled from common foods," *J Clin Endocrinol Metab*, 66:823, 1988

Baran, D., "Dietary modification with dairy products for preventing vertebral bone loss in premenopausal women: a three-year prospective study," *J Clin Endocrinol Metab*, 70:264, 1989

Greger, J., "Mineral utilization by rats fed various commercially available calcium supplements or milk," *J Nutr,* 117:717, 1987

Chan, G., "Effects of increased dietary calcium intake upon the calcium and bone mineral status of lactating adolescent and adult women," *Am J Clin Nutr,* 46:319, 1987

Schuette, S., "Effects on Ca and P metabolism in humans by adding meat, meat plus milk, or purified proteins plus Ca and P to a low protein diet," *J Nutr,* 112:338, 1982

143 —Beresteijn, E., "Relationship between the calcium-to-protein ratio in milk and the urinary calcium excretion in healthy adults—a controlled crossover study,"*Am J Clin Nutr,* 52:142, 1990

144 —Lloyd, T., "Calcium supplementation and bone mineral density in adolescent girls," *JAMA*, 270:841, 1993

Andon, M., "Spinal bone density and calcium intake in healthy postmenopausal women," *Am J Clin Nutr*, 54:927, 1991

Johnston, C., "Calcium supplementation and increases in bone mineral density in children," *N Engl J Med,* 327:82, 1992

Dawson-Hughes, B., "A controlled trial of the effect of calcium supplementation on bone density in postmenopausal women," *N Engl J Med*, 323:878, 1990

Smith, K., "Calcium absorption from a new calcium delivery system (CCM)," *Calcif Tissue Int*, 41:351, 1987

145 —Dawson-Hughes, B., "Calcium supplementation and bone loss: a review of controlled clinical trials," *Am J Clin Nutr*, 54:274, 1991

Dawson-Hughes, B., "Dietary calcium intake and bone loss from the spine in healthy postmenopausal women," *Am J Clin Nutr*, 46:685, 1987

Lee, C., "Effects of supplementation of the diet with calcium and calcium-rich foods on bone density of elderly females with osteoporosis," *Am J Clin Nutr*, 34:819, 1981

146 —Barger-Lux, M., "Effects of calcium restriction on metabolic characteristics of premenopausal women," *J Clin Endocrinol Metab*, 76:103, 1993

Smith, E., "Calcium supplementation and bone loss in middle-aged women," *Am J Clin Nutr*, 50:833, 1989

Polley, K., "Effect of calcium supplementation on forearm bone mineral content in postmenopausal women: a propective, sequential controlled trial," *J Nutr,* 117:1929, 1987

Freudenheim, J., "Relationship between usual nutrient intake and bone-mineral content of women 35–65 years of age: longitudinal and cross-sectional analysis," *Am J Clin Nutr*, 44:863, 1986

Thalassinos, N., "Calcium balance in osteoporotic patients on long-term oral calcium therapy with and without sex hormones," *Clin Sci,* 62:221, 1982

Chapuy, M., "Vitamin D3 and calcium to prevent hip fractures in elderly women," *N Engl J Med*, 327:1637, 1992

Hu, J., "Dietary calcium and bone density among middle-aged and elderly women in China," *Am J Clin Nutr*, 58:219, 1993

Prince, R., "Prevention of postmenopausal osteoporosis," *N Engl J Med*, 325:1189, 1991

147 —Smith, T., "Absorption of calcium from milk and yogurt," *Am J Clin Nutr*, 42:1197, 1985

148 —Spencer, H., "Effect of a high protein (meat) intake on calcium metabolism in man," *Am J Clin Nutr*, 31:2167, 1978

149 —Spencer, H., "Further studies of the effect of a high protein diet as meat on calcium metabolism," *Am J Clin Nutr*, 37:924, 1983

150 —Dawson-Hughes, B., as per note 144

Smith, K., as per note 144

151 —National Osteoporosis Foundation, *Osteoporosis Report*, 9(4), Winter 1993, pg 1
152 —Abelow, B., "Cross-cultural association between dietary animal protein and hip fractures: a hypothesis," *Calcif Tissue Int*, 50:14, 1992
Hegsted, D., "Calcium and osteoporosis," *J Nutr,* 116:2316, 1986
Lewinnek, G., "The significance and a comparative analysis of the epidemiology of hip fractures," *Clin Ortho Related Res,* 152:35, 1980
153 —Lemann, J., "The importance of renal net acid excretion as a determinant of fasting urinary calcium excretion," *Kidney Int,* 29:743, 1986
Lutz, J., "Calcium balance and acid-base status of women as affected by increased protein intake and sodium bicarbonate ingestion," *Am J Clin Nutr,* 39:281, 1984
Hegsted, D., "Urinary calcium and calcium balance in young men as affected by level of protein and phosphorus intake," *J Nutr,* 111:553, 1981
Linkswiler, H., "Protein-induced hyper-calciuria," *Federations Proc*, 40:2429, 1981
154 —Ibid
155 —Hegsted, D., as per note 153
156 —Kitt, D., *Nutr Quarterly*, 14:28, 1990
Martson, R., "Nutritional review," *Natl Food Supply*, 158:25, 1976
157 —Altchuler, S., "Dietary protein and calcium loss: a review," *Nutr Res,* 2:193, 1982
"High protein diets and bone homeostasis," *Nutr Reviews*, 39:11, 1981
Allen, L., "Protein-induced hypercalcuria: a long-term study," *Am J Clin Nutr,* 32:741, 1979
Hegsted, D., as per note 152
As per note 153
158 —Quoted in Rattenbury, J., "What's the score on osteoporosis?," *Veg Times*, Nov. 1992, pg 68
159 —Gordon, G., "Calcium and osteoporosis," *J Nutr,* 116:319, 1986
160 —As per note 152
Ibid
161 —Adapted from Hegsted, D., as per note 152
162 —Ibid
163 —Heaney, R., "Calcium intake requirement and bone mass in the elderly," *J Lab Clin Med*, 100:309, 1982
164 —Zemel, M., "Calcium utilization: effect of varying levels and source of dietary protein," *Am J Clin Nutr*, 48:880, 1988
Schuette, S., "Studies on the mechanism of protein-induced hypercalciuria in older men and women," *J Nutr,* 110:305, 1980
As per note 153
165 —Garrison, R., *The Nutrition Desk Reference*, Keats Publishing, 1985, pg 60
166 —Hegsted, D., as per note 152
167 —Goldin, B., "Effect of diet on excretion of estrogens in pre- and post-menopausal women," *Cancer Res*, 41:3771, 1981
168 —Marsh, A., "Vegetarian lifestyle and bone mineral density," *Am J Clin Nutr*, 48:837, 1988

Tylavski, F., "Dietary factors in bone health of elderly lactoovovegetarian and omnivorous women," *Am J Clin Nutr,* 48, 842, 1988

Goldin, B., "Estrogen excretion patterns and plasma levels in vegetarian and omnivorous women," *N Engl J Med*, 308:1542, 1992

Armstrong, B., "Diet and reproductive hormones: a study of vegetarian and nonvegetarian postmenopausal women," *JNCI*, 67:761, 1981

169 —Heaney, R., "Calcium absorption from kale," *Am J Clin Nutr*, 51:656, 1990

170 —Schuette, S., as per note 164

171 —Hu, J., "Dietary intakes and urinary excretion of calcium and acids," *Am J Clin Nutr*, 58:398, 1993

Brockis, J., "The effects of vegetable and animal protein diets on calcium, urate and oxalate excretion," *Br J Urology,* 54:590, 1982

Zemel, M., as per note 164

172 —Gorbach, S., "Dietary phyto-oestrogens and the menopause in Japan," *Lancet*, 339:1233, 1992

Wilcox, G., "Oestrogenic effects of plant foods in postmenopausal women," *Br Med J,* 301:905, 1990

Ferrando, R., "Hormones and antihormones," *Traditional and Non-traditional Foods*, Food and Agricultural Organization, 1981, pg 42

173 —National Research Council, *Recommended Dietary Allowances*, 10th ed., National Academy Press, 1989, pg 185

174 —Riggs, L., "Involutional osteoporosis," *N Engl J Med,* 314:1676, 1986

175 —Allen, L., "The role of insulin and parathyroid hormone in protein-induced calciuria of man," *Nutr Res*, 1:3, 1981

176 —Chen, J., *Diet, life-style, and mortality in China: a study of the characteristics of 65 Chinese counties*, Oxford University Press, Cornell University Press, China People's Medical Publishing House, 1991

177 —Quoted in Brody, J., "Huge study of diet indicts fat and meat," *New York Times* (western edition), May 8, 1990, pg B5

178 —Mazess, R., "Bone mineral content of North Alaskan Eskimos," *Am J Clin Nutr*, 27:916, 1974

179 —Danielson, C., "Hip fractures and fluoridation in Utah's elderly population," *JAMA*, 268:746, 1992

Cooper, C., "Water fluoridation and hip fractures," *JAMA*, 266:513, 1991

180 —Heaney, R., "Protein intake and calcium economy," *JADA*, 93:1259, 1993

Heaney, R., as per note 141, *Ann Rev Nutr*, pgs 305–6

181 —Recker, R., "Bone gain in young adult women," *JAMA*, 268:2403, 1992

182 —Kanis, J., "Calcium supplementation of the diet–II," *Br Med J*, 298:205, 1989

Lewis, N., "Calcium supplement and milk: effects on acid-base balance and on retention of calcium, magnesium and phosphorus," *Am J Clin Nutr,* 49:527, 1989

183 —Mazess, R., "Bone density in premenopausal women: effects of age, dietary intake, physical activity, smoking and birth-control pills," *Am J Clin Nutr,* 53:132, 1991

Riggs, B.L., "Dietary calcium intakes and rates on bone loss in women," *J Clin Invest*, 80:979, 1987

Stevenson, J., "Dietary intake of calcium and postmenopausal bone loss," *Br Med J,* 297:15, 1988

Riis, B., "Does calcium supplementation prevent postmenopausal bone loss?," *N Engl J Med*, 316:173, 1987

Nilas, L., "Calcium supplementation and postmenopausal bone loss," *Br Med J,* 289:1103, 1984

Kanis, J., Ibid

184 —Reid, I., "Effect of calcium supplementation on bone loss in postmenopausal women," *N Engl J Med*, 328:460, 1993

185 —Ibid, pg 463

186 —Recker, R., as per note 142

187 —Ibid, pg 261

188 —Colditz, G., "The use of estrogens and progestins and the risk of breast cancer in postmenopausal women," *N Engl J Med,* 332:1589, 1995

Toniolo, P., "A prospective study of endogenous estrogens and breast cancer in postmenopausal women," *JNCI*, 87:190, 1995

Stampfer, M., "Postmenopausal estrogen therapy and cardiovascular disease: ten-year follow-up from the Nurses' Health Study," *N Engl J Med*, 325:756, 1991

189 —Harrison, *Principles of Internal Medicine*, 12th ed., 1991, pg 1925

190 —Prior, J., "Progesterone and the prevention of osteoporosis," *Canad J Ob/Gyn*, 3:178, 1991

Lee, J., "Osteoporosis reversal—the role of progesterone," *Int Clin Nutr Rev*, 10:384, 1990

Chang, K., "Influences of percutaneous administration of estradiol and progesterone on human breast epithelial cell cycle in vivo," *Fertility and Sterility*, 63:785, 1995

191 —Lee, J., *Optimal Health Guidelines,* 2nd ed., BLL Publishing, 1993, pg 90

192 —Campbell, B., "Menstrual variation in salivary testosterone among regularly cycling women," *Hormone Res*, 37:132, 1992

Prior, J., "Spinal bone loss and ovulatory disturbances," *N Engl J Med*, 323:1221, 1990

193 —Feichtinger, W., "Environmental factors and fertility," *Human Reprod*, 6:1170, 1991

194 —US EPA, "Risk characterization of dioxin and related compounds," Bureau of National Affairs, May 3, 1994

195 —"Osteoporosis: alternatives to estrogen," *Harvard Health Letter*, Mar. 1994, pg 6

196 —"The bare-bone facts for avoiding osteoporosis," *Tufts U Diet Nutr Letter*, June 1994, pg 3

197 —"A lifelong program to build strong bones," *UC Berkeley Wellness Letter,* July 1993, pg 4

198 —"Should you take estrogens to prevent osteoporosis?," *John Hopkins Medical Letter,* Aug. 1994, pg 4

199 —Liebman, B., "Calcium: after the craze," *CSPI Nutr Action Healthletter,* June 1994, pg 1

200 —McBean, L., "Osteoporosis: visions for care and prevention—a conference report," *JADA*, 94:668, 1994

201 —National Osteoporosis Foundation, *Boning Up on Osteoporosis,* 1991, pg 22
202 —McClellan, W., "Prolonged meat diets with a study of the metabolism of nitrogen, calcium and phosphorus," *J Biol Chem,* 87:669, 1930
203 —National Osteoporosis Foundation, *How Strong Are Your Bones?*, 1994, pg 5
204 —As per note 158, pg 69
205 —American Medical Association, *Let's Talk About Food*, Publishing Services Group, 1974, pg 75
206 —Quoted in Woteki, C. and Thomas, P., *Eat For Life: The Food and Nutrition Board's Guide to Reducing Your risk of Chronic Disease*, National Academy Press, 1992, pg 103
207 —"Rock-solid bones," *Prevention*, Nov. 1991, pg 62
"Making the grade," *Prevention*, Nov. 1991, pg 68
208 —Quoted in Bloyd-Peshkin, S., "The health-fraud cops," *Veg Times*, Aug. 1991, pg 58
209 —Ibid
210 —National Osteoporosis Foundation letterhead, Oct. 27, 1993

Arthritis

211 —Quoted in Beck, M., "Living with arthritis," *Newsweek*, Mar. 20, 1989, pg 68
212 —Ibid, pg 65
213 —Centers for Disease Control, *Morbidity and Mortality Weekly Report*, Oct. 14, 1994
214 —National Institutes of Health, "How to cope with arthritis," NIH Pub. No. 82–1092,Oct. 1991
Verbrugge, L., "From sneezes to adieux: stages of health for American men and women," *Soc Sci Med*, 22:1195, 1986
215 —Steinbaum, E., "Tomarrow's health-care," *Arthritis Today,* Mar./April 1995, pg 41
"Ayurvedic formula may help some arthritis," *Better Nutrition*, Feb. 1995, pg 16
As per note 211, pg 65
216 —McCarthy, D., *Arthritis and Allied Conditions: A Textbook of Rheumatology*, 12th ed., Lea & Febiger, 1993, pg 15
217 —Short, C., "The antiquity of rheumatoid arthritis," *Arthritis Rheum*, 17:193, 1974
218 —Pincus, T., "Early mortality in RA predicted by poor clinical status," *Bull Rheumatic Dis*, 41:4, 1992
219 —Fuchs, H., "Evidence of significant erosions in rheumatoid arthritis within the first 2 years of disease," *J Rheumatol*, 16:585, 1989
220 —Beasley, R., "Low prevalence of rheumatoid arthritis in Chinese," *J Rheumatol*, 10:11, 1983
221 —As per note 216, pg 21
222 —Panush, R., "Nutritional therapy for rheumatoid diseases," *Ann Int Med,* 106:619, 1987
223 —Bahna, S., *Allergies to Milk*, Grune and Stratton, 1980

224 —Cunningham–Rundles, C., "Dietary antigens and immunologic diseases in man," *Rheum Dis Clin North Am,* 17:287, 1991

Moneret–Vautrin, A., "Food antigens and additives," *J Allergy Clin Immunol,* 5:1039, 1986

225 —Bjarnason, I., "Intestinal permeability and inflammation in rheumatoid arthritis: effects of non-steroidal anti-inflammatory drugs," *Lancet,* 1:1171, 1984

Ibid

226 —Paganelli, R., "The role of antigenic absorption and circulating immune complexes in food allergy," *Ann Allergy*, 57:330, 1986

227 —Darlington, L., "Placebo-controlled blind study of dietary manipulation therapy in rheumatoid arthritis," *Lancet*, 1:238, 1986

228 —Rowe, P., "Fat of the land and of the lab," *Lancet*, 346:46, 1995

Phinney, S., "Potential risk of prolonged gamma-linolenic acid use," *Ann Int Med*, 120:692, 1994

Kelley, D., "Dietary alpha-linoleic acid and immunocompetence in humans," *Am J Clin Nutr,* 53:40, 1991

Sperling, R., "Dietary omega–3 fatty acids: effects on lipid mediators of inflammation and rheumatoid arthritis," *Rheum Dis Clin North Am,* 17:373, 1991

229 —Kremer, J., "Effects of manipulation of dietary fatty acids on clinical manifestations of rheumatoid arthritis," *Lancet*, 1:184, 1985

230 —Cunningham–Rundles, C., as per note 224

231 —Kjeldsen–Kragh, J., "Controlled trial of fasting and one-year vegetarian diet in rheumatoid arthritis," *Lancet*, 338:899, 1991

Darlington, L., "Diets for rheumatoid arthritis," *Lancet*, 338:1209, 1991

Skoldstam, L., "Fasting and vegan diet for rheumatoid arthritis," *Scand J Rheum*, 15:219, 1987

232 —National Institutes of Health, *1993 Research Highlights. Arthritis, Rheumatic Diseases and Related Disorders,* NIH Pub. No. 93–3413, Jan. 1993

Markides, K., *Aging and Health: Perspectives on Gender, Race, Ethnicity and Class*, Springer, 1989, pg 23

233 —Davis, M., "Sex differences in osteoarthritis of the knee. The role of obesity," *Am J Epidemiol,* 127:1019, 1988

234 —Valkenburg, H., "Osteoarthritis in some developing countries," *J Rheumatol,* 10:20, 1983

As per note 216, pg 38

235 —Champion, B., "Immunity to homologous collagens and cartilage proteoglycans in rabbits," *Immunology*, 48:605, 1983

236 —Jasin, H., "Autoantibody specificities of immune complexes sequestered in articular cartilage of patients with rheumatoid arthritis and osteoarthritis," *Arthritis Rheum*, 28:241, 1985

237 —Collier, S., "The role of plasminogen in interleukin–1 mediated cartilage degradation," *J Rheumatol,* 15:1129, 1988

238 —Pizzorno, J., *Encyclopedia of Natural Medicine*, Prima Publishing, 1991

239 —Zollner, D., "Diet and gout," *Proc 9th Int Congress Nutr,* Mexico, 1:267, 1975

240 —Torralba, T., "The Filipino and gout," *Semin Arthritis Rheum*, 4:307, 1975
241 —Quoted in McDougall, J., *McDougall's Medicine*, New Century, 1985, pg 236
242 —Arthritis Foundation, *Diet Guidelines & Research*, 1987, pg 12
243 —National Institutes of Health, *Age Page: Arthritis Advice*, 1985–461–308/20003
244 —Arthritis Foundation, *Arthritis. The Basic Facts,* 1981
As per note 216, pg 1139
245 —Witter, D., "Never say diet," *Arthritis Today*, Nov./Dec. 1991, pg 23
246 —Lindner, L., "You call it bad, and that ain't good," *Arthritis Today*, July/Aug. 1993, pg 54
Nierenberg, C., "Grains take center stage," *Arthritis Today*, Mar./April 1995, pg 59
247 —Arthritis Foundation, *Diet & Nutrition: Facts To Consider,* 4280/9–85, pg 9
248 —Ibid
249 —Arthritis Foundation, "Unproven remedies," *Joint Movement*, Dec. 1989–Jan. 1990, pg 2
250 —Lee, J., *Optimal Health Guidelines*, 2nd ed., BLL Publishing, 1993, pg 131
251 —Harris, E., "Rheumatoid arthritis—pathophysiology and implications for therapy," *N Engl J Med*, 322:1272, 1990
As per note 216, pg 877
252 —Scott, D., "Long-term outcome in treating rheumatoid arthritis: Results after 20 years," *Lancet*, 1:1108, 1987
253 —Arthritis Foundation, *Arthritis Today*, Mar./April 1995, pg 5
254 —"Tenth annual lemon awards," *CSPI Nutr Action Healthletter,* Mar. 1995, pg 3
255 —As per note 253, pg 70
256 —As per note 253, pg 71
257 —Arthritis Foundation, "Corporate corner," *Arthritis Today*, Mar./April 1992, pg 13
258 —Arthritis Foundation, *Bull Rheum Dis*, 41(4), 1992

Diabetes

259 —Quoted in Bose, R., "Diabetes in the tropics," *BMJ*, 2:1053, 1907
260 —Quoted in Aesoph, L., "5 ways to prevent illness," *Delicious!*, Nov./Dec. 1992, pg 42
261 —"Vital statistics," *Health*, Jan./Feb. 1994, pg 14
262 —National Institutes of Health, "Diabetes Mellitus Trans-NIH Research," NIH Pub No. 84–1982, May 1984
263 —Matsumura, F., "Mechanism of action of dioxin-type chemicals, pesticides and other xenobiotics affecting nutritional indexes," *Am J Clin Nutr*, 61:695S, 1995
264 —World Health Organization, *Diet, Nutrition and the Prevention of Chronic Diseases*, Technical Report Series 797, WHO, Geneva, 1990, pg 108
National Research Council, Food and Nutrition Board, *Recommended Dietary Allowances,* 10th ed., National Academy Press, 1989, pg 40
265 —Marshall, J., "Dietary fat predicts conversion from impaired glucose tolerance to NIDDM," *Diabetes Care*, 17:50, 1993

Ward, G., "Insulin receptor binding increased by high carbohydrate, low fat diet in non-insulin-dependent diabetics," *European J Clin Invest*, 12:93, 1982

266 —Rifkin, H., *Diabetes Mellitus: Theory and Practice*, 4th ed., Elsevier, 1990, pg 129

Oettle, G., "Glucose and insulin responses to manufactured and whole-food snacks," *Am J Clin Nutr,* 45:86, 1987

267 —Adapted from *Fighting Disease*, Rodale Press, 1984, pg 109

268 —Kaplan, S., "Diabetes mellitus," *Ann Int Med*, 96:635, 1982

269 —*NIH News & Features*, July 1994

270 —Martin, B., "Role of glucose and insulin resistance in development of type 2 diabetes mellitus: results of a 25–year follow-up study," *Lancet*, 340:925, 1992

271 —DeFronzo, R., "Pathogenesis of NIDDM. A balanced overview," *Diabetes Care*, 15:318, 1992

272 —DeFronzo, R., "Fasting hyperglycemia in non-insulin-dependent diabetes mellitus: contributions of excessive hepatic glucose production and impaired tissue glucose uptake," *Metabolism*, 38:387, 1989

273 —As per note 271

274 —Lillioja, S., "Insulin resistance and insulin secretory dysfunction as precursors of non-insulin-dependent diabetes mellitus," *N Engl J Med*, 329:1988, 1993

275 —Ibid

276 —Bolton, R., "The role of dietary fiber in satiety, glucose and insulin: studies with fruit and fruit juce," *Am J Clin Nutr,* 34:211, 1981

277 —Editors of UC Berkeley Wellness Letter, *The Wellness Encyclopedia*, Houghton Mifflin, 1991, pg 130

Simmons, J., "Is the sand of time sugar?," *Longevity,* June 1990, pg 51

278 —Emmett, P., "Is extrinsic sugar a vehicle for dietary fat?," *Lancet*, 345:1537, 1995

"The fats of life," *Good Dietary Practice News,* 3:1, 1992

279 —American Diabetes Association, "How to head off an insulin reaction," *The Diabetes Advisor,* Mar./April 1993, pg 14

280 —American Diabetes Association, "Nutritional recommendations and principles for individuals with diabetes mellitus," *Diabetes Care*, 14:20, 1991

281 —Cavaiani, M., *The New Diabetic Cookbook*, Contemporary Books, 1994, pgs 302-312

282 —Nathan, D., "Ice cream in the diet of insulin-dependent diabetic patients," *JAMA*, 251:2825, 1984

283 —Chait, A., "Dietary management of diabetes mellitus," *Contemp Nutr,* Feb. 1984

Rivellese, A., "Effect of dietary fibre on glucose control and serum lipoproteins in diabetic patients," *Lancet*, 2:447, 1980

As per note 265

284 —Proctor, R., *Cancer Wars,* Basic Books, 1995, pg 289

285 —"Industry news," *CSPI Nutr Action Healthletter,* Sept. 1993, pg 3

286 —Quoted in "Sweet talk," *CSPI Nutr Action Healthletter,* Nov. 1993, pg 2

Hypertension

287 —Tobian, L., "The Volhard lecture: potassium and sodium in hypertension," *J Hyperten*, 6:S20, 1988

Elliott, P., "International studies of salt and blood pressure," *Ann Clin Res*, 16:67, 1984

288 —Liebman, B., "One nation, under pressure," *CSPI Nutr Action Healthletter*, July/Aug. 1995, pg 6

289 —Dahl, L., "Salt intake and salt need," *N Eng J Med,* 258:1152, 1958

290 —National Academy of Sciences, *Recommended Dietary Allowances,* 10th ed. National Academy Press, 1989, pgs 252–253

291 —American Heart Association, "Position statement: dietary guidelines for healthy American adults," *Circulation*, 77:721A, 1988

292 —As per note 290

293 —USDA Human Nutrition Information Service, *The Sodium Content of Your Food*, 1983, pg 3

294 —National High Blood Pressure Educational Program, "The Fifth Report of the Joint National Committee on Detection, Evaluation, and Treatment of High Blood Pressure," NHLBI, Oct. 30, 1992, pg 15

295 —"NAS on NA," *CSPI Nutr Action Healthletter,* May 1990, pg 13

296 —As per note 290

297 —American Diabetes Association, *Diabetes Forecast: Nutrition Notes,* June 1991, pg 65

298 —As per note 291

Personal communication with AHA, Nov. 5, 1992

299 —Grobbee, D., "Does sodium restriction lower blood pressure?," *Br Med J,* 293:27, 1986

Huttunen, J., "Dietary factors and hypertension," *Acta Medica Scand*, 701:72, 1985

Flanagan, P., "Dietary sodium restriction alone in the treatment of mild hypertension," *Clin Res*, 31:329A, 1983

300 —Matali, A., "Impaired insulin action on skeletal muscle metabolism in essential hypertension," *Hypertension*, 17:170, 1991

DeFronzo, R., "Pathogenesis of NIDDM. A balanced overview," *Diabetes Care*, 15:318, 1992

301 —From presentations at the AHA Scientific Sessions, "Plenary Session VI: Insulin Resistance, Hypertension, Dyslipidemia, Obesity and CAD," Nov. 1992

Zavaroni, I., "Risk factors for coronary artery disease in healthy persons with hyperinsulinemia and normal glucose tolerance," *N Engl J Med*, 320:702, 1989

302 —Landsberg, L., "Insulin and hypertension," *N Engl J Med,* 317:378, 1987

Matali, A., as per note 300

Zavaroni, I., Ibid

303 —O'Brien, J., "Acute platelet changes after large meals of saturated and unsaturated fats," *Lancet*, 1:878, 1976

Hamberg, M., "Thromboxanes: a new group of biologically active compounds derived from prostaglandins endoperoxides," *Proc Nat Acad Sci USA*, 72:2994, 1975

Malhotra, S., "Dietary factors causing hypertension in India," *Am J Clin Nutr,* 23:1353, 1970

304 —MacGregor, G., "Dietary sodium and potassium intake and blood pressure," *Lancet*, 1:750, 1983

Langford, H., "Dietary potassium and hypertension: epidemiologic data," *Ann Int Med*, 98:770, 1983

Kolata, G., "Value of low-sodium diets questioned," *Science*, 216:38, 1982

Ernst, E., "Blood rheology in vegetarians," *Br J Nutr,* 56:550, 1986

305 —Intersalt Cooperative Research Group, "Intersalt: an international study of electrolyte excretion and blood pressure. Results for 24 hour urinary sodium and potassium excretion," *Br Med J,* 297:319, 1988

306 —Bellin, L., "Vegetarian diet and blood pressure levels: incidental or causal association," *Am J Clin Nutr,* 48:806, 1988

Rouse, I., "Vegetarian diet and blood pressure," *J Hyperten,* 2:231, 1984

Rouse, I., "Blood-pressure lowering effect of a vegetarian diet, controlled trial in normotensive subjects," *Lancet*, 1:5, 1983

Ophir, O., "Low blood pressure in vegetarians: the possible role of potassium," *Am J Clin Nutr*, 37:755, 1983

307 —Gould, G. and Pyle, W., *Anomalies and Curiosities of Medicine,* The Julian Press, 1956, pg 407 (original copyright 1896)

308 —Henry, H., "Increasing calcium intake lowers blood pressure: the literature reviewed," *JADA*, 85:182, 1985

McCarron, D., "Dietary calcium and blood pressure: modifying factors in specific populations," *Am J Clin Nutr,* 54:215, 1991

McCarron, D., "Calcium, magnesium and phosphorus balance in human and experimental hypertension," *Hypertension*, 4(Suppl):III-27, 1982

McCarron, D., "The calcium paradox of essential hypertension," *Am J Med*, 82(Suppl 1B):27, 1987

Hatton, D., "Dietary calcium and iron: effects on blood pressure and hematocrit in young spontaneously hypertensive rats," *Am J Clin Nutr,* 53:542, 1991

Repke, R., "Pregnancy-induced hypertension and low birth weight: the role of calcium," *Am J Clin Nutr,* 54:237, 1991

Bukoski, R., "Calcium-regulating hormones in hypertension: vascular actions," *Am J Clin Nutr,* 54:220, 1991

Oparil, S., "Dietary Ca prevents NaCl-sensitive hypertension in sponaneously hypertensive rats via sympatholytic and renal effects," *Am J Clin Nutr,* 54:227, 1991

309 —Lyle, R., "Metabolic differences between subjects whose blood pressure did or did not respond to oral calcium supplementation," *Am J Clin Nutr*, 47:1030, 1988

310 —Ferrannini, E., "Insulin resistance in essential hypertension," *N Engl J Med,* 317:350, 1987

Melby, C., "Blood pressure and blood lipids among vegetarians, semivegetarians and nonvegetarian African Americans," *Am J Clin Nutr*, 59:103, 1994

Eye Protection

311 —"At first sight: phototoxicity and the eye," American Academy of Ophthalmology

312 —Robertson, J., "Vitamin E intake and risk of cataracts in humans," *Ann NY Acad Sci,* 570:372, 1989

"The ocular hazards of UV exposure," American Academy of Ophthalmology

313 —Taylor, H., "Effect of ultraviolet radiation on cataract formation," *N Eng J Med*, 319:1429, 1988

314 —As per note 311

315 —Young, R., "The Charles F. Prentice Metal Award Lecture 1992: optometry and the preservation of visual health," *Optom Vision Sci,* 70:255, 1993

Murphy, R., "Age-related macular degeneration," *Ophthal*, 93:969, 1986

316 —Young, R., "Solar radiation and age-related macular degeneration," *Surv Ophthal*, 32:252, 1988

Mainster, M., "Light and macular degeneration: a biophysical and clinical perspective," *Eye*, 1:304, 1987

Zigman, S., "Effects of near ultraviolet radiation on the lens and retina," *Doc Ophthal*, 55:375, 1983

317 —Taylor H., "Visible light and risk of age-related macular degeneration," *Trans Am Ophthal Soc*, 88:163, 1990

Sliney, D., "Standards for the use of visible and nonvisible radiation on the eye," *Am J Optom & Physiol Optics*, 60:278, 1983

Young, R., Ibid

318 —Schmidt, S., "Melanin concentration in normal retinal pigment epithelium—regional variation in age-related reduction," *Invest Ophthal Vis Sci*, 27:1063, 1986

319 —*FDA Consumer*, May 1991, pg 19

320 —Young, R., *Age Related Cataract*, Oxford Press, 1991, pg 6222

Young, R. as per note 316

321 —Robertson, J., "A possible role for vitamin C and E in cataract prevention," *Am J Clin Nutr,* 53:346, 1991

322 —Young, R. as per note 315, pg 258

323 —Quoted in Lemonick, M., "The ozone vanishes," *Time*, Feb. 17, 1992, pg 60

Chapter 7—Industry

1 —Quoted in "Soundings," *Earth Island Journal,* Winter 1994–95, pg 42

2 —Young, F., "A golden anniversary of consumer protection," *FDA Consumer*, June 1988, pg 4

3 —Grigg, W., "The making of a milestone in consumer protection," *FDA Consumer,* Nov. 1988, pg 30

4 —Davis, D., "Cancer prevention: assessing causes, exposures and recent trends in mortality for US males 1968–1978," *Teratogen Carcinogen Mutagen*, 2:105, 1982

5 —Stauber, J., "Going…going…green," *PR Watch*, April/June, 1994, pg 2

6 —Hoffman, R., "Health effects of long-term exposure to 2,3,7,8-tetrachlorodibenzo-p-dioxin," *JAMA*, 255:2031, 1986

7 —Whiteside, R., *The Pendulum and the Toxic Cloud*, Yale University Press, 1979, pg 134

8 —Regenstein, L., *How to Survive in America the Poisoned*, Acropolis Books, 1982, pg 74

Pesticides

9 —Quoted in Gallagher, C., *American Ground Zero*, MIT Press, 1993, pg 150

10 —Department of the Army Training Circular, "Employment of riot control agents, flame, smoke, antiplant agents, and personnel detectors in counterguerrilla operations," Antiplant Agent Operations, Section I Technical Aspects, TC 3-16, April 1969

11 —Quoted in "A plague on our children," NOVA, WGBH Educational Foundation, Boston, 1979

12 —Schechter, A., "Dioxins in humans and the environment. Biological basis for risk assessment of dioxins and related compounds," *Banbury Report*, 35:169, 1991

13 —USDA Agricultural Marketing Service, "Pesticide Data Program: Summary of 1992 Data," April 1994

14 —Sustainable Agriculture Committee, *Organic Food Matters,* Summer 1990

15 —Quoted in Associated Press, "New chief discusses disease center policy," *New York Times,* Dec. 13, 1983, pg III-7

16 —EPA Study, "Unfinished Business: A Comparative Assessment of Environmental Problems," Feb. 1987

17 —Lowe, C., *Toxic Food*, Avon Books, 1990, pg 8

18 —Committee on Agriculture, Nutrition and Forestry, "Hearing on the circle of poison: impact on U.S. consumers," Sept 20, 1991

19 —US GAO, "Better regulation of pesticide exports and pesticide residues in imported foods is essential," Report No. CED–79–43, June 22, 1979, pg 39

20 —Rapaport, R., "New DDT inputs to North America: atmospheric deposition," *Chemosphere*, 14:1167, 1985

Eisenreich, S., "Airborne organic contaminants in the Great Lakes ecosystem," *Environ Sci Technol,* 15:30, 1981

21 —Dewailly, E., "Inuit exposure to organochlorines through the aquatic food chain in Arctic Quebec," *Environ Health Perspect*, 101:618, 1993

22 —Hilman, B., "Environmental estrogens linked to reproductive abnormalities, cancer," *Chem Engineer News,* Jan. 31, 1994, pg 19

23 —Foundation for the Advancement of Science and Education, *FASE Reports*, 11:S1, 1993

24 —Hecht, K., "Notes from the front," *Mother Jones,* Nov./Dec. 1993, pg 14

25 —Marquardt, S., "On the trail of pesticide export controls in the US," *Global Pesticide Campaigner,* Aug. 1993, pg 6

26 —Weir, D., *Circle of Poison*, Institute for Food and Development Policy, 1981, pg 51

27 —Heifetz, R., "Mothers' milk or mothers' poison? Pesticides in breast milk," *J Pest Reform*, 9:15, 1989

Calabrese, E., "Human breast milk contamination in the United States and Canada by chlorinated hydrocarbon insecticides and industrial pollutants: current status, " *J Am Coll Tox*, 1:91, 1982

28 —Krieger, N., "Breast cancer and serum organochlorines: a prospective study among white, black and Asian women," *JNCI*, 86:589, 1994

Wolff, M., "Blood levels of organochlorine residues and risk of breast cancer," *JNCI,* 85:648, 1993

29 —Dewailly, E., "High organochlorine burden in women with estrogen-positive breast cancer," *JNCI*, 86:232, 1994

Falck, F., "Pesticides and polychlorinated biphenyl residues in human breast lipids and their relation to breast cancer," *Arch Environ Health*, 47:143, 1992

Mussalo-Rauhamaa, H., "Occurrence of beta-hexachlorocyclohexane in breast cancer patients," *Cancer*, 66:2124, 1990

Unger, M., "Organochlorine compounds in human breast fat from deceased with and without breast cancer and in a biopsy material from newly diagnosed patients undergoing breast surgery," *Environ Res,* 34:24, 1984

Wasserman, M., "Organochlorine compounds in neoplastic and adjacent apparently normal breast tissue," *Bull Environ Contam Tox*, 15:478, 1976

30 —Wasserman, M., "Organochlorine compounds in neoplastic and adjacent apparently normal gastric mucosa," *Bull Environ Contam Tox*, 20:544, 1978

Radomski, J., "Pesticide contamination in the liver, brain and adipose tissue of terminal hospital patients," *Food Cosmet Tox*, 6:209, 1968

Dacre, J., *Tox Applied Pharmacol*, 17:277, 1970

31 —Morrison, H., "Herbicides and cancer," *JNCI*, 84:1866, 1992

Blair, A., "Cancer among farmers," *Occupat Med*, 6:335, 1991

32 —Sharpe, R., "Are oestrogens involved in falling sperm counts and disorders of the male reproductive tract?," *Lancet*, 341:1392, 1993

Carlsen, E., "Evidence for decreasing the quality of semen during the past 50 years," *Br J Med,* 305:609, 1992

Brown, L., "Testicular cancer in the United States: trends in incidence and mortality," *Int J Epidemiol*, 15:164, 1986

Auger, J., "Decline in semen quality among fertile men in Paris during the past 20 years," *N Engl J Med,* 332:281, 1995

33 —Feichtinger, W., "Environmental factors and fertility," *Human Reprod*, 6:1170, 1991

Ginsburg, J., "Residence in the London area and sperm density," *Lancet*, 343:230, 1994

Dougherty, R., "Sperm density and toxic substances: a potential key to environmental health hazards," *Environ Health Chem*, 1981, pg 263

34 —Quoted in Stone, R., "Environmental estrogens stir debate," *Science*, 265:309, 1994

35 —Colborn, T., "Developmental effects of endocrine-disrupting chemicals in wildlife and humans," *Environ Health Perspect,* 101:378, 1993

Raloff, J., "That feminine touch," *Science News*, Jan. 22, 1994, pg 56

36 —US General Accounting Office, Report to the Senate Committee on Government Affairs, "Reproductive and Developmental Toxicants," Oct. 1991

37 —Schwartz, D., "Parental occupation and birth outcome in an agricultural community," *Scand J Work Environ*, 12:51, 1986

Schwartz, D., *Physician's Handbook on Pesticides*, UCSD Medical Center, 1980

38 —Quoted in *Newsweek,* April 23, 1990, pg 17

39 —Whelan, E. and Stare, F., *The Nutrition Hoax*, Atheneum, 1983, pg 141

40 —Green, N., *Poisoning Our Children,* Noble Press, 1991, pg 49

Tattersall, A., "Is EPA registration a guarantee of pesticide safety?," *J Pest Reform*, Spring 1986

41 —National Academy of Sciences, *Regulating Pesticides in Foods*, National Academy Press, 1987

42 —Westin, J., "The Israeli breast cancer anomaly," *Ann NY Acad Sci*, 609:269, 1990

43 —Goldman, B., *The Truth About Where You Live*, Random House, 1991

44 —Young, F., "Weighing food safety risks," *FDA Consumer,* Sept. 1989, pg 11

45 —Wasserman, H. and Solomon, N., *Killing Our Own*, Dell Publishing, 1982, pg 81

Fuller, J., *The Day We Bombed Utah: America's Most Lethal Secret,* New American Library, 1984

Keyes, K., *The Hundredth Monkey*, Vision Books, pg 27

46 —Quoted in Andrews, R., *The Concise Columbia Dictionary of Quotations*, Avon Books, 1987, pg 105

Chlorine

47 —Union of Concerned Scientists, "World scientists' warning to humanity," Dec. 1992

48 —Quoted in Henderson, C., "Chlorine Institute issues response to Greenpeace report on breast cancer," *Cancer Weekly*, Nov. 23, 1992, pg 8

49 —Rossberg, G., "Chlorinated hydrocarbons," *Ullman's Encyclopedia of Industrial Chemistry*, 5th ed., VCH Publishers, 1986, pg 233

50 —Braungart, M., *Halogenated Hydrocarbons: Principle Thoughts and Data About a Possible Ban and Substitution*, Hamburg Umwelt Institute, 1987

51 —Cooke, B., "Distribution and breakdown of DDT in orchard soil," *Pesticide Sci*, 13:545, 1982

52 —Howard, P., *Handbook of Environmental Fate and Exposure Data for Organic Chemicals*, Vol. II–Solvents, Lewis Publishers, 1990

53 —Jeffers, P., "Homogeneous hydrolysis rate constants for selected chlorinated methanes, ethanes, ethenes and propanes," *Environ Sci Technol,* 23:965, 1989

54 —Swain, W., "Human health consequences of consumption of fish contaminated with organochlorine compounds," *Acquatic Toxicol,* 11:357, 1988

55 —Vallentyne, J., Chairman, Great Lakes Science Advisory Board, Int. Joint Commision, Testimony and submission before the Alberta-Pacific Environmental Impact Assessment Review Board, Edmonton, Alberta, Dec. 1, 1989

Onstot, J., "Characterization of HRGC/MS unidentified peaks from the analysis of human adipose tissue," Vol. 1, US EPA Office of Toxic Substances, 560/6-87-002A, May 1987

56 —Coppolino, E., "Pandora's poison," *Sierra*, Sept./Oct. 1994, pg 42

57 —Dewailly, E., "Inuit exposure to organochlorines through the aquatic food chain in Arctic Quebec," *Environ Health Perspect*, 101:618, 1993

58 —Schechter, A., "Dioxins in humans and the environment. Biological basis for risk assessment of dioxins and related compounds," *Banbury Report*, 35:169, 1991

59 —US EPA, "Risk characterization of dioxin and related compounds," Bureau of National Affairs, May 3, 1994

60 —Walrath, J., "Causes of death among female chemists," *Am J Pub Health*, 75:883, 1985

61 —Thornton, J., *The Product Is The Poison: The Case for a Chlorine Phase-out,* Greenpeace, 1991, pg 33

62 —US EPA, "Effluent Limitations Guidelines, Pretreatment Standards and New Source Performance Standards: Pulp, Paper and Paperboard Category," 1993

Suntio, L., "A review of the nature and properties of chemicals present in pulp mill effluent," *Chemosphere*, 17:1249, 1988

Kroesa, R., *The Greenpeace Guide to Paper,* Greenpeace International, 1991

63 —As per note 61, pg 4

64 —International Joint Commission, Sixth Biennial Report on Great Lakes Water Quality, Windsor, ON, 1992

65 —American Public Health Association, "Recognizing and Addressing the Hazards of Chlorinated Organic Chemicals," San Francisco, CA, Oct. 28, 1993

66 —Clinton, W., "President Clinton's Proposal for the Clean Water Act," The White House, Feb. 1, 1994

67 —Hirl, R., quoted in Flam, F., "Chlor-alkali makers face up to marketplace realities," *Chemical Week*, Oct. 3, 1990, pg 21

68 —Verbonic, C., "Can chlorine and caustic recycle the good times?," (advertising section), *Chemical Business*, Sept. 1990, pg 23

69 —Quoted in Lewis, S., "Inconclusive by design," *Earth Island Journal,* Winter 1993, pg 19

70 —Garren, B., quoted in Mothers and Others, *The Green Guide,* June 21, 1995, pg 4

71 —Holloway, M., "A press release on dioxin sets the record wrong," *Scientific American*, April 1991, pg 24

Bailey, J., "Dueling studies," *Wall Street Journal*, Feb. 20, 1992, pg A-1

As per note 59

72 —Zurer, P., "Ozone depletion's recurring surprises challenge atmospheric scientists," *Chem Engineer News*, May 24, 1993, pg 8

Taubes, G., "The ozone backlash," *Science*, 260:1580, 1993

Schaum, J., "Sources of dioxin-like compounds and background exposure levels," 13th International Symposium on Chlorinated Dioxins and Related Compounds, *Organohalogens*, 14:319, 1993

73 —Charles River Associates, *Assessment of the Economic Benefits of Chlor-Alkali Chemicals to the United States and Canadian Economies,* Prepared for the Chlorine Institute, April 1993
74 —"Reilly calls pollution technology to expensive," Bureau of National Affairs' *Environment Watch*, Oct. 15, 1990, pg 4
75 —Thornton, J., *Transition Planning for the Chlorine Phase-out,* Greenpeace, Feb. 1994, pg 14
76 —As per note 73
77 —US Dept. of Commerce, as cited in Renner, M., *Jobs in a Sustainable Economy*, Worldwatch Paper #104, Worldwatch Institute, Sept. 1991
78 —US Office of Technology Assessment, *Serious Reduction in Hazardous Waste*, Washington DC, OTA–ITE–317, 1986
79 —Hilman, B., "Curbs on chlorine sought: EPA plan outrages chemical makers," *Chem Engineer News*, Feb. 7, 1994, pg 4
Galin, R., "Industry says cluster rules, based on inaccurate data, go too far," *Pulp & Paper*, April 1994, pg 99
80 —Gldwacki, J., "INCB meeting focuses on latest ECF/TCF innovations, closed-cycle technologies," *Pulp & Paper*, June 1994, pg 87
Beaton, A., "Developing markets push industry to consider using TCF process,"*Pulp & Paper*, Feb. 1994, pg 77
81 —Gldwacki, J., Ibid, pg 90
82 —Raloff, J., "Something's fishy," *Science News*, July 2, 1994, pg 8
83 —Ibid
84 —Anderson, D., "Red tides," *Scientific American*, Aug. 1994, pg 62
Stone, R., "Dioxins dominate Denver gathering of toxicologists," *Science*, 266:1162, 1994
85 —As per note 47
86 —As per note 75, pg 28
As per note 61, pg 49
87 —McGeehin, M., "Case-control study of bladder cancer and water disinfection methods in Colorado," *Am J Epidemiol,* 138:492, 1993
Morris, R., "Chlorination, chlorination by-products and cancer: a meta-analysis," *Am J Public Health*, 82:955, 1992

Fluoride

88 —Botta, J., "Fluoridation the cancer scare," *Consumer Reports*, 43:392, 1978
89 —"Water boom for industry," *Chemical Week*, July 7, 1951, pg 14
90 —Miller, G., "The effect of fluoride on higher plants," *Fluoride*, 26:4, 1993
National Academy of Sciences, *Fluorides*, National Academy Press, 1971, pg 66
91 —*Van Nostrand's Scientific Encyclopedia*, 7th ed., Van Nostrand Reinhold, 1989
92 —Shell, E., "Fluoride," *San Francisco Chronicle*, This World, Sept. 28, 1986, pg 9
93 —*Clinical Toxicology of Commercial Products*, Williams & Wilkins, 1984, pg II–4
94 —Foulkes, R., "Fluoridation of community water suplies: 1992 update," *Townsend Letter for Doctors,* June 1992, pg 455

95 —US EPA, "Final draft for the drinking water criteria document on fluoride," US EPA Report PB85–199321, April 1985, pg II–5
96 —Fels, H., "Fluoridation," *East West Journal,* Oct. 1989, pg 64
97 —Griffith, J., "Fluoride: commie plot or capitalist ploy," *Covert Action*, Fall 1992, pg 29
98 —Yiamouyiannis, J., *Fluoride The Aging Factor*, 3rd ed., Health Action Press, 1993, pg 141
99 —As per note 97, pg 30
100 —Colquhoun, J., "Is there a dental benefit from water fluoridation?," *Fluoride*, 27:13, 1994

Sutton, P., *Fluoridation: Errors and Omissions in Experimental Trials*, Melbourne University Press, 1960

101 —As per note 97, pg 63
102 —Foulkes, R., "The cost of fluoridation," *Townsend Letter for Doctors*, Nov. 1993, pg 1087

Hill, D., Paper presented to public forum sponsored by The Chemical Institute of Canada, Calgary, Sept. 29, 1992

103 —Government of Canada, *Inorganic Fluorides*, ISBN 0-662-21070-9, 1993
104 —Jerard, E., "The summing of fluoride exposures," *Int J Environ Studies*, 3:143, 1973
105 —USDA Handbook No. 380, *Air Pollutants Affecting the Performance of Domestic Animals*, Aug. 1970, pg 41
106 —US EPA, "Engineering and cost effectiveness study of fluoride emissions control,"EPA Report SN 16893.000, Jan. 1972, pg III–59
107 —Raloff, J., "The St. Regis syndrome." *Science News*, July 19, 1980, pg 42
108 —Miller, G., as per note 90
109 —US EPA, "Summary review of health effects associated with hydrogen fluoride and related compounds," EPA Report 600/8-29/002F, Dec. 1988, pg I–1
110 —Yiamouyiannis, J., *Lifesaver's Guide to Fluoridation*, Safe Water Foundation, 1983, pg 1
111 —Foulkes, R., "Impact of artificial fluoridation on salmon species in the Northwest USA and British Columbia Canada," *Fluoride*, 27:220, 1994
112 —Berk, R., *Aluminum: Profile of the industry,* McGraw-Hill, 1985, pg 148
113 —As per note 111
114 —Begley, S., "Don't drink the water?," *Newsweek*, Feb. 5, 1990, pg 61
115 —As per note 111
116 —Spittle, B., "Psychopharmacology of fluoride: a review," *Int Clin Psychopharm*, 9:79, 1994

Call, R., "Histological and chemical studies in man on effects of fluoride," *Public Health Reports*, 80:529, 1965

117 —As per note 104
118 —As per note 98, pg 5
119 —Liu, C., "Fluoride content of dairy milk from supermarket," *Fluoride*, 28:10, 1995

Stannard, J., "Fluoride levels and fluoride contamination of fruit juices," *J Clin Pediat Dent*, 16:38, 1991

120 —Kintner, R., "Dietary fluoride intake in the USA revisited," *Fluoride*, 24:8, 1991

Burk, B., "The changing pattern of systemic fluoride intake," *J Dent Res,* 71:1228, 1992

121 —Hilman, B., "Fluoridation of water," *Chem Engineer News*, Aug. 1, 1988, pg 33

122 —Burk, B., "The increase in fluorosis in the United States: should we be concerned?," *Pediat Dent*, 15:146, 1993

123 —US National Research Council, *The Health Effects of Ingested Fluoride*, Office of News and Public Information, Aug. 17, 1993, pg 37

124 —As per note 121, pg 39

125 —Ibid, pgs 35–38

126 —Ibid, pg 28

127 —Ibid, pg 28

128 —US National Research Council, *Diet and Health,* National Academy Press, 1989, pg 121

129 —Jacqmin-Gadda, H., "Fluorine concentration in drinking water and fractures in the elderly," *JAMA*, 273:775, 1995

Danielson, C., "Hip fractures and fluoridation in Utah's elderly population," *JAMA*, 268:746, 1992

Jacobsen, S., "The association between water fluoridation and hip fracture among white women and men aged 65 and older," *Ann Epidemiol*, 2:617, 1992

130 —Riggs, B., "Effect of fluoride treatment on the fracture rate in postmenopausal women with osteoporosis," *N Engl J Med*, 322:802, 1990

131 —Sogaard, "Marked decrease in trabecular bone quality after 5 years of sodium fluoride therapy," *Bone*, 15:393, 1994

132 —Carton, R., *The Fluoride Report*, Sept. 1994, pg 2

133 —US Public Health Service, *Review of Fluoride: Benefits and Risks*, Department of Health and Human Services, Feb. 1991, pgs F1–F7

US National Research Council, *Drinking Water and Health*, National Academy Press, 1977, pg 388

Cohn, P., "An epidemiological report on drinking water fluoridation and osteosarcoma in young males," New Jersey Department of Health, Environmental Health Services, Nov. 8, 1992

134 —Yiamouyiannis, J., "Fluoridation and cancer," *Fluoride*, 26:83, 1993

135 —As per note 91, pg 1196

136 —Marcus, W., "The EPA's toxic bedfellows," *New York Times*, June 17, 1994, pg A–15

137 —Spittle, B., as per note 116

138 —Freni, S., "Exposure to high fluoride concentrations in drinking water is associated with decreasing birth rates," *J Toxicol Environ Health*, 42:109, 1994

139 —Chinoy, N., "In vitro fluoride toxicity in human spermatozoa," *Repro Toxicol,* 8:155, 1994

Kanwar, K., "In vitro inhibition of testosterone synthesis in the presence of fluoride ions," *IRCS Med Sci*, 11:813, 1983

140 —Gibson, S., "Effects of fluoride on immune system function," *Comp Med Res,* 6:111, 1992

Sutton, P., "Is ingestion of fluoride an immunosuppressive practice?." *Med Hypoth*, 35:1, 1991

141 —Kumari, D., "Red cell membrane alterations in human chronic fluoride toxicity," *Biochem Int*, 23:639, 1991

142 —Wandt, M., "Fluoride concentrations in a collection of urinary calculi," *J Urology,* 138:664, 1987

143 —DeSwarte, R., "Drug allergy," *Alergic Diseases, Diagnosis and Management,* JP Lippincott, 1980, pg 452

144 —Shukla, N., "Fluoride level in cataract lenses in an urban area of India," *Fluoride*, 24:40, 1991

145 —Ai-hua, S., "Observations on fluorotic aortosclerosis," *Fluoride,* 24:121, 1991

146 —Yiamouyiannis, J., "Water fluoridation, tooth decay and cancer," *Fluoride,* 27:237, 1994

147 —Carton, R., *The Fluoride Report,* April 1994, pg 5

Carton, R., *The Fluoride Report*, Dec. 1993, pg 8

148 —As per note 96, pg 62

149 —As per note 121, pg 37

150 —Maurer, J., "Two-year carcinogenicity study of sodium fluoride in rats," *JNCI*, 82:1118, 1990

151 —Begley, S., "Is science censored?," *Newsweek*, Sept. 14, 1992, pg 63

As per note 98, pg 170

152 —As per note 123

153 —Hirzy, B., "Press Release," *Fluoride*, 26:280, 1993

Carton, R., "EPA accepts fluoride report from biased NCR panel," *The Fluoride Report,* April 1994, pg 2

154 —Grossman, D., "Fluoride's revenge," *The Progressive*, Dec. 1990, pg 31

Griffiths, J., "Fluoride report softened," *Med Tribune*, April 27, 1989

155 —Colquhoun, J., "A view of the Beijing Conference," *Fluoride*, 27:183, 1994

156 —As per note 121, pg 30

157 —Brunelle, J., "Recent trends in dental caries in US children and the effect of water fluoridation," *J Dent Res,* 69:723, 1990

DeCava, J., "The fallacious faith in fluorine," *J Nat Acad Res Biochem*, 8:1086, 1988

Glass, R., "The first international conference on the declining prevalence of dental caries," *J Dent Res,* 61:1301, 1982

158 —Jones, T., "An analysis of the causes of tooth decay in children in Tucson, Arizona," *Fluoride,* 27:238, 1994

Ziegelbecker, R., "WHO data on dental carries and natural water fluoride levels," *Fluoride,* 26:263, 1993

Yiamouyiannis, J., "Water fluoridation and tooth decay: results from the 1986–1987 national survey of U.S. school children," *Fluoride*, 23:55, 1990

Diesendorf, M., "The mystery of declining tooth decay," *Nature*, 322:125, 1986

159 —Yiamouyiannis, J., Ibid
160 —Hileman, B., "New studies cast doubt on fluoridation benefits," *Chem Engineer News,* May 8, 1989, pg 5

Natural Toxins and Risk

161 —Stenger, V., "Toxicity of 2,4-D," *Chem Engineer News*, Nov. 14, 1983, pg 4
162 —Quoted in Lefferts, L., "Carcinogens au naturel?," *CSPI Nutr Action Healthletter,* July/Aug. 1990, pg 5
163 —Quoted in Hooper, J., "Ode to Cheez Whiz," *Health*, Oct 1989, pg 44
164 —Ames, B., "Diet and cancer," *Science*, 224:757, 1984
Yetiv, J., *Popular Nutritional Practices*, Dell Publishing, 1988, pg 64
165 —Ames, B., "Ranking possible carcinogenic hazards," *Science*, 236:272, 1987
As per note 162
166 —Quoted in Bloyd-Peshkin, S., "The health-fraud cops," *Veg Times*, Aug. 1991, pg 55
167 —*Monsanto Speaks Up About Chemicals*, 1977 brochure, pg 7
168 —Fenner, L., "A hard look at what we're eating," *FDA Consumer*, April 1984, pg 11
169 —U.S. Department of Health & Human Services, *Environ Health Persp,* 87:258, 1990
170 —"The clean entrepreneurs: cleaner than thou?," *California*, June 1990, pg 88
Clemings, R., "Organic food scams," *Longevity*, June 1992, pg 58
171 —Lijinsky, W., "Benzopyrene and other polynuclear hydrocarbons in charcoal broiled meat," *Science*, 145:53, 1964
172 —Matossian, M., *Poisons of the Past: Molds, Epidemics, and History*, Yale Press, 1989
173 —Begley, S., "A guide to the grocery," *Newsweek*, Mar. 27, 1989, pg 23
174 —Ames, B., as per note 165
175 —*Dorland's Medical Dictionary,* 27th ed., WB Saunders Company, 1988, pg 1292
176 —Quoted in Toufexis, A., "Dining with invisible danger," *Time*, Mar. 27, 1989, pg 28
177 —Coon, J., *Present Knowledge in Nutrition*, 4th ed., Nutrition Foundation, 1976, pg 530
178 —National Research Council, Committee on the Role of Alternative Farming Methods in Modern Agriculture, *Alternative Agriculture*, National Academy Press, 1989
179 —Ames, B., "To many rodent carcinogens: mitogenesis increases mutagenesis," *Science*, 249:971, 1990
180 —Quoted in Farley, D., "Setting safe limits on pesticide residues," *FDA Consumer,* Oct. 1988, pg 8
181 —EPA, "Pesticides in Ground Water Data Base: 1988 Interim Report," 1988
Center for Policy Research, *Nutrition Week*, Dec. 2, 1994, pg 7
182 —Schmidt, K., "Dioxin's other face," *Science News*, 141:27, 1992
183 —Quoted in Brooks, W., "Why organic foods are not safer," *San Francisco Chronicle*, Aug. 23, 1989

184 —Stephenson, M., "The confusing world of health foods," *FDA Consumer,* July/Aug. 1978
185 —Hazell, T., "Minerals in foods: dietary sources, chemical forms, interactions, bioavailability," *World Rev Nutr Dietetics*, 46:35, 1985
Robertson, L., *The New Laurel's Kitchen*, Ten Speed Press, 1986, pg 435
186 —Robertson, L., Ibid
187 —Ames, B., "Six common errors relating to environmental pollution," testimony before California State Assembly, Oct. 1, 1986
188 —Vickey, D., *Lifeplan For Your Health*, Addison-Wesley, 1978, pg 26
189 —Blumenthal, D., "Deciding about dioxins," *FDA Consumer,* Feb. 1990, pg 11
Jacobson, M., *Safe Food*, CSPI and Living Planet Press, 1991, pg 7
190 —Schneiderman, M., "Estimating cancer risks to a population," *Environ Health Persp*, 22:117, 1978
Weisburger, J., *Chemical Carcinogens*, American Chemical Society, 1976, pg 8
191 —"Does everything cause cancer?," *Consumer Research*, May 1989, pg 12
192 —Seligmann, J., *Newsweek*, May 11, 1992, pg 69
193 —Kimbrough, R., "Environmental protection: theory and practice," *Environ Sci Technol*, 24:1443, 1990
Nat Toxicol Prog, Tech. Report 347, 1990
194 —Stone R., "Environmental estrogens stir debate," *Science*, 265:310, 1994
195 —US Public Health Service, *Review of Fluoride: Benefits and Risks*, Department of Health and Human Services, Feb. 1991, pg H–6
196 —Stroloff, L., "Carcinogenicity of aflatoxins," *Science*, 237:1283, 1987
197 —Young, F., "Weighing food safety risks," *FDA Consumer*, Sept. 1989, pg 13
Van Rensburg, S., "Primary liver cancer rate and aflatoxin intake in high cancer area," *South African Med J,* 48:2508, 1974
198 —Americans for Safe Food, CSPI, *Guess What's Coming to Dinner,* 1987, pg 39
Young, F., Ibid
199 —Campbell, T., "A study on diet, nutrition and disease in the People's Republic of China, Part II," *Contemp Nutr*, 14:6, 1989
200 —Hiatt, H., *Mechanisms of Carcinogenesis*, New York: Cold Spring Harbor Laboratory, 1977, pg 705
Young, F., as per note 197
201 —Davis, J., "Family pesticide use and childhood brain cancer," *Arch Environ Contam Toxicol*, 24:87, 1993
Lowengart, R., "Childhood leukemia and parents' occupational and home exposures," *JNCI*, 79:39, 1987
202 —American Cancer Society, "Cancer in children," *Cancer Facts and Figures 1993*, pg 14
203 —Quoted in "Medical news," *American Health*, Dec. 1990, pg 8
204 —Gartrell, M., "Pesticides, selected elements and other chemicals in adult total diet samples," *J Assoc Anal Chem*, 69:146, 1986
Ames, B., as per note 165

205 —Colborn, T., "Developmental effects of endocrine-disrupting chemicals in wildlife and humans," *Environ Health Persp,* 101:378, 1993

206 —Quoted in Abelson, P., "Testing for carcinogens with rodents," *Science*, 249:1357, 1990

207 —Coats, J., "What happens to degradable pesticides?," *Chemtech*, Mar. 1993, pg 25

208 —Felton, J., "Accelerator mass spectrometry for measuring low-dose carcinogen binding to DNA," *Environ Health Persp,* 102:450, 1994

209 —Duke, S., "Herbicide-resistant crops," *Sci Food Agricul*, July 1991, pg 12

210 —Texas Agricultural Extension Service, "Neuropeptides for pest control," *Sci Food Agricul*, Jan. 1990, pg 5

New York State Agricultural Experiment Station, "Pheromones could replace some insecticides," *Sci Food Agricul*, July 1991, pg 11

University of California, "Lasers guard food against insects and microbes," *Sci Food Agricul*, July 1993, pg 6

Montana State University, "Weed control using lasers," *Sci Food Agricul*, July 1993, pg 2

211 —Quoted in Doyle, J., "Court ruling could ban many pesticides in food," *San Francisco Chronicle*, July 9, 1992, pg A4

212 —American Medical Association, *Let's Talk About Food*, Publishing Services Group, 1974, pg 251

213 —FDA and The International Food Information Council Foundation, *Food Risks: Perception vs. Reality*, HHS Pub. No. (FDA) 93–2253, pg 9

214 —Quoted in Proctor, R., *Cancer Wars*, Basic Books, 1995, pg 153

215 —Quoted in *Newsweek*, Jan. 12, 1976, pg 47

Organic vs. Conventional

216 —Quoted in Fumento, M., "Are pesticides really so bad?," *Investors' Business Daily,* April 1, 1993, pg 2

Quoted in Brooks, W., "Why organic foods are not safer," *San Francisco Chronicle*, Aug. 23, 1989

217 —Fumento, M., Ibid

218 —Quoted in Armstrong, D. and E., *The Great American Medicine Show,* Prentice Hall, 1991, pg 226

219 —US EPA, *Pesticide Industry Sales and Usage: 1992 and 1993 Market Estimates*, Washington DC, June 1994

Reid, C., "Little known insecticide dangers," *Total Health*, Feb. 1995, pg 14

220 —Reid, C., Ibid

221 —Food & Water, "The toxic tap," *Safe Food News*, Winter 1995, pg 5

222 —Ibid

223 —US EPA, Office of Pesticide Programs, *Pesticides in Ground Water Data Base: 1988 Interim Report*, Washington DC, 1988

224 —Lefferts, L., "Eating as if the Earth mattered," *E Magazine,* Jan./Feb. 1992, pg 33

Pimentel, D., *Handbook of Pest Management in Agriculture*, 2nd ed., CRC Press, 1990

CSPI Nutr Action Healthletter, July/Aug. 1990, pg 7

US News & World Report, April 20, 1992, pg 13

225 —Ibid
226 —Ausubel, K., *Seeds of Change,* Harper San Francisco, 1994, pg 74
"Failing soil threatens food supply," *Boston Globe*, Feb. 14, 1993
227 —USDA Study Team on Organic Farming, *USDA Report and Recommendations on Organic Farming*, July 1980
228 —National Research Council, Board of Agriculture, Committee on the Role of Alternative Farming Methods in Modern Agriculture, *Alternative Agriculture*, National Academy Press, 1989, pgs 5–23
229 —Faeth, P., "Paying the farm bill: US agricultural policy and the transition to sustainable agriculture," World Resources Institute, Washington DC, 1991
230 —Hightower, J., interview in *E Magazine* , Jan./Feb. 1995, pg 17
Lefferts, L., "A commonsense approach to pesticides," *CSPI Nutr Action Healthletter*, Sept. 1993, pg 7
231 —Pimentel, D., "Environmental and economic effects of reducing pesticide use," *BioScience*, 41:402, 1991
Pimentel, D., *Handbook of Pest Management in Agriculture,* CRC press, 1991, pg 679
232 —Smith, B., "Organic foods vs. supermarket foods: element levels," *J Applied Nutr,* 45:35, 1993
233 —Ministry of Agriculture, Fisheries and Food, *Living Earth and the Food Magazine*, 25:3, 1994
234 —Pimentel, D., "Environmental and economic costs of pesticide use," *BioScience*, 42:750, 1992
Hornick, S., "Factors affecting the nutritional quality of crops," *Am J Altern Agricul*, 7(1 and 2), 1992
Lairon, D., "Effects of organic and mineral fertilization on the contents of vegetables in minerals, vitamin C and nitrates," IFOAM Conference, University of Kassel, Germany, 1984
235 —Krizmanic, J., "Managing those pesky pests," *Veg Times*, Oct. 1994, pg 21
236 —Stauber, J., "Let them eat sludge," *PR Watch*, July/Sept. 1995, pg 1
237 —Procter & Gamble, "You may never clean produce the same again," *FIT brochure*, 1995
Procter & Gamble, "FIT Produce Rinse: a helpful guide from Procter & Gamble," Bulletin No. 25102
238 —USDA Agricultural Marketing Service, "Pesticide Data Program: Summary of 1992 Data," April 1994
239 —Pelkie, C., "Unsafe produce?," *Veg Times,* Nov. 1992, pgs 22–24
Ambrosio, D., *Eating Well,* Jan./Feb. 1992

Seed Wars

240 —Quoted in Weir, D. and Schapiro, M., *Circle of Poison*, Institute for Food and Development Policy, 1981, pg 42
241 —Gore, E., *Earth in the Balance*, Houghton Mifflin, 1992, pg 144
242 —Parr, J., "Diversity dearth," *Veg Times*, Feb. 1994, pg 14
243 —Ausubel, K., *Seeds of Change,* Harper San Francisco, 1994, pg 63
244 —Fowler, C. and Mooney, P., *Shattering: Food, Politics, and the Loss of Genetic Diversity*, University of Arizona Press, 1990
Ibid, pg 89

245 —As per note 243, pg 78
246 —As per note 243, pg 17
247 —National Academy of Sciences, *Genetic Vulnerability of Major Crops*, 1972
248 —As per note 243, pg 86
249 —Crapo, T., Organic Foods Production Association of North America Reports, May 1993
250 —Rhoades, B., as reported in note 240, pg 36
251 —Butler, R., "Patents: a gradual learning process," *Seed World*, Sept. 1992
252 —Henkes, R., "Tomarrow's seeds: patent pending," *The Furrow*, Sept. 1992
253 —As per note 243, pg 200
254 —Randolph, E., "Seed patents: fears sprout at grass roots," *Los Angeles Times*, June 2, 1980, pg 1
255 —As per note 241, pg 140
256 —Romney, L., "Seeds of creation?," *California*, June 1990, pg 96
257 —Doyle, J., *Altered Harvest: Agriculture, Genetics, and the Fate of the World's Food Supply,* Viking, 1985, pgs 139, 289
258 —Ibid, pg 141
259 —National Academy of Sciences, *Task Force on Genetic Alterations in Food and Feed Crops*, 1973
260 —Gorbachev, M., speech to the Global Forum of Spiritual and Parliamentary Leaders, Kyoto, Japan, April 20, 1993

Industrial-Grade Hemp

261 —Quoted in Friedman, M., "Whatever happened to hemp?," *Veg Times*, Aug. 1994, pg 71
262 —Bock, A., *Orange County Register,* Oct. 30, 1988
263 —Herer, J., *The Emperor Wears No Clothes,* HEMP/Queen of Clubs Publishing, 1992, pg 8
264 —Ibid, pg 6
265 —Ibid, pg 1
266 —Roulac, J., *Industrial Hemp*, Hemptech, 1995, pg 5
Conrad, C., *Hemp: Lifeline to the Future*, Creative Xpressions, 1993, pg 3
267 —Ibid
268 —As per note 263
269 —As per note 261
270 —Young, J., "It's time to reconsider hemp," *Pulp & Paper*, June 1991, pg 7
Dewey, L., *Hemp Hurds as Paper-Making Material*, USDA Bulletin No. 404, Washington DC, Oct. 14, 1916
271 —As per note 261
272 —"New billion-dollar crop," *Popular Mechanics*, Feb. 1938, pg 238
273 —Colby, J., *DuPont Dynasties*, Lyle Stewart, 1984
Conrad, C., as per note 266, pg 55
As per note 263, pg 22
274 —Ibid
275 —Brewer, J., "Has the golden goose gone up in smoke?," *Perceptions*, Summer 1993, pg 6
Roulac, J., as per note 266, pg 12
As per note 263, pg 25

276 —DuPont Corporation, *Annual Report*, 1937, Wilmington DE, pg 25
277 —Meijer, E., "Hemp variations as pulp source researched in the Netherlands," *Pulp & Paper*, July 1993, pg 42
278 —Ibid
279 —Lyford, J., "Trade uber alles," *Propaganda Review*, Number 11, 1994, pg 22
280 —Conrad, C., "Euro hemp," *Hemp World*, June/July 1994, pg 10
281 —Ibid, pg 11
282 —"Suisse hemp," *Hemp World*, Jan./Feb. 1995, pg 13
283 —Wigley, T., University Corporation for Atmospheric Research, *Weather Guide Calendar,* Accord Publishing, 1994, pg 1
284 —Pimentel, D., "Natural resources and an optimum human population," *Earth Island Journal*, Summer 1994, pg 26
285 —As per note 263, pg 43
286 —As per note 263, pg 44
287 —Weinberg, C., "Energy from the sun," *Scientific American*, Sept. 1990, pg 152
288 —"Radioactivity from burning coal," *Science News*, Oct. 1, 1994, pg 223
289 —Osburn, L., "To the editor," *Hemp World*, April/May 1994, pg 4
290 —Rosenthal, E., "Hemp as biomass?," *Hemp World*, Feb./Mar. 1994, pg 5
291 —Executive Order 12919 of June 3, 1994, filed in the *Federal Register*, 59(108), June 7, 1994, pg 29532
292 —Roulac, J., as per note 266, pg 39
293 —"Oregon economy thrives despite spotted owls," *Sprectrum*, Jan./Feb. 1995, pg 13
294 —USDA film, *Hemp for Victory,* 1942
295 —University of Kentucky, *Agriculture Extension Leaflet 25*, March 1943
296 —As per note 272

National Media

297 —Quoted in Cohen, J., "Rush Limbaugh's reign of error," April 5, 1995, c/o Alternative Radio, PO Box 551, Boulder, CO 80306
298 —Quoted in Mintz, M., "Media coverups of corporate crime," *Propaganda Review*, Number 9, 1992, pg 18
299 —Lapham, L., "And now a word from our sponsor," *San Francisco Chronicle,* This World, Jan. 16, 1994
300 —Moss, R., "The cancer establishment's propaganda machine," *Propaganda Review*, Number 9, 1992, pg 7
301 —Paganelli, G., "Effect of vitamin A, C, and E supplementation on rectal cell proliferation in patients with colorectal adenomas," *JNCI*, 84:47, 1992

Murray, R., "Physicians and healers—unwitting partners in health care," *New Engl J Med*, 326:61, 1992
302 —Brody, J., "Tricks to ease the side effects of cancer drugs," *New York Times*, Jan. 22, 1992, pg C–12
303 —US Congress, Office of Technology Assessment, *Unconventional Cancer Treatments*, OTA–H–405, US Government Printing Office, Sept. 1990
304 —As per note 300

305 —As per note 298
306 —Lyford, J., "Trade uber alles," *Propaganda Review*, Number 11, 1994, pg 22
307 —Schneider, K., "How a rebellion over environmental rules grew from a patch of weeds," *New York Times,* Mar. 24, 1993, pg A–16
308 —Montague, P., "Flack to greens: grow up and take the cash," *PR Watch,* April/June 1994, pg 7
309 —Montague, P., *Rachel's Hazardous Waste News*, April 15, 1993
310 —Spencer, M., The New York Times and environmental cleanup: green is the color of money," *EXTRA!*, July/Aug. 1993, pg 21
311 —Stauber, J., "Shut up and eat your 'Frankenfoods,'" *PR Watch*, Jan./Mar. 1994, pg 8
312 —"Sound bites back," *PR Watch,* July/Sept. 1994, pg 12
313 —FAIR, "GE irrelevancies," *EXTRA!,* Jan./Feb. 1991, pg 4
314 —"Gallup poll," *In Health*, Nov. 1991, pg 46
315 —Goulart, F., "15 ways to cancerproof your diet," *Total Health,* April 1990, pg 28
316 —Frankl, S. and D., "Women: decrease your health risks," *Total Health,* Dec. 1993, pg 26
317 —Ibid, pg 12
318 —Katzenstein, L., "Udder nonsense," *American Health*, July/Aug. 1994, pg 46
319 —Katzenstein, L., "Food irradiation," *American Health*, Dec. 1992, pg 62
320 —Weiss, R., "Breast cancer," *American Health*, Sept. 1992, pg 49
321 —Conkling, W., "Pesticide perspectives," *American Health*, Oct. 1994, pg 46
322 —Ibid, pg 96
323 —Epstein, S., "Evaluation of the National Cancer Program and proposed reforms," *Int J Health Services*, 23:23, 1993
Moss, R., *The Cancer Insustry*, Paragon House, 1989, pg 78
Wolk, M., "Reader's Digest discloses finances," *Washington Times*, Dec. 20, 1989, pg C–8
324 —Coppolino, E., "Pandora's poison," *Sierra*, Sept./Oct. 1994, pg 43
"What's riskier: PCBs or peanut butter?," *Hippocrates*, July/Aug. 1987, pg 11
325 —Coppolino, E., Ibid
326 —Bloyd-Peshkin, S., "The health-fraud cops," *Veg Times,* Aug. 1991, pg 57
327 —Bleifuss, J., "Journalist, watch thyself: keeping tabs on the messengers," *PR Watch*, Jan./Mar. 1995, pg 10
Stauber, J., "Burning books before they're printed," *PR Watch*, Oct./Dec. 1994, pg 1
Carter, L., "Raisin hell," *California*, Dec. 1990, pg 19
Ibid
328 —Meadows, D., "Freedom from disinformation," *Amicus Journal*, Fall 1991, pg 11
Stauber, J., Ibid
As per note 326
329 —Stauber, J., as per note 327

330 —Shuchman, L., "'Green' Ninja turtles have farmers steamed," *San Francisco Chronicle*, Sunday Punch, Sept. 15, 1991, pg 2
"Carrot and Stick," *Veg Times*, Dec. 1991, pg 77
331 —Bagdikian, B., *The Media Monopoly*, Beacon Press, 1992, pg 38
332 —Bleifuss, J., as per note 327
333 —Ibid
334 —Stauber, J., "Ketchum helps Clorox keep its image whiter than white," *PR Watch*, April/June 1995, pg 11
Cox, R., "Ketchum if you can—Clorox Corporation versus Greenpeace," *Propaganda Review*, No. 8, Fall 1991, pg 27
335 —Colby, M., "Agribusiness leads effort to silence activists," *Safe Food News,* Summer 1994, pg 16
336 —Ibid

Chapter 8—Government

1 —Wallechinsky, D. and Wallace, I., *The People's Almanac*, Doubleday, 1975, pg 710
2 —Reid, C., "Little known insecticide dangers," *Total Health*, Feb. 1995, pg 15
3 —Coppolino, E., "Pandora's poison," *Sierra*, Sept./Oct. 1994, pg 41
4 —"GATT threatens U.S. food safety, report claims," *Nutrition Week*, April 22, 1994, pg 3
Lyford, J., "Trade uber alles," *Propaganda Review*, Number 11, 1994, pg 63
Bauerlein, M., "GATTzilla?," *Utne Reader*, Jan./Feb. 1994, pg 19
5 —Roberts, J., "Food and Drug Administration under assault," *British Med J,* 310:82, 1995
6 —Jehl, D., "Clinton outlines health-care plan paid by employers," *New York Times,* Aug. 17, 1993, pg A–1
7 —Dowie, M., "A lighter shade of green," *Utne Reader*, July/Aug. 1994, pg 77
8 —Reported by Jerry Brown, *We The People*, 650 AM Radio, Oakland CA, Aug. 1, 1994
9 —Grossman, K., "A nuclear conflict of interest?," *EXTRA!,* Jan./Feb. 1994, pg 12
10 —Rosenberger, J., "Compromising safe food?," *Veg Times,* Jan. 1995, pg 18

Campaign Finance Reform

11 —Interview on KGO Radio, San Francisco, Oct. 4, 1991
Interview on the Larry King Show, New York, Mar. 2, 1993
12 —Rifkin, J., *Beyond Beef*, Plume, 1992
13 —Snell, B., "American Ground Transport," Hearings before the Subcommittee on Antitrust and Monopoly, Committee on the Judiciary, US Senate, US Government Printing Office, 1974, pg A–30
14 —Ibid, pg A–32
15 —Quoted in Walford, R., *The 120 Year Diet*, Pocket Books, 1986, pg 195
16 —Quoted in Williams, G., "Swearing off the miracle," *Veg Times,* Feb. 1994, pg 79

17 —Editorial, "The infant formula controversy: an international health policy paradigm," *Ann Intern Med*, 95:383, 1981

18 —Gerth, J., "Bush tried to sway a tax rule change but then withdrew," *New York Times,* May 19, 1982

19 —*US News & World Report,* April 30, 1990, pg 60

20 —Quoted in "Health system reform: medicine's litmus test for change," *The Commonwealth*, Nov. 22, 1993, pg 673

21 —Levine, A., "How the drug lobby cut cost controls," *The Nation*, Dec. 13, 1993, pg 730

22 —*UC Berkeley Wellness Letter,* Aug. 1991, pg 1
Castro, J., "Paging Dr. Clinton," *Time*, Jan. 18, 1993, pg 24

23 —Howell, J., "Real campaign finance reform must contain key essential elements," *Common Cause News*, Mar. 1993, pg 6

24 —Quoted in "Whatever happened to campaign finance reform?," *Common Cause News*, June 1994, pg 2

25 —As per note 23, pg 7

26 —"A happy marriage: cut the budget, help environment," *USA Today,* Jan. 31, 1995, pg 7–A
Dowie, M., "Greens outgunned," *Earth Island Journal,* Spring 1995, pg 26
US Public Interest Research Group, *USPIRG,* Fall 1994, pg 5

27 —"A big fuss of a visit," *Newsweek*, Nov. 6, 1989, pg 54
"Eight days in Japan earn Ron and Nancy $2 million—now that's Reagonomics," *People Weekly*, Nov. 6, 1989, pg 52

28 —Perry, J., "Young guns: a second generation of political handlers outduels forebears," *Wall Street Journal*, Jan. 10, 1994, pg A–1

29 —Stauber, J., "Smokers' hacks: the tobacco lobbys' PR front groups," *PR Watch*, July/Sept. 1994, pg 2
Lucas, G., "Smoking petition is suspect," *San Francisco Chronicle,* June 2, 1994, pg A–1
Elsner, R., "Another tobacco industry smokescreen," *California Physician*, June 1994, pg 16

30 —Ibid

31 —"Public-interest pretenders," *Consumer Reports*, May 1994, pg 320

32 —Quoted in Augarde, T., *The Oxford Dictionary of Modern Quotations*, Oxford University Press, 1991, pg 119
Quoted in Cutler, J., *Honey Fitz*, 1962, pg 306

Health-Care Reform

33 —Quoted in Hoar, W., "The Clinton cure-all," *The New American,* Nov. 1, 1993, pg 4

34 —Quoted in Sherrill, R., "Dangerous to your health: the madness of the market," *The Nation*, Jan. 9/16, 1995, pg 48

35 —Ibid

36 —Ibid

37 —Ibid

38 —Jehl, D., "Clinton outlines health-care plan paid by employers," *New York Times,* Aug. 17, 1993, pg A–1

39 —Pear, R., "Health-care costs may be increased $100 billion a year," *New York Times,* May 3, 1993, pg A–1

40 —Eisenberg, D., "Unconventional medicine in the United States," *N Engl J Med,* 328:246, 1993
41 —Dean, W., "Dr. Dean's health-care reform plan," *Forefront Health Investigations*, Aug. 1994, pg 7
42 —Nelson, C., "Oncology nursing: major changes needed to meet changing U.S. health-care needs," *JNCI*, 87:6, 1995
43 —Teisberg, E., "Making competition in health-care work," *Harvard Business Review*, July/Aug. 1994, pg 133
44 —US General Accounting Office, Special Supplemental Food Program for Women, Infants and Children, 1995, reported by Physicians Committee on Childhood Hunger, Tufts University School of Medicine

The EPA

45 —Quoted in "Warning: your food, nutritious and delicious, may be hazardous to your health," *Newsweek*, Mar. 27, 1989, pg 16
Quoted in "Is our food safe?," *Mother Earth News*, Sept. 1989, pg 87
46 —"Pesticides," *Nutrition Week*, Dec. 10, 1993, pg 7
47 —Walsh, M., "The lake that's a photo lab," *San Francisco Chronicle*, Sunday Punch, Nov. 25, 1990, pg 2
48 —National Resources Defense Council, *Think Before You Drink: 1992–1993 Update*, reported in *Amicus Journal*, Fall 1994, pg 3
49 —*Townsend Letter for Doctors*, May 1993, pg 408
50 —EPA, "Pesticides in Ground Water Data Base: 1988 Interim Report," 1988
Center for Policy Research, *Nutrition Week*, Dec. 2, 1994, pg 7
51 —Turner, T., *Wild by Law*, Sierra Club Legal Defense Fund, 1990, pg 125
52 —Marquardt, S., "On the trail of pesticide export controls in the U.S.," *Global Pesticide Campaigner*, Aug. 1993, pg 5
53 —Fleogel, M., *The Medium is the Message: Water Pollution, Time Magazine and Opportunities for Clean Production,* Greenpeace, 1994, pg 3
54 —Quoted in Hirzy, B. and Morison, R., "Carpet / 4-PC toxicity: the EPA headquarters case," Proceeds from the Society of Risk Analysis, Nov. 1989
55 —EPA Atmospheric Research and Exposure Assessment Laboratory, "Indoor air quality and work environment study: EPA headquarters buildings," 4:21M–3004, June 1991
Duehring, C., "Unraveling the carpet toxicity problem," *Environment & Health*, Winter 1993, pg 8
Highsmith, V., "An indoor air quality measurement study at the headquarters facility in Washington DC," US EPA, July 15, 1988
56 —*Indoor Air Quality and New Carpet—What You Should Know*, EPA 560/2-91/003, Mar. 1992
57 —Beebe, G., *Toxic Carpet III,* 1991, pg 66; c/o Glenn Beebe, P.O. Box 399086, Cincinnati, OH 45239
58 —Duehring, C., "Industry strategizing memorandum comes to light," *Informed Consent*, Sept./Oct. 1994, pg 44
59 —Nordmark, S., "Environmental health network conference," *Environment & Health*, 4(1), Winter 1993, pg 16
60 —Heuser, G., "Diagnostic markers in immunotoxicology and neurotoxicology," *J Occupat Med Tox*, 1(4):v–x, 1992

Metcalf, P., "EEG, psychological and neurological alterations in humans with organophosphorus exposure," *Ann NY Acad Sci,* 160:357, 1969
61 —"Ex-EPA head leads inquiry," *New York Times,* Aug. 21, 1985, pg A-20
62 —Quoted in Shabecoff, P., "Concern growing over unclear threat of dioxin," *New York Times,* Feb. 15, 1983, pg A-1
63 —Bailey, J., "Dueling studies," *Wall Street Journal*, Feb. 20, 1992, pg A-1
64 —Proctor, R., *Cancer Wars,* Basic Books, 1995, pg 100
65 —Meadows, D., "Freedom of disinformation," *Amicus Journal*, Fall 1991, pg 11
"News release: EPA bows to industry pressure, pulls consumer handbook," Environmental Action Foundation, April 23, 1991
66 —Roth, R., "Two years later: what's been done to the ozone layer—and for whose benefit?," The Atmosphere Alliance, *No Sweat News,* Summer 1994, pg 1
67 —Ozone Action press release, Dec. 20, 1993
Ibid
68 —Efron, E., *The Apocalyptics,* Touchstone, 1984, pg 97
69 —Thrasher, J., *Informed Consent*, Nov./Dec. 1993, pg 2
70 —National Institute of Health, "Issues and challenges in environmental health," NIH Publication No. 87–861
Board of Environmental Studies and Toxicology, National Research Council, reported in *Amicus Journal*, Winter 1989
71 —Sussman, G., "Allergy to latex rubber," *Ann Intern Med*, 122:43, 1995
"Fear of latex," *Newsweek*, Nov. 21, 1994, pg 81
72 —Quoted in *E Magazine*, Nov./Dec. 1994, pg 33

The USDA

73 —US Department of Agriculture, *USDA Today*, PA–1503, pg 3
Taylor, J. and McGraw, M., "Failing the grade," *Kansas City Star,* Dec. 8–14, 1991, pg 1
74 —Taylor, J. and McGraw, M., Ibid
75 —*The 48th Annual Congressional Quarterly Almanac, 102nd Congress, 2nd Session,* Congressional Quarterly, 1993, pg 214
76 —McNamara, D., "Heterogeneity of cholesterol homeostasis in man," *J Clin Invest*, 79:1729, 1987
Vorster, H., "Egg intake does not change plasma lipoprotein and coagulation profiles," *Am J Clin Nutr,* 55:400, 1992
Kestin, M., "Effect of dietary cholesterol in normolipidemic subjects is not modified by nature and amount of dietary fat," *Am J Clin Nutr,* 50:528, 1989
77 —Wargovich, M., "Inhibition of the promotional phase of azoxymethane-induced colon carcinogenesis in the F344 rat by calcium lactate: effect of stimulating two human nutrient density levels," *Cancer Letters*, 53:17, 1990
78 —Matkovic, V., "Factors that influence peak bone mass formation: a study of calcium balance and the inheritance of bone mass in adolescent females," *Am J Clin Nutr*, 52:878, 1990
79 —McCarron, D., "Dietary calcium and blood pressure: modifying factors in specific populations," *Am J Clin Nutr,* 54(Suppl):215, 1991

80 —Benenson, B., "House OKs agriculture spending with most grants unscathed," *Congressional Quarterly Weekly Report,* July 3, 1993, pg 1725

81 —Friedman, M., "It's nutrition, stupid," *Veg Times*, Nov. 1993, pg 70

82 —"Children get fat, agribusiness gets rich," *Spectrum*, July/Aug. 1993, pg 14

83 —"De la Garza, Stenholm top funding recipients list," *Nutrition Week*, Aug. 12, 1994, pg 2

84 —As per note 74, pg 20

85 —Harris, G., "Combating pesticide residues," *Complementary Med*, Summer 1988, pg 30

Smith, J., "Hawaiian milk contamination creates alarm, a sour response by state regulators," *Science*, 217:137, 1982

86 —As per note 73

87 —As per note 74, pg 9

88 —Riley, M., "The dangers of foul fowl," *Time*, Nov. 26, 1990, pg 78

Hall, B., "Chicken empires," *Southern Exposure*, Summer 1989

89 —Ibid

90 —As per note 74, pg 9

Food Safety

91 —Quoted in Lyons, R., "Trouble over drugs on the market," *New York Times*, Jan. 4, 1970, pg IV–5

92 —Quoted in Whiteman-Jones, M., "Are pesticides poisoning our children?," *Delicious!*, Oct. 1993, pg 10

93 —Leonard, R., "Food safety report card: Espy fumbles first year," *Nutrition Week*, Feb. 25, 1994, pg 4

"GAO examines inspection resources, effectiveness," *Nutrition Week,* June 17, 1994, pg 4

94 —Leonard, R., "Chicken feces fine to eat, says new USDA proposal," *Nutrition Week,* July 22, 1994, pg 4

95 —US General Accounting Office, "Food safety: risk-based inspections and microbial monitoring needed for meat and poultry," GAO/RCED–94–110, 1994

96 —Ames, B., "Ranking possible carcinogenic hazards," *Science*, 236:272, 1987

97 —*Perceptions*, Summer 1994, pg 52

98 —Smith, J., "Hawaiian milk contamination creates alarm, a sour response by state regulators," *Science*, 217:137, 1982

99 —Garland, A., *For Our Kids Sake*, Natural Resources Defense Council, 1989, pg 21

100 —Harris, G., "Combating pesticide residues," *Complimentary Medicine*, Summer 1988, pg 31

101 —Marwick, C., "Pesticides pose concern about children's diet," *JAMA*, 270:802, 1993

National Academy of Sciences, *Regulating Pesticides in Foods*, National Academy Press, 1989

102 —US General Accounting Office, "Changes needed to minimize unsafe chemicals in food," GAO/RCED–94–192, 1994

US General Accounting Office, "FDA strategy needed to address animal drug residues in milk," 1992

103 —US House of Representatives, Committee on Government Operations, "Problems Plague the EPA's Pesticide Registration Program," Oct. 1984

104 —"FDA's food safety effort criticized at house hearing," *Nutrition Week,* June 13, 1994, pg 2

105 —Leonard, R., as per note 93, pg 6

106 —Quoted in Rymer, R., "The mission," *In Health,* Mar./April 1990, pg 76

Food Labels

107 —Quoted in *Veg Times*, Mar. 1993, pg 18

108 —Quoted in Jacobson, M., "1991 Strategic issues survey," Center for Science in the Public Interest, 1991, pg 2

109 —Quoted in Kradjian, R., *Save Yourself from Breast Cancer*, Berkley Books, 1994, pg 218

110 —*Time*, July 15, 1991, pg 55

111 —*CSPI Nutr Action Healthletter*, July/Aug. 1991, pg 9

112 —*CSPI Nutr Action Healthletter*, July/Aug. 1990, pg 10

113 —*CSPI Nutr Action Healthletter,* Oct. 1989, pg 8

114 —*CSPI Nutr Action Healthletter*, May 1995, pg 8

The RDA

115 —Quoted in *PCRM Update*, May/June 1991, pg 8

116 —Campbell, T., "Mortality Rates in Transition in the People's Republic of China," International Congress of Nutrition, Seoul, Korea, Aug. 25, 1989, pg 13

117 —Council for Responsible Nutrition, Washington DC, 1990

118 —Murphy, S., "Demographic and economic factors associated with dietary quality for adults in the 1987–88 Nationwide Food Consumption Survey," *JADA*, 92:1352, 1992

119 —Yetiv, J., *Popular Nutritional Practices,* Dell Publishing, 1986, pg 173

120 —*Wholesome Diet,* Time-Life Books, 1981, pg 49

121 —Garrison, R., *The Nutrition Desk Reference*, Keats Publishing, 1985, pg 60

122 —Quoted in Note 120

123 —National Research Council, Food and Nutrition Board, *Recommended Dietary Allowances,* 10th ed., National Academy Press, 1989

124 —Passmore, R., *Handbook of Human Nutritional Requirements*, World Health Organization, Geneva, 1974, pg 17

125 —"Proposed nutrient and energy intakes for the European Community: a report of the Scientific Committee for Food of the European Community," *Nutr Rev*, 51:209, 1993

Index

NOTES

NOTES

NOTES 

NOTES

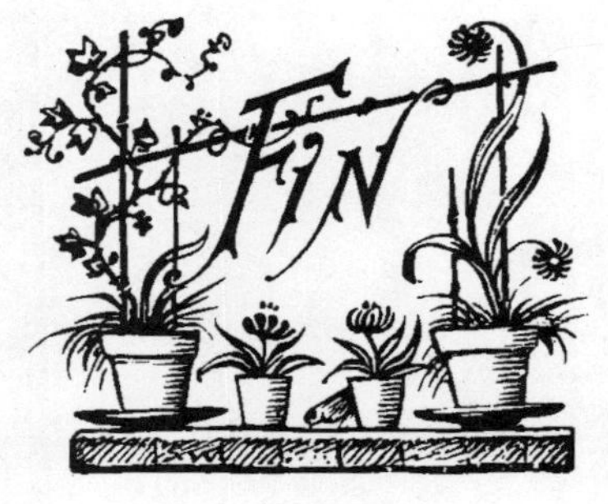
FIN